The
Family Nutrition Book

Also by William Sears, M.D., and Martha Sears, R.N.

The Pregnancy Book
(with Linda Hughey Holt, M.D., F.A.C.O.G.)
Parenting the Fussy Baby and High-Need Child
The Discipline Book
The Birth Book
The Baby Book
Nighttime Parenting
Becoming a Father

Also by William Sears, M.D.

The A.D.D. Book (with Lynda Thompson, Ph.D.)
SIDS: A Parent's Guide to Understanding and Preventing Sudden Infant Death Syndrome

The
Family Nutrition Book

Everything You Need to Know About Feeding
Your Children — From Birth Through Adolescence

WILLIAM SEARS, M.D., AND MARTHA SEARS, R.N.

LITTLE, BROWN AND COMPANY
Boston • New York • London

To our picky eaters, kitchen helpers,
and garden growers, who helped us
learn the connection between
good food and good health

James

Robert

Peter

Hayden

Erin

Matthew

Stephen

Lauren

FIRST EDITION

Library of Congress Cataloging-in-Publication Data

Sears, William, M.D.
    The family nutrition book : everything you need to know about feeding your children — from birth through adolescence / William Sears and Martha Sears
        p.   cm.
    Includes index.
    ISBN 0-316-77716-1 hc
    ISBN 0-316-77715-3 pb
    1. Children — Nutrition — Popular works.   2. Infants — Nutrition — Popular works.   I. Sears, Martha.   II. Title.
RJ206.S49   1999
613.2'083 — dc21   98-51879

10 9 8 7 6 5 4 3 2 1

MV-NY

Designed by Jeanne Abboud
Drawings by Deborah Maze

PRINTED IN THE UNITED STATES OF AMERICA

Contents

A Big Helping of Thanks

THE FIRST PLATEFUL of thanks goes to the parents in our pediatrics practice who demonstrate the connection between healthy eating habits and their children's better health, especially Kathy Kroe, Stephanie Mayo, and Jeane Scott. Special thanks to my research assistants, Tracee Zeni and Gwen Gotsch; to our office registered dietitian, Lynda Morita-Chan, for her scientific review of the manuscript and assistance with Chapter 30, "The ABC's of Teaching Nutrition to Your Kids"; and to our editor, Jennifer Josephy, and our copyeditor, Pamela Marshall, for their patience and dedication to improving the finished product.

A Word from Dr. Bill

THIS IS A BOOK about feeling good. When you eat right, you are more likely to feel right. Feeding your family good, nutritious foods is a wise investment, for the present and for the long term. Our goal in writing this book is to help you make wise food choices, foods that not only smell good, taste good, and are convenient but also help you feel good. Much of what is in this book was learned on the job — in thirty-two years in the Sears family kitchen preparing food for our eight children and in more than twenty-five years of nutrition counseling in our pediatrics practice. We have discovered which ways of eating work and which don't; why some families have healthy eating habits and some don't. These secrets we will share with you throughout this book.

To help you learn how to become your own family nutritionist, I want to tell you the story of how I became convinced of the importance of nutrition. No, it wasn't in medical school, where "nutrition" study consisted of a few hours each week spent chasing test tubes around the biochemistry laboratory. My career as a nutritionist began out of necessity in my pediatrics office when parents began asking me questions about what their kids should eat. Often I didn't have the answers. So I took the advice of my mentor, Dr. Richard Vanpraagh, Professor of Pediatrics at Harvard Medical School's Children's Hospital: "Surround yourself with informed parents and have the wisdom to listen to them."

I started paying attention to experienced parents and their children. I asked myself which children seemed to be the healthiest. What did these children eat? After years of observation, I became convinced that the children who ate the healthiest foods were the healthiest kids. They were sick less often, had fewer discipline problems, and achieved better in school. They not only had healthier bodies, they had healthier minds. I noticed that parents who consistently did not allow junk foods to pollute the bodies of their children had healthier children. I dubbed these children "kids of 'pure' parents." Over the years, I collected a lot of nutrition tips from these parents, and many of them appear in this book.

As I was starting to think about writing this book, I wondered why it is that children usually don't eat right. It gradually became clear to me that if parents aren't passionate about nutrition, they won't convey to their children the importance of eating right. So I decided to expand the scope of this book from its original premise, how to feed children, to how all family members can eat right.

Then a medical crisis occurred in my life that made me personally passionate about family nutrition. In April of 1997, I was diagnosed with colon cancer. As I lay in my hospital bed after surgery, I wondered what went wrong. I was a reasonably fit guy — my eating habits were okay and I didn't overindulge in stuff that was bad for my health. One problem was that I began this relatively healthy lifestyle late in life. Instead of making changes in my thirties, or even earlier, I waited until my fifties and, even now, there was certainly room for improvement.

Realizing that colon cancer, and all major diseases for that matter, are influenced by diet, I was determined not to let my medical problem repeat itself. So I began devouring scientific literature on the connection between diet and health. During the year following my surgery, I read volumes about nutrition, subscribed to every nutrition journal I could find, put together a collection of over five hundred file folders about food, and became what my friends tagged a "health nut."

About three months into my new style of eating, I noticed some amazing changes. My energy level skyrocketed, prompting my wife, Martha, to call me "Zip." We stepped up our ballroom dancing, and we even beat some of the younger couples in the swing contest. My mind was working better, too. I just plain felt good all over — mind and body — and finally learned what it is to experience real well-being. It was as if I had been introduced to a new life, a richer life, perhaps a second chance to live the way my mind and body were designed to live.

Why was I feeling so good? As a doctor, taught to analyze what happens in the body, I gave this a lot of thought. The answer seemed clear: I was putting the fuel into my body that made it run better. Too bad I, like many others, had to discover this after a life-changing catastrophe. Too bad I had to get sick in order to learn to eat right instead of eating right to keep from getting sick.

During medical school I learned about a principle called "the wisdom of the body," which says that under the right circumstances the body will crave what is healthy for itself and intuitively steer away from what's wrong. Years of indulgence had kept my body from being so wise, but now this wisdom had returned. After a year into the eating program I recommend in this book, I noticed that not only was I feeling great and thinking more creatively, but I now actually craved what was good for me and shunned the foods that threatened my well-being. Occasionally I would "sin," indulging in some treat that didn't meet my usual standards. But then both my mind and body would give me the clear message, "You shouldn't have eaten that." For the first time in my life I began to look at labels while shopping, trying to outsmart food manufacturers who tout the "purity" of their product on the front of the package but confess the real nutritional truth on the back.

In the first part of this book, we will help you make wise food choices. We not only want to give you the right information about different foods but also want to correct much of the misinformation that has been spoon-fed to unsuspecting consumers. This book is meant to empower you with the knowledge you need to feed your body better so it will work better for you.

To improve your own nutrition, and your family's, here are six steps you will need to take:

1. **Start now.** Don't wait until a medical crisis, such as cancer, diabetes, or a heart attack, forces you to adopt a healthier eating style. You don't have to almost die to keep yourself from dying prematurely.

2. **Be passionate.** Have you ever believed in a cause so much that it consumes every free moment? You think about it constantly and read everything you can find about it. Believe in your body and the need to feed it right. Unless you are really *hungry* for nutritional information, you won't devour enough of it.

3. Know your nutrition. The more you know about nutritious food, the better the good food will taste. Increasing your nutritional knowledge will make healthy foods more appealing to you, not only because of the taste but also because of their nutritional content. Before you eat, you will evaluate how a food affects your body — for better or for worse. As you sink your teeth into your salad, all those green, yellow, and red colors will take on a richer meaning. It's more fun to eat when you truly understand what you're putting into your body. When you see a red tomato, you'll remember why tomatoes are red and why that red stuff is good for you. As one of our nutrition-savvy children said, "I'm eating my lycopene today."

4. Change your mind-set about food. Sure, food needs to look and taste appealing, but you deserve more than that. *Think of food as medicine* — the best preventive pill you'll ever swallow, and a tasty one at that. "Health foods" are not about self-denial but rather about the promise of enjoying good health.

5. Shape young tastes. Parents, in the first three years of your child's life, you have a window of opportunity to instill lifelong eating patterns. The food you serve and the habits you promote become your child's nutritional norms. Throughout this book we'll show you how to help your children crave the foods that are healthy for them.

6. Model good nutrition for your children. Since you teach mostly by example, you have to evaluate and change your own eating habits before you can shape your children's. That is why this book begins with a crash course on nutrition for parents. Yet, information about the nutritional value of foods is not enough. Let's face it, we all, especially children, often eat for pleasure. We'll show you how to make healthy eating fun for your whole family.

When families start eating right, the benefits are clear — physically, emotionally, and mentally. Health is a blessing, one that is a direct result of the efforts parents make to provide what is best for their children. And your children will bless you for your efforts in years to come. What a wonderful legacy you are leaving when you establish healthy eating habits for yourselves and your children.

I

Becoming Your Own Family Nutritionist

The food you offer your family members has a profound effect on their physical, emotional, and intellectual health. The more you learn about the nutritional value of different foods, the more excited you will be about serving the best foods to your family. In Part 1 of the book, we'll give you a crash course on everything you need to know about the six essential nutrient groups required for optimal health: fats, carbohydrates, proteins, vitamins, minerals, and fiber. We'll also teach you about the benefits of drinking water and take you on a trip through the digestive system to learn about the magical metabolic processes that take place as food becomes you. Once you understand how different foods work in different ways in your body and what you can do to make them work better, you'll look at your food differently. When you sit down for an appetizing meal, you will not only anticipate the pleasure of eating but also become excited about the health benefits of the food on your plate. When you learn how to feed yourself wisely, you'll become more passionate about your children's nutrition, too. You are as healthy as the foods you eat, so learn about what it takes to eat well.

1

Facts About Fats

HERE'S A SURPRISE: Fat is a healthy nutrient — if you eat the right kinds and the right amounts. Medical problems, such as heart disease, stroke, and diabetes, that have been linked to a fat-filled diet are caused by eating too much of the wrong kinds of fat. Yes, most Americans need to lower the amount of fat in their diets. But, in addition to a lower-fat diet, they need a "right-fat" diet. This chapter on fat is one of the fattest ones in the book because dietary fat is a popular topic — and one that is obese with misinformation. Here are the facts on fat that every eater should know.

WHY YOU NEED FATS

Naturally today's consumers are confused by all the marketing hype on food packaging: "no fat," "low fat," "no cholesterol," "low saturated fat," and so on. Which fats are good, which are bad, and how much fat do we really need? Fat *is* an important nutrient. Here are the facts about why you need fat in your diet.

Fats provide energy. Gram for gram fats are the most efficient source of food energy. Each gram of fat provides 9 calories of energy for the body, compared with 4 calories per gram of carbohydrates and proteins. Fat is a more energy-efficient fuel because it contains less oxygen than carbohydrates or proteins do, and it contains no water. Fat is also the most efficient way for the body to store energy, although most of us store more fat than we really need. One pound of stored fat provides eight times more energy than the same pound of carbohydrates.

Fats build healthy cells. Fats are a vital part of the membrane that surrounds each cell of the body. Without a healthy cell membrane, the rest of the cell couldn't function.

Fats build brains. Fats provide structural components for many of the body's vital organs, especially the brain. Fat provides the structural components not only of cell membranes in the brain, but also of myelin, the fatty insulating sheath that surrounds each nerve fiber, enabling it to carry messages faster (see Chapter 31, "Feeding the Brain").

Fats help your body use vitamins. Vitamins A, D, E, and K are fat-soluble vitamins, meaning that the fats in foods help the intestines absorb these vitamins into the body.

Fats make hormones. Fats are structural components of some of the most important substances in the body, including prostaglandins, hormone-like substances that regulate many of the body's functions. Fats regulate the production of sex hormones, which explains why some teenage girls who are too lean experience delayed pubertal development and amenorrhea.

Fat provides for healthier skin. One of the more obvious signs of fatty-acid deficiency is dry, flaky skin. In addition to giving skin its rounded appeal, the layer of fat just beneath the skin (called "subcutaneous fat") acts as the body's own insulation to help regulate body temperature. Thin people tend to be more sensitive to cold; obese people tend to be more sensitive to warm weather.

Fat forms a protective cushion for your organs. Many of the vital organs, especially the kidneys, heart, and intestines, are cushioned by fat that helps protect them from injury and hold them in place. As an example of the body's own protective wisdom, this protective fat is the last to be used up when the body's energy reserves are being tapped.

Fats are pleasurable. Besides being a nutritious energy source, fats add to the appealing taste, texture, and appearance of food. Fats carry flavor. Fats are the reason that cookies melt in your mouth, french fries are crispy, and mom's apple pie has a flaky crust.

A FIRST HELPING OF FAT FACTS: MUFA'S, PUFA'S, AND SATFA'S

To make wise choices about what you eat, you first need to understand the three basic types of fats: monounsaturated fats (MUFA's), polyunsaturated fats (PUFA's), and saturated fats (SATFA's).* MUFA's and PUFA's are good fats; SATFA's are

* The FA's stand for "fatty acids," but we simply call them "fats."

bad fats. How do you tell a good fat from a bad one? Look at the food on your plate. A good fat flows like oil; a bad fat just sits there, like the fat that marbles a piece of sirloin. And these fats behave similarly in your body: The good fats (MUFA's and PUFA's) are like oil, flowing through your arteries. The bad fats (SATFA's) are like sludge, sticking to your arteries.

What makes a good fat a healthy fat and a bad fat an unhealthy one has to do with the chemical structure of the fat, called "saturation." The fat molecule is composed mostly of hydrogen atoms attached to carbon atoms in a carbon chain. On this molecule there are open spaces, like parking spots. When all the available spots, or parking spaces, on the carbon atom are filled (that is, saturated) with hydrogenated atoms, the fat is said to be saturated. If one or more places on the carbon are not filled with hydrogen, the fat is called "unsaturated." A fat molecule with one empty space is called a "monounsaturated fat," or "monounsaturated fatty acid," and is found in such foods as olive oil, canola oil, and nut oils. If two or more spots on the atom are empty, the fat is known as a "polyunsaturated fat," or "polyunsaturated fatty acid" (PUFA), which is found primarily in vegetable oils and seafood.

Whether or not fats help or harm the body depends upon their degree of saturation. Here's why. Unsaturated fat molecules (MUFA's and PUFA's) are curved molecules with negative charges that repel each other so they don't stick together, sort of like little bits of popcorn in a popper. Because these molecules don't stick together, they flow — both in the food and in the arteries. The molecules of a saturated fat are flat. They pile up like pages in a book and stick to each other. MUFA's and PUFA's are liquid at room temperature; SATFA's, such as butter and shortening, are solid at room temperature. Consider for a moment the fat molecules in your bloodstream. Do you want them to flow like oil or clump together like butter?

NUTRITIP
The Two F's of Healthy Skin — Fish and Flax

Your skin may reflect a fatty-acid deficiency. If your skin feels dry and flaky and has an unhealthy look, add flax oil, salmon, and tuna to your diet — at least several times a week. If a few months of eating more of these foods high in essential fatty acids makes your skin feel smoother and softer, your skin is telling you that your body needs more EFA's.

Another interesting fat fact is that your body makes all the SATFA's it needs. You don't have to eat any saturated fats. Is your body trying to tell you something? Yet the body needs oiling. It needs essential PUFA's. Your body can't live without them. While it can't live without MUFA's and PUFA's, we will live a lot longer if we eat less SATFA's.

> **Fat Tip #1: Eat more MUFA's and PUFA's and less SATFA's.**

A SECOND HELPING OF FAT FACTS: ESSENTIAL FATTY ACIDS

Fatty acids are the basic building blocks and the main nutritional component of fats. The body requires about twenty fatty acids in order to live and operate. It can make all but two of these: linolenic and linoleic. These are two of the essential fatty acids (EFA's), so called because they are essential for life and health. They can be supplied only by food or supplements. EFA's are essential to the body because they form the building blocks of vital cell membranes and are used to manufacture

BEST FATS

Now that you understand why you need fats, here's how fats rank:

- fats from seafood and plant sources (e.g., soy, nuts, and vegetable oils) are the healthiest
- fats from food factories (i.e., hydrogenated oils) are the worst
- fats from animal sources fall somewhere in between — healthy in moderation, unhealthy in excess

The following ranks the categories of fats — from best to worse — according to their effects on fat circulating in the bloodstream.

1. omega-3 fatty acids: decrease cholesterol; decrease total fats or triglycerides
2. monounsaturated fats: decrease total fats; decrease LDL (bad cholesterol); no effect on HDL (good cholesterol)
3. polyunsaturated fats: decrease total cholesterol; decrease LDL; decrease HDL
4. saturated fats: increase total cholesterol; increase LDL
5. trans fatty acids (see page 6): increase total fats; increase cholesterol; increase LDL; may decrease HDL

important substances, such as hormones. EFA's occur mostly in seafood and plant foods, with only trace amounts found in meat.

> **Fat Tip #2: It's essential to eat EFA's.**

All about omegas. The two essential fatty acids that you will be hearing about throughout this book are *linolenic acid* (also known as an "omega-

AMERICANS DON'T EAT ENOUGH FAT

You may be surprised to learn that most American children and many American adults don't eat enough fat — healthy fats, that is. The SAD (Standard American Diet) has a double fault: too much of the wrong fats and too little of the right fats. Most Americans eat an excess of unhealthy fats (animal and hydrogenated fats) and not enough healthy fats (plant and fish fats). Vegetable and fish fats are mostly MUFA's, PUFA's, and EFA's. Animal fats also have a double fault: They are low in EFA's and high: in SATFA's. Do your health a favor: Eat less animal fat and more veggie fat and fish fat.

ESSENTIAL FATTY ACIDS — ESSENTIAL FOR WELL-BEING

American families need more than a low-fat diet. They need a "right-fat" diet that includes essential fatty acids. Essential fatty acids benefit the body in the following ways:

- lower the risk of breast and colon cancers
- improve learning and attention span in schoolchildren
- improve cognitive function in the elderly
- elevate mood, resulting in less depression
- lower the risk of cardiovascular disease
- promote healthy skin
- improve vision, especially night vision

3 fatty acid") and *linoleic acid* (also known as an "omega-6 fatty acid"). The omega number describes where the important carbon atom is located on the fat molecule. If this atom is third from the end, the fatty acid is known as an "omega-3 fatty acid" (*omega* is the last letter of the Greek alphabet, and so, means "end"). If it is sixth from the end, it is known as an "omega-6 fatty acid." Omega-3 fatty acids especially have a valuable role in reducing the risk of heart disease and building healthy brain cells. The Standard American Diet (SAD) is sadly deficient in omega 3's, found mainly in plant foods (especially canola oil and flax oil, soybeans, and walnuts) and seafood.

Fat Tip #3: Don't be SAD: Eat more omega 3's.

A THIRD HELPING OF FAT FACTS: TRIGLYCERIDES, PHOSPHOLIPIDS, AND CHOLESTEROL

"Lipids" is a chemical name for fats. For practical purposes, all the lipids we eat are from the triglyceride category, which means they are formed by three ("tri-") fatty acids plus glycerol. "Triglyceride" is a term you may see in the ingredients list on food packaging. It sounds complicated, but all it refers to are ordinary fats. Triglycerides make up 95 percent of the fat in food and the fat stored in the human body. The other 5 percent of fats are called "phospholipids" and "cholesterol." The "fat" listed on food labels refers to triglycerides. A phospholipid is simply a fat that contains phosphorus. The most common phospholipid that is present in our bodies and in many of the foods we eat is lecithin, which is one of the important ingredients in sauces, salad dressings, mayonnaise, and in nonstick cooking sprays. Cholesterol is not really a fat, but rather, chemically, a sterol. It combines with fats in the bloodstream. Even though it's an important nutrient, it's not classified as essential, since the body can make its own. Both phospholipids and cholesterol form important structural components of cell membranes throughout the body. (See also "Cholesterol Facts You Should Know," page 21, and "Factory Fats: Hydrogenated Fats," below.)

Saturated vs. Unsaturated Fats. At room temperature, some fats are solids (e.g., butter and lard), and some are liquids. The liquids are usually called "oils." Whether a fat is solid or liquid depends upon its chemical structure, or its *saturation*. A saturated fat is solid at room temperature; an unsaturated fat is liquid at room temperature.

FACTORY FATS: HYDROGENATED FATS

The nutritional "bad word" every label reader should be aware of is "hydrogenated." Zapping an unsaturated oil with high-pressure hydrogen turns the oil into saturated fat. (Hydrogen is forced into the empty parking spaces on the fat molecule.) This hydrogenation process is how vegetable oil is turned into margarine. Hydrogenated fats have two major economic advantages over natural saturated fats: They are cheaper and they have a longer shelf life. Hydrogenated fats and partially hydrogenated fats are everywhere in processed foods — added to cookies, crackers, and peanut butter, for example. Hydrogenated fats are also used instead of oil for frying in many restaurants and fast-food establishments because they stand up better to heat and so can be used longer.

Despite their origins as unsaturated oils, hydrogenated oils are saturated fats and behave that way in the body. Crackers or cookies made with hydrogenated fats may proclaim themselves to be cholesterol free, but a closer look at the label will show that the product still contains plenty of artery-clogging saturated fat. And there's another problem with these fats that the label won't tell you about.

Hydrogenated fats contain another kind of fat that falls outside the saturated and unsaturated categories. This kind is called "trans fatty acids," or trans fats, so named because the hydrogenation process transports hydrogen atoms across the fat molecule to a new location. Dr. Udo Erasmus in his book *Fats That Heal, Fats That Kill* aptly describes a trans fatty acid as a "molecule that has its head on backwards." For your arteries trans fats are as bad as (or worse than) saturated fats. A number of studies have shown that trans fats raise cholesterol levels in the blood. However, current label laws in the United States do not require food manufacturers to include information about trans fats in nutrition labeling. So, a product whose label says it is low in heart-damaging saturated fat may still contain a large amount of trans fats and be no better for you than a fast-food cheeseburger or grandma's fried steak. You would never know this from the label. Hydrogenated fats are also widely used in restaurants for deep-fat frying, so the french fries so popular with children may be full of cholesterol-raising trans fats even if the establishment claims it uses "100 percent vegetable oil" for cooking.

DUMB FATS

Just as there are fats that improve how the brain functions, there are fats that hinder the brain's work. The dumbest fats are those that are man-made through the process of hydrogenation. These fats are referred to on package labels as "hydrogenated" or "partially hydrogenated." A diet rich in these fats not only deprives the eater of the smart fats but actually can interfere with the action of smart fats on brain function.

bel Loopholes

ne real irony is that this labeling loophole also eps consumers from being able to recognize ods that are low in trans fats. Most of the hyogenated fats used by food manufacturers are nly partially hydrogenated. Some of these parally hydrogenated fats contain less saturated fat nd fewer trans fats than others, but there is no vay of knowing how heart-threatening a particuar food product is. One of the difficulties with putting information about trans fats on the nutrition label is that different batches of hydrogenated oils may contain different amounts of trans fats. Food manufacturers would have to standardize the hydrogenation process and the oils they use to be able to give consumers accurate information.

Trans fats have found their way into most of the packaged foods bought by uninformed and unsuspecting consumers. Butter, which has gotten a bad rap because of its saturated fat and cholesterol, has been replaced by margarine, but, ironically, because the trans fats in margarine can raise cholesterol levels in the blood, some margarines are worse than butter. True, foods made with hydrogenated fats are cheaper and last longer, but consumers pay a higher price in the long run,

---

NUTRITIP
Chips That Clog

Potato chips are one of the most heart-unfriendly foods. Most are high in fake fats, which gives them an enticing flavor. To keep one fat ahead of chip-savvy consumers, some potato chip manufacturers are beginning to add the fakest of fats — the indigestible ones. This marketing ploy may take our plump little fat lovers from the nutritional frying pan into the fire.

---

since trans fats provide little nutritional benefit to the body, except as an energy source. What's good for business in the short run is often bad for the body in the long run. When manufacturers chemically change a food, all sorts of unanticipated problems may result. This is especially true of hydrogenated fatty acids. Here's a summary of what the literature says about hydrogenated fats and trans fats:

- Hydrogenated fats act biochemically in the body like saturated fats.

- Trans fats elevate blood cholesterol levels, similar to the cholesterol-raising effects of saturated fats.

- Trans fats raise the level of LDL (bad) cholesterol, while reducing the level of HDL (good) cholesterol. Raising the bad cholesterol and lowering the good cholesterol in the blood spells double trouble.

- Trans fats have been shown to decrease the body's ability to produce natural anti-inflammatory prostaglandins, those hormone-like substances that regulate many of the body's functions.

- Eating a diet high in nutritionally worthless hydrogenated fats may reduce a person's daily intake of other fats, especially essential fatty acids, which are important for the growth and function of vital organs, such as the brain. This is of concern especially in children and frequent fast-food consumers whose daily diet is high in processed and fat-fried foods and snacks.

- Trans fats and hydrogenated fats may interfere with the ability of the cells of the body to metabolize the fats that are good for you. This may damage cell membranes of vital structures, such as the brain and nerve cells. Cell membranes contain receptor sites for fat molecules, sort of like parking places, which are specifically designed to receive certain molecules. When the right fatty acid arrives, it fills its assigned parking spot and contributes to the health of the membrane. However, trans fatty acid "cars" can also come along and squeeze into a space that doesn't really fit these biochemical impostors. A sort of biochemical traffic jam occurs, and the right cars cannot get to where they need to be.

Or, think of cell membranes as having millions of tiny locks that nutrient molecules can open like keys. Changing the shape of the molecule, which is what happens when a fat is hydrogenated, changes the shape of the key, so it doesn't fit properly into the lock. Two problems can occur. Either the misfit molecular keys are left to wander throughout the body, causing damage in other places, or they push their way into the locks, damaging them, so that the right keys, the natural nutrients, no longer fit. At least in theory, hydrogenated fats can weaken cell membranes, keeping out needed nutrients and also allowing harmful ones to leak in. This may set the body up for chronic, degenerative diseases. This is why fake fats are becoming known in the medical community as "the silent killer."

We can take a tip from physiology that trans fatty acids are not good for the body. Both the placenta and the brain have a biochemical way of filtering most trans fatty acids out, although the protection is not complete. If a diet is not overwhelmed with trans fatty acids, it can deal with them by metabolizing these fats as energy sources before they have a chance to do any cellular damage and then use the good fats (the essential fatty acids) as healthy nutrients for the cells. A few trans fatty acids (which may occur naturally in some foods anyway) might not harm the body but, like all other fats, an excess will.

- Trans fatty acids may be linked to other health problems as well, including decreased testos-

terone, abnormal sperm production, prostate disease, obesity, immune-system depression, and diabetes.

Here are some commercial foods that are notoriously high in hydrogenated fats:

cookies	airline snack foods
some crackers	french fries
pies	shortening
pot pies	deep-fried burgers
pretzels	deep-fried fish
doughnuts	fried chicken
muffins	fried potatoes
stuffings	corn chips
potato chips	spoonable dressings
candy bars	some peanut butters
nondairy creamer	fast-food shakes
cinnamon buns	some cereals
cakes	margarine
biscuits	

Avoiding Hydrogenated Fats

Consumers can improve the quality of the food they buy. If enough consumers demand less hydrogenated fat and more truthful labeling, food packagers will take action. Here's what you can do:

- Write the Food and Drug Administration (FDA) and ask that regulations be changed to require food manufacturers to list grams of trans fats on nutrition labels. At present, hydrogenated fats are lumped into the "Total Fat" amount on the "Nutrition Facts" box. Truthfully, they should be listed on a line of their own as well as on the "Saturated Fat" line. Consumers have a right to know exactly how much of the most harmful fats are in a given food. Claims such as "low cholesterol" or "low saturated fat" should be prohibited on packaging of foods with high levels of cholesterol-raising

SMART FATS

Fats make up 60 percent of the brain and the nerves that run every system in the body. It stands to reason that the better the fat in the diet, the better the brain. So, with all the fat eaten by the average American, why don't we have millions more geniuses in this country? The problem is not that the average American brain does not get enough fat; the problem is that it doesn't get the right kind of fat.

Think of your brain as the master gland that sends chemical messengers throughout the body, telling each organ how to work. An important group of these chemical messengers are the prostaglandins (so called because they were originally discovered in the prostate gland). Prostaglandins initiate the body's self-repair system. The body needs two kinds of fat to manufacture healthy brain cells (the message senders) and prostaglandins (the messengers). These are omega-6 fatty acids (found in many oils, such as safflower, sunflower, corn, and sesame oils) and omega-3 fatty acids (found in flax seeds, pumpkin seeds, walnuts, and cold-water fish, such as salmon and tuna). The foods from which oil can be extracted are generally the foods highest in essential fatty acids. Most important to brain function are the two essential fatty acids linoleic (or omega 6) and alphalinolenic (or omega 3). These are the prime structural components of brain cell membranes and also are an important part of the enzymes within cell membranes that allow the membranes to transport valuable nutrients in and out of the cells. When the cells of the human body — and the human brain — are deprived of the omega-3 fatty acids they need to grow and function, they try to build replacement fatty acids that are similar but may actually be harmful. Higher blood levels of *replacement fatty acids* are associated with diets that are high in hydrogenated fats and diets that contain excessive amounts of omega-6 fatty acids. Elevated levels of replacement fatty acids have been found in persons suffering from depression or Attention Deficit Disorder (A.D.D.). A diet rich in omega-3 fatty acids, such as the alphalinolenic (ALA) from flax oil or the eicosapentaenoic (EPA) and docasahexaenoic (DHA) from fish oils, not only provides the body with healthy fats but also lowers the level of potentially harmful substances in the blood, such as cholesterol, possibly even reversing the effects of excess trans fatty acids.

Using the "lock and key" analogy will help you understand how the brain communication system works. Neurotransmitters are biochemical messengers that carry information from one brain cell to another, sort of like sparks flying across the gap between nerve cells. Each cell membrane contains a series of locks. The various message carriers (prostaglandins and neurotransmitters) are like keys. The keys and the locks must match. But, when the cell membrane is unhealthy because it is made of the wrong kind of fatty acids, the keys won't fit, and brain function suffers. Nutrients may also fail to fit into a mismade lock.

The eye is a perfect example of the importance of getting the right kind of fat. The retina of the eye contains a high concentration of the fatty acid DHA, which the body forms from nutritious fats in the diet. The more nutritious the fat, the better the eye can function. And since most people are visual learners, better eyes mean better brains.

Most Western diets contain too much of the omega-6 fatty acids and too little of the omega-3. Omega-3 fatty acids are found in ground flax seeds and flax oil, cold-water fish (primarily salmon), canola oil, soybeans, walnuts, wheat germ, pumpkin seeds, and eggs. (For more discussion of smart fats, see Chapter 31, "Feeding the Brain.")

NUTRITIP
Fats and Fibers

Because fiber gives you a sense of fullness sooner, eating a fiber-filled meal is likely to prompt you to eat less fat. On the other hand, you are likely to consume more fat when the menu is low in fiber.

---

trans fats. A consumer nutrition advocacy group that has done an excellent job of making the public more aware of this issue, as well as other nutrition concerns, is the Center for Science in the Public Interest. CSPI publishes the "Nutrition Action Newsletter."

- Look for newer labels, such as on some margarines, that proudly say "saturated-fat free" or "contains no trans fatty acids."

- Shun foods that contain the words "hydrogenated" or "partially hydrogenated" in their ingredients list. Terms like "vegetable oil" or "cholesterol free" tell you nothing about the amount of trans fat in the food.

- Avoid deep-fried foods, especially those at fast-food restaurants. If you must indulge, ask if the food is immersed in oils containing hydrogenated or trans fats. Don't settle for claims that the food is cooked in "100 percent vegetable shortening." That label lie camouflages a lot of hydrogenated fat. Can you imagine if people across the country walked into a McDonald's or Burger King and asked the manager if the oil in the fryer was truly polyunsaturated or if it was really hydrogenated vegetable fat? Imagine how the marketing departments of fast-food chains would react. Soon there would be an advertising war over which french fries had the lowest amount of trans fatty acids.

- Be suspicious of doughnuts from doughnut shops, since they don't come with nutrition labels. Inquire about the oil the doughnuts were fried in. You can bet doughnuts will continue to be high in saturated fats and trans fats unless consumers complain. One popular doughnut chain's old-fashioned cake doughnut contains an artery-clogging 310 calories, 19 grams of total fat, 5 grams of saturated fat, and 6 grams of trans fats.

- If you use margarine instead of butter, choose one that boasts low levels of trans or hydrogenated fats. In general, whipped or tub margarines tend to be lower in saturated and trans fats than sticks. Some products contain a blend of butter and vegetable oil to provide the consistency of margarine but with no trans fats.

- Even trendy restaurants that provide the nutritional breakdown of popular entrees list only the amount of fat a food contains, not the type. Ask what oil is used and if it contains trans fats (see "Ranking Oils: The Good, the Bad, and the In Between," page 208).

Food manufacturers argue that health concerns about the hydrogenation of fats are more theoretical than real. Yet, a study of eighty thousand women by the Harvard School of Public Health proved that the kind of fats a person eats is more important than the amount. In this study, women who consumed the most trans fats increased their chance of suffering a heart attack by 53 percent. However, the total amount of fat in their diet did not appear to pose any extra risk: The women who ate 46 percent of their dietary calories in fat were no more at risk for heart disease than those who ate 28 percent of their calories in fat.

SWEET FATS

We all know that if we eat too much fat, most of us will get fat. What many people do not realize is

FACTORY FATS

Tastes like fat . . . looks like fat . . . but it's not fat! A dieter's dream? Read on:

The newest factory fat (i.e., olestra) is so fake that the body rejects it even though the mouth seems to get the pleasure of fat. This fat substitute is made by joining together molecules of vegetable oil and sugar into a compound with molecules so big that they are not absorbed through the intestines and into the bloodstream. They just slide through on a calorie-free trip. So far, so good. You get the taste of fat without the calories. Sound like a great deal? *Wrong!* Since this fake fat can't get into the bloodstream, it has to get out of the body somehow, so it makes its greasy way through the intestines, taking along some of the fat-soluble vitamins (vitamins A, D, E, and K) and other nutrients, such as carotenoids (plant phytonutrients that fight against cancer and heart disease and may contribute to better vision), that depend upon fat for absorption. These nutrients that should have gotten into the body go out with the waste. So, even though the fat you may not want is not absorbed, some of the nutrients in the foods you do want are not absorbed either.

"No problem," say the food chemists. "We'll just add more of the nutrients to the food you eat." In May of 1998 the FDA began requiring snack-food packagers to put the following warning (in small print on the back of the package, of course): THIS PRODUCT CONTAINS OLESTRA. OLESTRA MAY CAUSE ABDOMINAL CRAMPING OR LOOSE STOOL. OLESTRA INHIBITS THE ABSORPTION OF SOME VITAMINS AND OTHER NUTRIENTS. VITAMINS A, D, E, AND K HAVE BEEN ADDED.

So to a bag of potato chips the manufacturer of olestra must add 3,400 IU of vitamin A, 240 IU of vitamin D, 56 IU of vitamin E, and 160 mcg. of vitamin K. The problem with decreased absorption of carotenoids seems to have been discounted.

Besides causing bloating, diarrhea, and crampy abdominal pain in some people, these synthetic fats allow people to simply change brands without changing their eating habits. They believe they can eat more fat without guilt, which further contributes to the development of a "fat tooth," the need to taste fat in food in order for it to be satisfying. These synthetic substitutes encourage eaters to overdose on fat-filled foods that have no nutritional value. In a study reported in *Pediatrics,* the official journal of the American Academy of Pediatrics, children ate more food when olestra was substituted for ordinary dietary fat in the food they were eating. The potato chips contain half as much fat, so you may feel you have the license to eat twice as many, but our advice is, don't be a guinea pig. Wait a while to see the long-term health risks of this new experiment.

---

that even eating excess sugar can make them fat. Here's how.

Sugar is a prime energy source for the body. Sugar molecules are constantly traveling to each cell to provide energy. Within each cell is a tiny furnace, called the "mitochondria." The sugar or glucose molecules enter the furnace and are burned as energy for the cell. This energy-conversion process creates carbon molecules that are building blocks for both cholesterol and saturated fatty acids. When you eat more sugar than your body needs for energy, excess carbon molecules are produced. If carbon is produced faster than it can be converted by the body into carbon dioxide, water, and energy, the excess saturated fatty acids and cholesterol are then deposited as fat or

TASTES GREAT, EAT MORE

Burgers and fries from fast-food chains can't honestly be called complete "junk food," since they do contain some nutritious foods in addition to harmful ones. But remember: The goal of fast-food chains is to create a taste in their food that makes you want more. Besides being more economical, hydrogenated oils give food a fatty taste that makes you want to eat more. The same craving cycle occurs with sugar. When you eat a high-junk-sugar food, your insulin levels rise, which causes your blood sugar to plummet from high to low. Even when the blood sugar is low, the insulin release may continue keeping blood insulin levels high, which increases your cravings for more sugar, and the cycle continues. As a result of the chemistry of cravings, people who eat more junk food crave more junk food; those who eat more nutritious foods crave more nutritious foods. The nutritionally rich get richer, and the nutritionally poor get poorer.

carried in the bloodstream as cholesterol. The body does this because the excess carbon molecules themselves would otherwise be toxic to its metabolic processes. However, while the body can turn excess sugar into fat, it can't turn fat back into sugars. It must burn off the excess fat as fuel through exercise. Another side to the "sugar becomes fat" story is the body's "feast or famine" survival mechanism. When you feast on excess high-carbohydrate foods, the body stores these excess calories as fat as a way of storing energy in case of famine.

NUTRIMYTH

Low-fat food is healthier for your heart and reduces your weight. Not necessarily. Overeating any food, whether it's fats or carbohydrates, will put on the body fat. "Low-fat" snacks and fast foods tend to be loaded with carbohydrates and often junk sugars. Without the fat to fill up on, it's easier to overdose on carbs. If you eat more carbohydrates than the body can burn, the excess carbs will not only be deposited as fat but also raise the level of triglycerides in the bloodstream, which in itself increases the risk of heart disease and stroke. A low-fat diet can lead to a lean body *only* if it's part of an overall low-calorie diet.

A FOURTH HELPING OF FAT FACTS

If you really want to both trim the amount of fat in your diet and eat the right kinds of fats, here are some important fat facts to consider:

Fishy fats. Ever wonder why cold-water fish contain more polyunsaturates and are healthier to eat than warm-water swimmers? The fat in the fish is adapted to the temperature of the water. The colder the water, the more fluid — therefore, the less saturated — the oil needs to be. So, cold-water fish are naturally higher in unsaturated, healthier fats, called "omega fatty acids." The fat an animal contains is perfectly suited for its survival. If a fish contained the same fat as a steer, and the steer was loaded with fish oil, the steer would feel like Flubber, and the fish would sink.

THE FAT OF THE LAND OR THE FRUITS OF THE SEA?

Fats from fish or algae are nutritionally preferable to animal fats for several reasons. Fish and algae fats are much higher in unsaturated fatty acids, whereas most animal fats are around 50 percent saturated and 50 percent unsaturated. Another factor is the difference in the essential-fatty-acid content of fish and animals. Fish and algae fats contain essential fatty acids primarily of the omega 3 variety, which are important to the formation of anti-inflammatory prostaglandins, which help the body repair and heal itself, replacing old tissue with new. It is interesting to speculate about a connection between the rising incidence of inflammatory and degenerative diseases, such as arthritis, multiple sclerosis, and colitis, as well as many neurological disorders, such as depression and A.D.H.D., and the predominance of animal fats over fish fats in the average American diet. It is also interesting that cultures that eat a lot of fish have a lower incidence of these diseases.

Also, consider the fish skins. The healthiest fish oils are found under the skin. Unlike poultry, it's best to eat the fish with the skin on.

Fattening fats. If you are trying to lose weight or stay lean, be especially vigilant about counting fat calories, since these are absorbed and stored as fat more quickly than calories from carbohydrates or proteins. Calories from fat are more fattening than those from carbohydrates or proteins for three reasons. First, each gram of fat contains over twice as many calories as the same amount of protein or carbohydrate. Second, the body stores the

NUTRITIP
The Healthiest Fats Award

The two F's, fish and flax, win our Best Fats Award because they are the richest sources of essential fatty acids, such as omega 3. Add a tablespoon of ground flaxseed or flaxseed oil to smoothies or salads. Cold-water fish, especially salmon and tuna, are two of the best seafood sources of essential fatty acids.

calories from dietary fat as body fat more easily than calories from other nutrients. Third, when you eat a food, the body burns some of the calories from that food just to metabolize it. The body uses only 3 percent of the calories from fat to metabolize it, yet burns 20 to 25 percent of the calories from carbohydrates to convert them into sugars. The body prefers to burn carbohydrates as

FAT CALORIES ARE FATTER

While an excess of any calorie-containing food can turn to body fat, an excess of fat calories is more likely to find its way to your waistline than an excess of calories from carbohydrates and proteins. There are two reasons for this. First, the body uses two main fuels, carbohydrates and fats, but the body prefers to burn carbohydrates and store fat. A second reason is that the body burns fewer calories during the digesting and metabolizing of fats than it burns with carbohydrates. Not only are fat calories more costly, but the wrong fats carry an even greater price. The body burns unsaturated fats more easily than it burns saturated fats. This means that saturated fat is even more likely to be stored as body fat.

a quick energy source, burning fat for energy only when the carbohydrate stores are exhausted. Also, the body burns the healthier fats (unsaturated fats) for fuel more easily than it burns saturated fats, which are more likely than unsaturated fats to make their way onto your waistline.

Fowl fats. Most fowl fat lies just under the skin. Once you remove that flavorful fatty stuff, the underlying meat, especially the white, is fairly lean — around 7 percent fat. As an added fat perk, fowl fat is rich in omega fatty acids. So, choose the whiter chicken breast over the darker chicken thighs, bake instead of frying the bird, and remove the skin. Also, pick your poultry. Turkey is leaner than chicken, and its white meat is leaner than dark. Dark meat contains almost twice as much fat as white meat.

Green fats. While we don't think of plants as rich sources of fat, some are. Although it is true that plants do not contain a lot of fat, what little fat they contain is high in essential fatty acids. Plants use omega-3 fatty acids to store sunlight energy. The darker and greener the leaves, the more essen-

tial fatty acids these leaves usually contain. So, do your brain and your body a favor: Choose spinach, collards, mustard greens, and kale for your salad makings and leave the iceberg lettuce at the store.

Slimming fats. Essential fatty acids (omega 3 and 6) are the fascinating fats that are least likely to succeed in making their way to the thighs and waist. Essential fatty acids actually stimulate metabolism by speeding up the rate at which the body burns fats and glucose. I noticed this interesting fat perk when I began my L.E.A.N. program (see Chapter 35). I consumed most of my daily fat requirements in fish and flax, and my craving for fattening fats was reduced.

Farm fats. Fish that swim and fowl that run have healthier fat profiles than those that live in a cage or pond, for two reasons. It's common sense that meat that exercises is leaner than meat that just

---

NUTRITIP
An Omega Salad

Want to make a "right fats" salad? The following salad makings are high in omega-3 fatty acids: 1 tablespoon of flax oil; seeds and nuts, especially walnuts. Flax seed, pumpkin seed, canola, and soy are common oils that are high in omega 3's, and a good combination with omega 3-rich green, leafy vegetables such as spinach.

NUTRITIP
The Chicken and the Egg

What a chicken eats shows up in her eggs. Eggs from free-range chickens contain more omega-3 fatty acids and a lower ratio of omega-6 to omega-3 fatty acids than cage-raised chickens, which are fed lower omega-3 fatty acids and a higher omega-6-to-omega-3 ratio. The yolk of Greek eggs (which come from hens fed fish meal) contains six times the amount of omega-3 fatty acid found in the usual U.S. supermarket eggs. Similarly, ocean-caught fish contain more DHA than farm-raised fish do. This is because the fish eat the algae, which are the primary producers of DHA on our planet.

```
┌─────────────────────────────────────┐
│              NUTRITIP                │
│       The Mother and the Infant      │
│                                      │
│  As with the proverbial chicken and  │
│  egg, the amount of DHA in a         │
│  mother's breast milk depends on the │
│  amount of DHA in her diet. A        │
│  recent study from Australia showed  │
│  that infants nursing from mothers   │
│  who had higher levels of DHA in     │
│  their diets also had better mental  │
│  development at one year of age.     │
└─────────────────────────────────────┘
```

```
┌─────────────────────────────────────┐
│              NUTRITIP                │
│             Easy Mixing              │
│                                      │
│  To help mix in the oil that rises   │
│  to the top of the jar of            │
│  unhydrogenated peanut butter,       │
│  store the jar upside down. That     │
│  way, the oil rises to the bottom of │
│  the jar. Remember to screw the top  │
│  on tightly when you turn it         │
│  upside down.                        │
└─────────────────────────────────────┘
```

sits. Also, plants that grow in the field or foods that grow in the sea are nutritionally better than factory-made feeds. In fact, farm-raised meat may contain as much as 40 percent more fat than free-range or free-swimming varieties.

Fertile fats. The amount of estrogen in the blood seems to be dependent on the amount of fat in a woman's body. If less than 15 percent of a female's normal body weight is fat, menstruation is likely to be delayed or stop temporarily. Gymnasts in training, women with anorexia, and overly lean teens are likely to have delayed or interrupted menstruation.

Polluted fats. Chemical pesticides and pollutants tend to be stored in body fat. So, theoretically, the higher the fat content of the food, the more pesticides and pollutants it could contain. For this reason be careful of high-fat foods, such as beef. For high-fat foods, buying organic varieties makes nutritional sense.

Blood fats. Healthy fats, especially omega-3 fatty acids found in flax and fish oils, can be thought of as blood thinners. Saturated fats are blood thickeners, clogging the arteries and leading to cardiovascular disease.

Nut fats. If you're a peanut butter lover, as I am, be sure to look at the label to detect whether or not it contains the bad fat word — "hydrogenated." Hydrogenating the peanut oil solidifies it so it doesn't separate from the solids and float to the top. In old-fashioned, unhydrogenated peanut butter, the oil has to be stirred back into the peanut butter when you open the jar. Sure, it's a little bit of work, but your arteries will thank you.

Cooking fats. Remember, oils higher in monounsaturates spoil more quickly. Fat-savvy eaters consume antioxidants (literally anti-rust or anti-spoiling nutrients), such as vitamin E, along with vitamin C and beta carotene with their healthy fats and oils. Cooking such foods as onions and garlic (rich in antioxidants) may lessen the damaging effect of heat on oils. Mediterranean cooks who start every dish by slicing onions, mincing garlic, and cooking it all in olive oil may be onto something.

A little bit of fat. Don't burn extra calories worrying about eating all of your fats as essential fatty acids every day. A tablespoon of flax oil or one serving of fish each day should do it. Plant oils and fish oils are much richer sources of essential fatty acids than meat, while meat is a rich source of essential amino acids and protein.

Less of a fat tooth. The Western taste bud is programmed to enjoy the fatty taste and feel of foods in the mouth. Reprogram your taste buds. The more you lower the total fat in your diet, the less your taste buds will crave fat. You may even begin to find that slippery fat feeling on your tongue unpleasant.

Sluggish fats. Don't feel you have to eat a high-fat meal in order to have plenty of energy. Because fat is slower to digest, high-fat meals make you feel full longer, but they also make you feel more sluggish. High-fat meals don't leave you feeling energetic — they make you want to sit rather than run.

Brain fats. The principal fat in the brain is DHA, and the best sources of this fat are products from the sea (seafood and seaweed).

TEN TIPS TO REDUCE YOUR DIETARY FAT

The less fat goes into your mouth, the less fat is deposited in your body. The healthiest diet not only has less total fat but also more of the right kind of fats.

1. **Eat the right amount of fat.** How much fat is the right amount depends upon the age of the eater. Here is a general guide:

   - During the first year, infants need *40 to 50 percent* of their daily calories from fat, since growing brains and bodies need a lot of extra energy.
   - For most children and teens, *30 percent* of daily calories from fat is plenty.

BABY FATS

Babies need fat — lots of it. Adult fat restrictions should not be applied to infants. Human milk contains around 50 percent of its calories in fats. Not only do infants need more fats, but they need more of the right kind of fats, such as DHA for brain growth. Since the brain grows more in the first two years than at any other time in a person's life, it's most important to provide the infant with the right amount of the right fats at this crucial time. Breastfeeding is your best bet for delivering exactly what your baby needs. Infant formulas available in the United States today do not contain DHA, which is the most abundant omega-3 long-chain fat in breast milk.

- Most adults, depending on their general health, activity level, and body type, need *15 to 25 percent* of their total calories from fat. As people get older, the percentage of total daily calories they need from fat usually declines.

FAT AGES

The optimal percentage of fat in a person's diet varies with age. Infants require around 50 percent of their calories from fat. Children and adolescents require around 30 percent; and moderately active adults do not require more than 25 percent of their total daily calories as fats. Many adults can get by with even 10 to 15 percent as long as the fats come mainly from plant and fish sources.

2. **Eat the right kinds of fat.** What kind of fats is as important as the total amount of fat. *Two-thirds* of the fats eaten daily should be unsaturated, and *one-third or less* saturated. (In fact, it's not essential that you eat any saturated fats, since your body makes all the saturated fats it needs.) In a diet with 30 percent of calories from fat, less than 10 percent of the total daily calories should be in the form of saturated fats. There are 9 calories per gram of fat, so a person needing 2,500 calories a day, with 20 percent of those calories coming from fat (i.e., 500 calories), should consume less than 55 to 60 grams (500 calories ÷ 9 grams) of total fat in a day. Of that total, no more than 15 to 20 grams should be saturated fats (i.e., animal fats), and around 40 grams should be unsaturated fats, half of which should be monounsaturated fatty acids, found in vegetable oils, and half polyunsaturated fats, primarily from seafood and plant-food sources.

3. **Avoid hydrogenated and partially hydrogenated fats.** Fats that flow or swim (primarily polyunsaturated fats, such as oil and fish fats) are better for you than fat that just sits there (primarily saturated fats, such as animal fats). Hydrogenated fats have been shown to lower HDL ("good cholesterol"), raise LDL ("bad cholesterol"), raise harmful fats in the bloodstream (called "apolipoprotein B"), and generally raise the risk of cardiovascular disease.

4. **Emphasize fats from plants rather than from land animal sources.** Fats derived from plants contain more essential fatty acids and are predominantly unsaturated fats. Also, plants contain more fiber than animal foods, which gives you a feeling of fullness sooner and tends to reduce the total number of calories consumed.

5. **Use low-fat or nonfat alternatives, especially in dairy products.** Adults and teens should eat fat-free or low-fat yogurt, frozen yogurt, low-fat cheeses, and nonfat or 1-percent milk. Some kinds of cheese, for example, skim-milk mozzarella, have less fat than others. Besides low-fat dairy products, use reduced-fat salad dressings, mayonnaise, and margarine.

6. **Choose leaner cuts of meat and poultry.** Trim the skin off the poultry before cooking. Choose white meat over dark, which contains more than twice as much fat as white meat. Turkey meat is lower in fat than chicken. In most cases, a ground-turkey burger contains less fat than a lean ground-beef burger, but read the label to be certain. To serve a lower-fat beef patty, buy a very lean cut of meat and ask the butcher to grind it up into hamburger. (See page 219 for a ranking of fat content of various cuts of meat.)

7. **Use lower-fat toppings.** Opt for yogurt or "lite" sour cream instead of regular sour cream on baked potatoes and in dips and sauces.

8. **Shun fast-food restaurants.** Children especially eat for pleasure, without regard for the nutritional consequences. It's up to parents to be in charge of the nutritional content of the meal.

9. **Try alternatives to frying.** Instead of making french fries, sprinkle potato slices (even sweet potato slices) with olive oil and bake them. Poach fish and chicken in broth or bake them.

10. **Avoid fat substitutes.** These man-made molecules may taste like fat to the tongue, but they don't act like fat in the intestines, leading consumers to believe they can indulge in fat-laden foods without getting fat. But fake fats foster fat cravings instead

RATING FATS*

Green light. Fats in this category contain at least 80 percent unsaturated fats. Most contain some essential fatty acids, and all of them contribute to the health and well-being of the mind and body. (*Note:* The green light is not a license to overeat fat. Eating too much fat regardless of the type can cause obesity, which itself raises blood cholesterol levels.)

Food	Comment
Human milk	Richest overall source of healthy fats
Algae oil	Richest source of DHA
Flax seeds, flax oil	Richest plant source of essential fatty acids
Fish (cold-water, especially Atlantic salmon and tuna)	Rich source of DHA and other omega-3 fatty acids
Seeds (sunflower, pumpkin)	Rich source of essential omega-6 fatty acids; mostly unsaturated fats
Canola oil	Rich in essential omega-3 fatty acids
Soy products (e.g., soy milk, tofu, tempeh)	Rich in essential omega-3 and omega-6 fatty acids, similar to fish oils; contains lecithin; can reduce cholesterol
Olive oil	Mostly unsaturated fats
Nuts	Almonds and walnuts contain 90 percent unsaturated fats; cashews are lower in total fat, which is mostly unsaturated; walnuts are rich in omega-3 fatty acids
Avocado	Rich in monounsaturated fats
Peanut butter	Mostly unsaturated fats; buy organic and unhydrogenated; good source of protein. Healthy alternatives are soybean butter, sesame seed paste (tahini), and almond butter
Hummus (a spread made from chickpeas)	Approximately 85 percent of fat is unsaturated; good source of protein, folic acid, many vitamins and minerals
Wheat germ	Mostly unsaturated fats; rich source of many other vitamins and minerals

* *Rating foods in order of priority has inherent problems, since the key word to healthy nutrition is what grandmother always said: balance. It is best to eat a balanced diet containing many kinds of these fats, not just one or two of the top ten.*

RATING FATS (CONTINUED)

Yellow light. Fats in this category contain a balance of saturated and unsaturated fatty acids, which, if eaten in moderation, contribute to the health and well-being of the body. Look for low-fat varieties. Many of these foods are also rich sources of other nutrients.

Food	Comment
Yogurt (low fat)	Like all dairy products, mostly saturated fats
Milk (1 or 2 percent)	Around 50 percent the fat content of whole milk
Egg	More unsaturated than saturated fats; yolk is high in cholesterol; use only egg white if you are cholesterol sensitive
Beef (sirloin, trimmed)	High cholesterol; about 50-50 saturated and unsaturated fats
Turkey (breast, skinless)	Around 50-50 saturated and unsaturated fats
Veal (loin)	About 50-50 saturated and unsaturated fats
Cocoa butter	Even though it is a saturated fat, it is metabolized like a monounsaturated fat similar to olive oil

Red light. You could eliminate all the fats in this category and you would be healthier for it. Any nutrient that might be in any of these fats can be obtained from other fats with better nutritional credentials.

Food	Comment
Tallow (chicken or beef)	90 percent saturated fats
Lard	High in saturated fatty acids
Palm kernel oil	Mostly saturated fats; contains palmitoleic acid, a fat that, if eaten in excess, can interfere with essential-fatty-acid metabolism and prostaglandin formation
Coconut oil	Over 90 percent saturated fats
"Hydrogenated," or "partially hydrogenated"	Tops the list of fats that are bad for you
Margarines high in hydrogenated fats	Especially those with a lot of coconut, palm kernel, and hydrogenated oils
Shortening	Especially those with lard, hydrogenated oils, palm kernel, coconut oils, or tallow
Cottonseed oil	More unsaturated than saturated fat but usually hydrogenated and may contain pesticide residues

---

NUTRITIP
Better Butter

As a healthier alternative to butter, mix butter with canola oil. Put two sticks of butter into a food processor and blend until smooth. While the processor is running, slowly pour in 1 cup of canola oil. Continue to blend until smooth. Drizzle in 1 tablespoon of liquid lecithin. Store it in the refrigerator in a covered container.

NUTRITIP
Mixed Messages

Just don't buy junk foods. If your children see junk food in the pantry, they get a confusing message: "If these foods are bad for me, why do Mom and Dad buy them?" The same message can be said for using junk food as rewards, leaving children to wonder, "If they are so bad for me, why are they treats?"

---

of lowering the appetite and raising appreciation for low-fat foods. You can't fool your intestines without paying a nutritional price.

In determining how much of the right kinds of fat, take some tips from your body. Ideally, fat makes up 15 to 22 percent of your body's weight, so these same percentages should fit your diet. Also, the most important organs (brain, heart, kidneys) contain the most unsaturated fats and essential fatty acids; so should your diet. If your diet fat matches your ideal body fat, you're on the right fat track.

2

Controlling Your Cholesterol

EVER SINCE researchers discovered a connection between high-cholesterol diets and a high incidence of heart disease in adults, cholesterol has had a bad reputation. "Low cholesterol" or "no cholesterol" claims appear in red letters on food packaging, and everyone is encouraged to follow a low-cholesterol diet — and rightly so. Yet cholesterol is not really the nutritional gremlin that hides in the American diet, waiting to lash out at you as middle age approaches. It's an excess of cholesterol that is harmful.

CHOLESTEROL FACTS YOU SHOULD KNOW

Since you will see the word "cholesterol" on just about every food package you buy, it's important to know what it is, what it does, and how much is safe.

What Cholesterol Is

Cholesterol is not a fat. Biochemically it's called a "sterol." It contains no calories, so the body cannot derive any energy from it. Cholesterol forms an integral part of the cell membranes throughout your body, sort of like the mortar that holds a

brick wall together. It is particularly important in the cellular structure of the brain and central nervous system and is an important component of the myelin sheath that provides insulation to the nerves. The body uses cholesterol to make bile (hence, "chole- sterol"), which is necessary for proper fat digestion. Cholesterol is also a vital part of the adrenal and sex hormones (estrogen, progesterone, testosterone), and it helps the body manufacture vitamin D.

Only the cell membranes of animal tissue contain cholesterol; plants do not. Cell membranes of plants are composed of fiber, not cholesterol. When you see "no cholesterol" on a package of fruit, vegetables, grains, or even vegetable oil, don't believe that the manufacturer has done you a favor by removing the cholesterol. There was no cholesterol in these foods in the first place. While cholesterol is essential to life, the body makes all the cholesterol it needs. You can live well eating little or no cholesterol.

What Cholesterol Does

Cholesterol enters the body from saturated fats in foods from animal sources, such as meat, poultry, egg yolks, liver, butter, cheese, and other dairy products. This cholesterol goes to the liver, where

COUNTING CHOLESTEROL NUMBERS

Here are some cholesterol numbers you should know so that if your doctor presents them to you, you will understand what they mean:

Total cholesterol
- Desirable: less than 200 milligrams (preferably 180)
- Borderline: 200–239 milligrams
- High: 240 milligrams and above

LDL cholesterol
- Desirable: less than 130 milligrams
- Borderline: 130–159 milligrams
- High: 160 milligrams or above

HDL cholesterol
- Low: less than 35 milligrams
- Desirable: 50 or above

Heart-Healthy Numbers

Triglycerides: under 150 mg.
Cholesterol: under 200
LDL: under 130
HDL: over 50
Cholesterol/HDL < 3.5

What the numbers mean and what you should shoot for. Doctors use these numbers both as a guide to predicting a person's risk of heart disease and to monitor the effects of treatment. Rather than using absolute numbers, cardiologists emphasize ratios, both of LDL to HDL and of total cholesterol to HDL. An ideal ratio is 3.5 to 1 or less. For example, if your LDL is 130 and HDL is 40, your ratio is 3.3 to 1. As the ratio rises above 3.5 to 1, the risk of coronary artery disease increases. The number that seems to be the most predictive of heart disease is the ratio of total cholesterol to HDL. For example, a total cholesterol of 200 and an HDL of 50 would give you a cholesterol-to-HDL ratio of 4 to 1. A cholesterol-to-HDL ratio greater than 4.5 to 1 increases a person's risk of coronary artery disease. The risk doubles at a ratio of 5 to 1 and doubles again at a ratio of 7 to 1. Best is a ratio of less than 3.5 to 1.

The heart-healthy magic number is 3.5 or less

Cardiologists pay a lot of attention to the level of HDL as a predictor of heart disease. One study showed that the risk of heart disease was 38 percent higher in men with HDL under 35, even if their total cholesterol was below 200. So, shoot for a high HDL and a low total cholesterol.

COUNTING CHOLESTEROL IN FOODS

Here are some of the more common cholesterol-containing foods:

Food	Cholesterol (milligrams)	Food	Cholesterol (milligrams)
Human milk (3.5 ounces)	32 (varies)	Dairy products:	
Meats (3 ounces):		Milk (1 cup)	
Liver	400–500	nonfat	<5
Lean ground beef,	78	1 percent	10
lamb, chicken breast,		2 percent	18
pork		whole (3.3–3.7	33–35
Egg, whole or yolk (1 large)	213	percent)	
Fish (3 ounces):			
Catfish	49	Yogurt (1 cup)	
Clams	29	nonfat	<5
Cod	37	low-fat	15
Crab	36–50	whole	29
Halibut	35	Cheese (1 ounce)	
Lobster	81	cheddar	30
Mackerel	62	cheddar, low-fat	6
Orange roughy	17	Cottage cheese (½ cup)	
Salmon	47–60	nonfat	10
Shrimp	130–166	1 percent	10
Snapper	40	2 percent	15
Tuna	42–50	Butter (1 tbsp.)	10

Note: The recommended maximum dietary allowance for cholesterol is less than 300 milligrams per day. There is no RDA minimum for cholesterol. Since your body makes all it needs, it's not essential that you eat any.

it joins the cholesterol that is made there. The cholesterol is transported from the liver to the cells by low-density lipoproteins, or LDL, which acts like a nutritional ferryboat, loading up the cholesterol and navigating through the bloodstream, stopping at cells and depositing cholesterol to the cells that need it. If a cell already has enough cholesterol, it "refuses delivery" of the cholesterol cargo, and the excess LDL stays in the bloodstream, and the cholesterol is deposited in the walls of the arteries, causing atherosclerotic plaque. The more plaque that builds up, the narrower the arteries become, until eventually the blood supply to vital organs is reduced. This is why LDL is known as the "bad cholesterol."*

But take heart — a nutritional rescuer is also present in the bloodstream, the high-density lipoproteins, or HDL, which is known as "good cholesterol," since it travels like a vacuum cleaner through the bloodstream, picking up excess cholesterol in the bloodstream and also possibly sucking the cholesterol from the fat-laden plaques. The HDL carries excess cholesterol back to the liver, where it is converted into bile, which is eliminated in the intestines. How your liver handles cholesterol is determined primarily by genetics and secondarily by your diet.

While this is an oversimplification of a complicated biochemical process, it helps us understand two facts:

1. Any diet that raises cholesterol and LDL and/or lowers HDL is bad.
2. Any diet that lowers cholesterol and/or raises HDL is good.

---

* The cholesterol that is attached to the LDL's is actually the same as the cholesterol that is joined to the HDL's. There are not two different kinds of cholesterol, "good" and "bad." These terms are used to refer to the possibly helpful or harmful effects of the lipoprotein-cholesterol combination.

> ## NUTRIMINDER
> To remember which cholesterol is "good" and which is "bad," think of LDL as "*l*ousy" cholesterol, and HDL as "*h*ealthy" cholesterol. As a further reminder, "lousy fats," the ones that are saturated or hydrogenated, contribute to lousy cholesterol.

How Much Cholesterol Do You Need?

If your body has just the right amount of cholesterol, HDL, and LDL, it is in cholesterol balance. But how much is the right amount?

Homemade versus dietary cholesterol. Your body needs cholesterol so much that it makes around 3,000 milligrams per day; that's ten times the maximum recommendation for daily cholesterol intake from food. For most people, about 80 percent of the cholesterol in their blood is made by their own body, with the rest coming from diet. It is estimated that around 30 percent of people are sensitive to the cholesterol-raising effects of dietary cholesterol. Normally, when a healthy person eats high-cholesterol foods, the liver reduces its own cholesterol production to keep blood cholesterol at a healthy level. In cholesterol-sensitive individuals, this internal monitoring mechanism doesn't operate, so that their blood-cholesterol level goes up when they eat high-cholesterol foods.

One theory that explains cholesterol sensitivity is that humans were originally vegetarians. Originally, human bodies were not genetically equipped to metabolize dietary cholesterol, since plants are cholesterol free. As the human diet began to include animal products, some people's bodies developed metabolic ways to dispose of excess cholesterol and some didn't. People who

CONTROLLING KIDS' CHOLESTEROL

Why worry about cholesterol in children? Aren't heart disease and stroke diseases of older persons? Wrong! You don't get heart disease all of a sudden, even though the heart attack or stroke may be a surprise. Cardiovascular disease begins slowly, one cholesterol molecule at a time. The importance of controlling cholesterol in kids is supported by evidence from the Korean War era, when autopsies of soldiers in their late teens and early twenties revealed a buildup of cholesterol-related plaque and narrowing of the arteries, even though these men appeared to be healthy. Fatty streaks have been found in autopsies of children as young as three years of age, and autopsy studies have shown fatty accumulations in the coronary arteries in more than half of children between the ages of ten and fourteen. Also, studies have shown that in countries with high rates of coronary artery disease, both children and adults have higher cholesterol levels. Studies have also shown that children and adolescents with elevated cholesterol levels are three times more likely to have high levels as adults. Autopsy studies in children have also shown a relationship between LDL cholesterol levels obtained before death and the presence of fatty streaks in coronary arteries. (High cholesterol and fat deposits in the arteries upon autopsy also correlate well in adults.) Even though there have been no long-term studies proving that lowering children's cholesterol levels prevents coronary artery disease in adulthood, we can rely on common sense: Children growing up with a healthy diet are more likely to grow up to be adults with healthy hearts. As a general guide, children shouldn't eat more than 100 milligrams of cholesterol per 1,000 calories in their diet.

Should children have routine cholesterol testing? Currently the Committee on Nutrition of the American Academy of Pediatrics (AAP) recommends the following:

- No infants under one year of age, regardless of family history, should be put on a low-cholesterol diet. (We believe under *two years* of age would be wiser.)
- If there is a family history of hypercholesterolemia (a metabolic quirk causing very high cholesterol and fatty deposits in the skin), children should have their cholesterol checked beginning at age two years and rechecked annually.
- Children whose parents or grandparents (under fifty-five years of age) have a history of coronary artery or cerebrovascular disease should have their cholesterol checked before entering school and every few years thereafter.
- Children with parents whose cholesterol level is 240 milligrams or more should be tested any time after age two and then again five years later.

For school-age children, an acceptable blood, or serum, cholesterol level is below 170 milligrams. In a child with a serum cholesterol above this level or with a positive family history for any of the above risk factors, a complete blood lipoprotein panel (i.e., HDL, LDL, total cholesterol, and triglycerides) should be done on blood samples drawn in the morning after a twelve-hour fast. (To avoid the discomfort of fasting, do a routine nonfasting blood-cholesterol-level test first. If the result is borderline or high, get the complete profile, which needs to be done after fasting.)

The AAP does not believe that routine cholesterol tests are necessary for every child. Every child over two should be on a low-

---

CONTROLLING KIDS' CHOLESTEROL (CONTINUED)

cholesterol diet anyway, and foods high in cholesterol (e.g., a Big Mac, at 103 mg., a Whopper, at 90 mg., and a Double Whopper with cheese, at 195 mg.) should be discouraged for all kinds of nutritional reasons. The foods that children should eat more of (fruits, vegetables, grains, low-fat dairy, and fish) tend to be low in cholesterol anyway.

Though it's not healthy to have a choles-

terol phobia, the earlier you can help your children learn to be cholesterol conscious, the better for their adult hearts. Eating habits developed in childhood are likely to carry over into adulthood. Children who grow up on a high-fat, high-cholesterol diet are likely to continue this fat preference, whereas children who grow up with a healthy diet are more likely to choose healthy foods as adults.

---

descended from the ones that didn't adapt are the cholesterol-sensitive ones.

Gender differences and cholesterol. Women tend to have higher levels of HDL than men, since female sex hormones release HDL and male sex hormones lower HDL. At menopause, estrogen production drops, and so does HDL — just another midlife biochemical quirk that should stimulate menopausal-age women to start an HDL-raising exercise program.

TEN WAYS TO CONTROL YOUR CHOLESTEROL

With every 1-percent reduction of total blood cholesterol, there is about a 2-percent reduction in the risk of heart attack. Getting your total cholesterol down and your HDL, or good cholesterol, up is good medicine. Here's what you can do to control your cholesterol.

1. Eat less fat. Keep your total daily fat intake below 20 percent of your daily calories. If you average 2,250 calories a day, eat no more than 450 calories from fat, or 50 grams of fat (there are 9 calories per gram of fat).

2. Eat the right fats. Eat foods that are low in saturated fats, that contain mostly monounsaturated fats, and that are high in essential fatty acids. This means eating fats from seafood and plant sources. Minimize foods of animal origin, which are high in saturated fats. Keep your saturated fats to less than 10 percent (better is 7 percent) of your total daily calories.

Get used to checking package labels for grams of saturated fat per serving. Avoid hydrogenated or partially hydrogenated oils and shortenings. New insights into the fatty food–heart disease correlation reveal that the amount of saturated fats and hydrogenated fats in a food may actually do more harm to the fats in your blood than the cholesterol itself in the food. The trans fatty acids in hydrogenated fats do all kinds of bad things to

---

NUTRITIP
How Much Cholesterol Every Day?

The American Heart Association recommends that people keep their total daily cholesterol intake under 300 milligrams.

NUTRITIP
Eat Your Eggs.

Because eggs are high in cholesterol, they have been lumped together with meat as nutritional no-no's. Wrong! Studies show that for most people who do not have high cholesterol or who are not particularly sensitive to dietary cholesterol, consuming an egg a day does not significantly elevate serum cholesterol. Most nutrition experts suggest that one egg three times a week can be part of a healthful diet.

NUTRITIP
Prepare for Your Test.

Several things can affect the accuracy of cholesterol blood tests, such as fluctuations in weight, changes in diet, pregnancy, and excessive alcohol intake. The most accurate results are obtained when your weight has been stable for at least two weeks and you are eating your usual diet. While total cholesterol and HDL are fairly accurate without fasting, the most accurate measurements of triglycerides and LDL can be obtained first thing in the morning after a twelve-hour overnight fast. (To avoid the discomfort of fasting, do a routine nonfasting blood-cholesterol-level test first. If the result is borderline or high, get the complete profile, which needs to be done after fasting.)

blood fats, such as increase LDL (bad) cholesterol, decrease HDL (good) cholesterol, increase triglycerides, and increase lipoprotein A — the blood fat that contributes to plaque in the arteries. Look for labels that claim "contains no saturated fats" or "contains no hydrogenated oils."

Eat more fish that contain omega-3 fatty acids (i.e., cold-water fish, such as sea bass, salmon, and albacore tuna), which help lower blood fat levels and reduce the risk of blood clots, which can clog arteries and cause strokes and heart attacks. Replacing saturated fats in your diet with unsaturated ones (e.g., vegetable and fish oils) can reduce blood LDL levels. Also, avoid tropical oils, such as palm-kernel and coconut, that may promote atherosclerosis (see "Rating Fats," page 19). Choose monounsaturated fats instead, such as olive oil, canola oil, and nut oils. These monounsaturated fats do not lower HDL levels.

3. Cut cholesterol-containing foods. Too much cholesterol in the diet increases the amount of LDL, the bad cholesterol. As we said above, cholesterol is found only in animal products, not in plant foods. Therefore, eating fewer animal foods and more plant foods will lower the blood cholesterol. While eating lean beef and peeling the skin

off chicken reduces the cholesterol in these foods, cholesterol and saturated fat are still present within even lean meat and poultry. Organ meat, such as liver, is particularly loaded with cholesterol. (Remember, making cholesterol is the liver's job.) Lean beef, lean lamb, lean pork, and lean chicken all contain about the same amount of cholesterol. Egg yolks, milk fat, and shellfish (shrimp and lobster), though healthful, are high in cholesterol. Other oily fish, such as salmon and tuna, are much lower. White-fleshed fish tend to be the lowest in saturated fat. (For a list of common cholesterol-containing foods, see page 23.)

While your goal may be to raise the level of your good cholesterol, you can't get HDL directly from foods. If you have a high-cholesterol problem, switching to a vegetarian eating style (with fish and nonfat dairy products, such as nonfat yogurt) will lower your levels quickly. People who go

IS CHOLESTEROL REALLY THE CARDIAC CULPRIT?

The health-care industry has built a whole cardiovascular complex (almost a religion) around heart disease and cholesterol, and certainly experimental evidence seems to indicate that there is a cause-and-effect relationship between high-cholesterol diets and a high incidence of heart disease. But is it really the cholesterol in the food that causes problems, or could there be something else present (or absent) in high-cholesterol foods that affects heart disease? Why do plant-food eaters have lower cholesterol than animal-food eaters? While the obvious answer is that plant food doesn't contain cholesterol, and animal food does, could there be another explanation? Plant foods are high in phytonutrients and antioxidants, such as vitamin C, and fiber. Meat, on the other hand, is low in vitamin C and fiber. Our belief is that while it's easier to blame heart disease on one chemical, cholesterol, the connection is more complex. Switching from a primarily animal-based diet to one based on plant and seafood sources may be just what the heart doctor ordered.

on a vegetarian diet in which they reduce their fat intake by 26 percent have shown a significant drop in blood-cholesterol levels in just six weeks. One study showed that switching from whole milk to nonfat milk lowered the total cholesterol of people in the study by 7 percent and the LDL (bad) cholesterol by 11 percent after six weeks.

4. Eat cholesterol-lowering foods. Besides avoiding cholesterol-containing foods, you can eat plant foods that actually lower blood cholesterol. Plant foods have chemicals in them called "sterols," which, like cholesterol, hold the cell membranes together. By a fortunate biochemical quirk, plant sterols are not absorbed through the intestines and into the bloodstream, but they do decrease the absorption of the sterols in animal foods (cholesterol). The following are some plant foods in everyday use that lower blood cholesterol.

OVERWEIGHT CHOLESTEROL

We think of fatty foods as the cause of high cholesterol, yet eating more calories than we need from any food (fats or carbohydrates) can raise blood cholesterol, since being overweight itself raises blood cholesterol and increases the risk for heart disease. So, controlling your intake of all foods is important in controlling your cholesterol.

READ THE FINE PRINT

While some food packaging boasts "cholesterol free" on the front, the fine print on the back may tell you the food it contains is full of saturated and hydrogenated fats. Highly saturated tropical oils, such as palm kernel oil, may have a worse effect on cholesterol levels than foods that contain cholesterol. Hydrogenated fats also push cholesterol levels higher. Some cereals, for example, are labeled "cholesterol free" on the front of the package, but the fine print will reveal that they contain cholesterol-raising hydrogenated tropical oils.

- *Soy protein.* Switch from sirloin to soy. Replacing animal protein with soy protein reduces blood-cholesterol levels, even when the total amount of fat in the diet remains the same. A recent review of thirty-eight studies concluded that eating soy protein lowered blood cholesterol by an average of 32 milligrams (9 percent), LDL cholesterol by 22 milligrams (13 percent), and concentrations of triglycerides (total fats) by 10 percent. As an added perk, the HDL cholesterol increased a bit. Soy protein worked best in the people who needed it most. While the amount of soy protein it takes to lower cholesterol varies considerably among individuals, as a general guide, if half of your daily protein comes from soy (between 30 and 40 grams of soy protein a day), there should be a cholesterol-lowering effect. This can be accomplished simply by changing from cow's milk to soy milk, or from meat or dairy products to soy substitutes, such as tempeh or tofu. As an added health benefit, soy products contain phytonutrients called "isoflavones," which reduce the risk of some cancers.

NUTRIPERK
Can Yogurt Lower Cholesterol?

While results are inconclusive about whether or not yogurt lowers cholesterol, there is some evidence from experiments done on swine to suggest that byproducts of *Lactobacilli* fermentation (which is what turns milk into yogurt) reduce the body's production of cholesterol. The cholesterol-lowering effect was greatest with nonfat yogurt. Since swine seem to metabolize cholesterol in a way similar to humans, it is possible that yogurt may lower cholesterol in humans, too.

- *Fiber.* Soluble fiber slows the absorption of the cholesterol from animal foods and acts as an intestinal broom to sweep the cholesterol out. Top billing for research-backed cholesterol-lowering effects of fiber goes to oat bran. Eating 1 to 2 ounces a day (30–60 grams) along with a low-fat, low-cholesterol diet can reduce blood cholesterol by 10 to 15 percent. Similar benefits can be obtained from other soluble fiber–rich foods, such as beans, cruciferous vegetables, apricots, prunes, and a super-soluble fiber-rich food, psyllium, a branlike grain that has been shown to lower your cholesterol by 15 percent within two to four months if you eat an average of 10 grams (3 tsp.) per day.

- *Nuts.* A recent study showed that people who got 30 percent of their daily calories from fat, of which two-thirds were from walnuts, lowered their cholesterol by 12 percent within four weeks. The cholesterol-lowering effect of nuts was thought to be due to the combination of fiber, B vitamins, and vitamin E, and to the fact that these fats are primarily unsaturated ones. But don't go too nutty — nuts are high in fat, so it's important not to eat too many.

- *Garlic.* The jury is still out on whether or not garlic will lower your cholesterol. Powdered garlic supplements probably will not. Eating one clove of garlic per day may. Watch your local health columns for a garlic update. Until then, stick to the proven cholesterol-lowering foods, soy and fiber, and eat garlic because you enjoy it.

- *Alcohol.* You may also read that one or two drinks of alcohol a day can raise HDL cholesterol. In fact, the jury is still out on whether the HDL-raising effect is significant enough to lower the risk of heart disease and to outweigh the potential harmful effects of alcohol, at least in some individuals.

5. Get lean. Trimming excess body fat can increase the levels of good cholesterol (HDL). It is not only excess body fat that influences cholesterol levels, it's where you carry it. Studies show that men who carry excess fat around the middle (a body type we refer to as "apples") are at a higher risk of coronary artery disease than those who carry excess weight around the hips and buttocks ("pears"). Research has shown that apple-shaped people should pay even more attention to staying lean through a combination of exercise and a low-fat diet. Being fat increases LDL and decreases HDL, just the reverse of what you want, and this effect seems to be more aggravated in "apples" than in "pears."

6. Exercise. Aerobic exercise (the kind that gets your heart rate up) raises the level of HDL cholesterol and may also reduce levels of LDL. In fact, since there is no such thing as eating foods high in HDL cholesterol, the only two ways you can raise HDL cholesterol are by exercising and by reducing your body fat. (For more on the benefits of exercise, see Chapter 35.) Exercise is one of the few cholesterol-lowering activities that accomplish all three goals: lowering total cholesterol, raising HDL, and lowering LDL. Exercise stimulates the body to manufacture more HDL. The cholesterol level of athletes is much lower than that of sedentary individuals.

7. Relax. Stress releases the stress hormones, such as adrenaline, which can elevate blood-cholesterol levels. A daily relaxation program, such as meditation, deep breathing, or mental imagery, can lower blood cholesterol.

8. Graze. Grazing on many mini meals throughout the day rather than eating three big meals can lower cholesterol. In studies comparing frequent snackers to three-meals-a-day eaters, the grazers had lower cholesterol.

9. Don't smoke. Smoking makes everything that's bad for the heart worse.

10. Raise low-cholesterol kids. Children who grow up with a plant-and-seafood-based diet rather than one high in animal-based foods are more likely to grow up with healthier hearts.

3

Sweet Facts About Sugar

SUGAR, LIKE FAT, gets a lot of sour press, some deserved, some not. Babies are born with a sweet tooth. Human milk is quite sweet, so a child begins life making the connection between eating and drinking sweet food and pleasure. Sugars are one form of carbohydrates, and carbohydrates are good for you, as long as you eat the right kinds in the right amounts. Carbohydrates are your body's main source of energy. You couldn't live or work without them. Your body needs a lot of carbohydrates — around 60 to 70 percent of your total calories should be in the form of carbohydrates. But before you reach for the carbs in a candy bar, take some time to learn about sugar and other kinds of carbs. Overprocessed, factory-made sugars and starches have given carbohydrates a bad reputation. Once you understand which carbs are good for your body and which aren't, you can indulge a sweet tooth and still enjoy sweet health.

SUGAR SCIENCE

Carbohydrates appear in many forms in many foods, and there are also many different kinds of sugar besides the familiar white grains in the sugar bowl. Following are some carbohydrate terms you should know.

TOP NINE COMPLEX CARBS

- chickpeas
- lentils, beans, peas
- nut butters
- oatmeal (without added sugar)
- pasta
- soy
- sweet potatoes
- whole grains: whole wheat, brown rice
- whole-grain cereals

- *Carbohydrates* are the group of nutrients that contain *carbon atoms* that have been *hydrated* by adding water molecules. Carbohydrates are actually built of sugar molecules, called "saccharides." They're arranged like beads on a necklace. Carbohydrates include sugars, starches, and fiber. Both sugars and starches are broken down by the body into the simple sugar glucose. Glucose molecules then circulate in the bloodstream, supplying cells with fuel on an as-needed basis. Extra glucose is converted into glycogen, which is sugar that is stored in the muscles and the liver. If the body is already storing enough glycogen, glucose gets changed into fat. Your body prefers to burn glucose, or

31

glycogen, for energy, but when these reserves are depleted, it draws on fat, the reserve fuel. Carbohydrates are an important part of the diet, since your body needs energy to grow, to work, and to repair itself.

• *Simple carbohydrates* are those that contain only one or two saccharides. These include sucrose, which is table sugar (made of one molecule of glucose and one of fructose), and lactose, the sugar found in milk (made up of glucose and galactose). Simple carbohydrates all end in the suffix *-ose,* a tip-off that the substance is a sugar. A simple carb that contains one sugar is known as a "monosaccharide." Monosaccharides include glucose and fructose, the sugar in fruits. If the carbohydrate contains two sugar units, it is known as a "disaccharide." In general, the simpler the sugar, the more sweet it is. Fructose, the sugar found in fruit and honey, is the sweetest.

• *Complex carbohydrates* are known as "polysaccharides." They are made of long, complicated strings of simple sugars, and there are many different kinds. As a general rule, complex carbohydrates — what grandmother called "starches" — are the ones that are most nutritious, since they are usually part of foods that contain a variety of other nutrients and not much fat. Starches, like simple sugars, are broken down into glucose fuel by the body, but it takes longer to digest most starches, so they don't cause blood-sugar fluctuations the way simple sugars do. Fiber is also a complex carbohydrate, but human intestines do not contain the enzymes necessary to break down the fiber's long carbohydrate necklace into individual sugar molecules so that it can be absorbed in the bloodstream. Carbohydrates don't count as calories in the diet unless they are burned for energy, so fiber is really a calorie-free food. Fiber in a food slows the digestion of other carbohydrates, especially soluble fibers (e.g., citrus fruits, oats, and legumes). The extra fiber in whole grains also slows the digestion and absorption of sugar, which explains why whole grains in cereal are digested more slowly than high-carb refined pasta.

RATING THE SUGARS

Nutritionally speaking, there is no such thing as a bad sugar, since all digestible sugars provide en-

---

NUTRITIP
Satisfying Carbs

Beginning a meal with a complex carbohydrate food, such as pasta, and eating it slowly will lessen your craving for fats during the rest of the meal. You'll start to feel full and won't want as much of higher-fat foods. So use pasta (with low-fat sauce) to curb overeating.

SWEETEST SUGARS

Carbohydrates differ in their degree of sweetness, and complex carbohydrates, such as starches, while being the least sweet, are the best for your body. Carbs ranked from most sweet to least sweet are:

• honey
• fructose sugar (fruits, fruit concentrate)
• table sugar (sucrose)
• complex carbohydrates (starches)

Complex carbs taste less sweet because, being a larger molecule, they don't fit as easily into the sweet receptors of the taste buds as do the more simple sugars.

ergy to the body. It doesn't matter to an individual cell whether the glucose it is using for fuel entered the body as a starch or as a sugar. Yet, simple and complex carbohydrates behave differently in the body and are part of different nutritional packages. The best carbs are those that not only provide a steady supply of energy but also bring other nutrients the body needs. The worst carbs come in packages with few other nutrients, except perhaps fat, and cause the blood sugar, and often a person's mood, to be unstable.

Best Carbs

Here's how to cash in on your carbs. The best source of energy are complex carbohydrates, better known as "starches." It takes the body a long time to disassemble these elaborate necklaces of sugar molecules. Enzymes in the intestine work steadily to break the bonds between the sugars until they are changed into simple molecules of glucose, which enter the bloodstream at an even pace. Complex carbohydrates are like a time-released capsule. They provide slow, constant energy. The stomach feels full longer, and the body does not experience the highs and lows of blood-sugar swings.

NUTRITIP
Leaner Calories

You're less likely to get fat from the calories in complex carbohydrates than you are from the same number of calories in fat. The body uses a small number of the calories in the food to provide energy to digest that food. Depending on their body type, most people burn a higher proportion of the calories from carbs during the digestion process than they do from the same amount of fat.

Complex carbohydrates are found in grains, vegetables, and legumes — foods that provide vitamins, minerals, and fiber as well as energy. You get a lot of nutritional bang for your buck with complex carbs.

Next Best Carbs

Fructose sugars are simple monosaccharides rather than complex carbohydrates. They come in packages — fruits — that contain important nutrients and fiber. Fruit sugars provide quick energy, but do not excite the blood-sugar roller coaster because the fiber slows absorption of the sugars. Unlike the simple sugar glucose, which quickly enters the bloodstream, fructose sugar has to go to the liver before it is released into the bloodstream and carried to the body's cells. Since fructose is the preferred source of glycogens (sugars stored in the liver and muscle), it is a valuable energy food before and after long periods of exercise.

Carbs to Consume with Caution

Conventional wisdom says that since all carbohydrates are eventually digested and absorbed as glucose anyway, the original food source of the sugar, whether it's a bean or a candy bar, matters little. Sugar is sugar. Sucrose is sucrose. Not exactly! New insights into how various sugars behave in the body have revealed otherwise. While it is true that the sucrose in an orange is chemically the same as the sucrose in the much-maligned table sugar, the fact that the sucrose in the orange is packaged along with other nutrients makes it biochemically more friendly in the body. When you eat sucrose as part of a fruit or vegetable, you get not only vitamins and minerals in the package but also fiber and other complex carbohydrates that steady the absorption of the sugar. Take the sugar away from the rest of the fruit or vegetable and refine it into a powder, and the sucrose gets down-

SWEET NAMES

While there are many types of sugars, some are sweet somethings, while others are sweet nothings. Here are the more common sugars you will see in the ingredients list on a product label. Knowing what they are and their nutritional value will help you make better choices.

- **Glucose** is the simplest sugar and the one most rapidly absorbed into the bloodstream. Glucose is often called "dextrose" when it is added to foods. The body eventually breaks down all sugars and carbohydrates into glucose, which is the form in which sugar enters cells to be used for energy.

- **Sucrose** (otherwise known as "table sugar") is composed of one molecule of glucose and one molecule of fructose. This white sugar comes in many forms, such as powdered or granulated. It is usually made from refining extracts of sugar beet or sugarcane.

- **Fructose** is one of the main sugars found in fruits and honey. It is often preferred to straight glucose and sucrose as an energy source, since it is absorbed more slowly into the bloodstream and, therefore, has a less erratic effect on blood-sugar levels. It is a popular sweetener. But don't be fooled by fructose. Consumers associate this sugar with fruit, which is highly nutritious, but on its own, fructose is like any highly refined sugar — just a bunch of empty calories.

- **Lactose** is the primary sugar in dairy products and is composed of one molecule of glucose and one of galactose. Because of its galactose content, it is more slowly absorbed into the bloodstream than pure glucose and is therefore more blood-sugar friendly. Unlike glucose, which is quickly and easily absorbed through the intestines, lactose requires an enzyme in the intestines, lactase, to break down the sugars and allow absorption. People who are lactose intolerant don't produce enough lactase to break down milk sugars. The lactose ferments, causing gas and diarrhea.

- **Maltose** is composed of two molecules of glucose and is the sugar found in barley malt and some cereals. The maltose in beer causes a rapid rise in blood sugar.

- **Corn syrup** is a sugar extracted from corn. Being extracted from corn doesn't make it any healthier than ordinary table sugar. Syrups are really sugar concentrates, and 1 tablespoon of syrup, corn or maple, contains about twice the number of calories as 1 tablespoon of granulated sugar. While syrups do contain traces of a few minerals, such as calcium, phosphorus, iron, potassium, and sodium, they essentially have the same nutritional value as table sugar. Because corn syrup is cheap to produce, it is the most popular sweetener for beverages and even some juices. Because of its high calorie content, it is seldom found in diet drinks. People who are allergic to corn should check labels carefully, since corn syrup will trigger their allergies.

- **High-fructose corn syrup** is a sweetener containing 40 to 90 percent fructose and is a carbohydrate extract from corn. This popular and inexpensive sweetener is used widely in cereals and sodas.

- **Molasses** is a thick syrup, a by-product of the sugar-refining process. Yet, unlike ordinary table sugar, molasses contains other valuable nutrients besides carbohydrates. The darker the molasses, the greater its nutritional value. Blackstrap molasses, for example, is a valuable

---

SWEET NAMES (CONTINUED)

source of calcium, iron, and potassium and also contains traces of B vitamins.

- **Brown sugar** is simply ordinary table sugar made brown by adding molasses. Because of the added molasses, brown sugar contains a trace more nutritional value than white sugar, but not enough to make it any more valuable as a source of nutrients.

- **"Raw" sugar** is more about a marketing gimmick than about a nutritional difference. The term "raw" implies a more natural sugar. Yet, raw sugar is nothing more than crystallized, refined white sugar with a touch of molasses left in. Because raw sugar appears in larger crystals than the refined granules of ordinary table sugar, it seems more healthful. But this belief has no basis in fact.

---

graded from the health-food to the junk-food category. So it's the company the sugar keeps with other nutrients in the food that affects its absorption from the intestines and its consequent behavior in the body.

To understand why these sugars merit the label "junk sugars," let's take a ride with these sugars from the mouth to the bloodstream to see how they affect the body. Junk sugars are called "simple carbohydrates" because they are short, uncomplicated molecules. Because simple sugars are already so small, they require little or no breaking down in the intestines. The sucrose molecule is quickly broken down into glucose and fructose, and all that glucose is actively pumped through the intestinal cells quickly into the bloodstream. A sprinkle of sugar that hits the intestines enters the bloodstream almost immediately, and the roller-coaster ride begins.

After the refined sugars rush into the bloodstream, blood-sugar levels rise, pressuring the pancreas to release insulin, the hormone needed to escort these sugars into the body's cells. Lots of insulin helps the sugar get used up rapidly, but then the blood-sugar level plunges. The body hits a sugar low, also known as "hypoglycemia" or "sugar blues." Now, just as insulin was released when the blood-sugar level was too high, adrenal hormones are released when the blood-sugar level is too low. These stress hormones want to restore the blood

sugar to normal levels, so they squeeze stored sugar from the liver, sending the blood-sugar level back up. These adjustments work better in some people than in others and better in some circumstances than others. Sugar-sensitive individuals experience the ups and downs of blood-sugar levels as a roller-coaster ride, and their moods and behavior go up and down with their blood sugar.

GLYCEMIC INDEX

An important characteristic of sugars and starches is the glycemic index (GI), which is a measure of how quickly a carbohydrate is digested, enters the bloodstream, and raises the blood-sugar level. Foods with a low glycemic index enter the bloodstream slowly and trigger the insulin response less quickly, contributing to a steadier blood-sugar level, and, consequently, a steadier mood. On the other hand, foods with a high glycemic index enter the bloodstream quickly and jolt the insulin response into action, quickly leading to large blood-sugar swings — from high to low — which can cause irritability, anxiety, and jitteriness. When you eat a variety of carbohydrates together at a meal, the glycemic index is not that important. The effect of one food offsets that of another. Here's how different kinds of carbohydrates rank from lowest to highest in glycemic index:

SWEET SUBSTITUTES

Want to satisfy your sweet tooth yet get more nutritional bang for your calorie buck? Instead of heaping tablespoons of the white stuff, try these suggestions:

- *Fruit concentrates.* Fructose sugar is sweeter than table sugar, and because of its more steady absorption and metabolism in the bloodstream, it doesn't produce the roller-coaster effect of refined sugars. Fruit concentrates, such as pear and apple, are the best, because fructose is the primary sugar in these fruits. While the amount of fruit concentrate you choose to use depends upon your own sweet or tart preferences, as a general guide, use half as much fruit concentrate as sugar in a recipe.

- *Cinnamon.* Cinnamon is a sweet spice, and a small amount goes a long way. Two teaspoons of cinnamon can change a tart apple pie to a sweet one, lessening the amount of sugar needed. As an added nutritional perk, 1 teaspoon of cinnamon contains 28 milligrams of calcium and traces of B vitamins, fiber, and iron.

- *Other sweet spices.* Spicing up a dish with distinct flavors will lessen your temptation to add sugar. Try these herbs and spices to accent the flavor in foods: mint, cloves, anise, and ginger. A sprinkle of nutmeg is an additional sweet complement to cinnamon. A twist of lemon peel spruces up the look and flavor of almost any beverage, including plain water.

- *Fruit toppings.* Use crushed pineapple, applesauce, strawberries, or blueberries instead of syrup on pancakes and waffles. Sprinkle on some cinnamon or nutmeg to bring out the fruit's natural sweetness.

- *Plain yogurt flavored with fresh fruit.* The result is less sweet and contains better sugars than the yogurt with the added syrupy fruit preserves.

- *Unsweetened canned or frozen fruit packed in water or its own juices.* Check the label and avoid those to which syrups have been added.

- *Reducing the sugar called for in recipes by at least half.* Add some cinnamon, nutmeg, vanilla, or fruit concentrate to perk up the sweetness. (This may not work well in traditional recipes for cookies and cakes. You may have to experiment to discover how low you can go and still produce results you find acceptable.) If you substitute honey or molasses, use half or less of the recommended amount for sugar. If the recipe calls for 1 cup of sugar, try using ¼ cup to ½ cup of honey.

- *A cinnamon stick in coffee or tea.* The swirling is fun and gives you something to do with your hands. Many people find the cinnamon stick helpful after a meal for breaking not only the sugar habit but also the smoking habit.

1. legumes
2. dairy products
3. vegetables
4. fruits
5. whole grains
6. refined sugars and grains

The glycemic index is more important when eating carbohydrates alone as snacks. For example, an apple, because of its lower GI, is more blood sugar friendly than a banana. It would be better to eat the banana, which has a higher GI, with yogurt for breakfast or with peanut butter for lunch.

The foods with a lower GI will slow the absorption of the sugar in the banana.

Fat and fiber slow sugar absorption, so the sugar in ice cream enters the bloodstream more slowly than the sugar in soda. The sugar from a baked potato eaten without sour cream gets in the bloodstream faster than one loaded with sour cream or butter. Because of the fiber, the sugar in a whole orange enters the bloodstream more slowly than the sugar in orange juice. (Orange juice is often used as a quick perk-up for diabetics suffering a sudden bout of low blood sugar.) Fiber also is a factor in why apples have a lower glycemic index than bananas.

Sugary soft drinks have a more immediate effect on the blood sugar if they are consumed on an empty stomach than if taken with a meal. Anything that breaks down food into finer particles makes the sugar more quickly digestible, so cooking vegetables and mashing potatoes raises the glycemic index.

The glycemic index may seem like an obscure concept, important only to food chemists, but it actually affects everyone's general health and well-being. For example, one study found that persons who tend to eat diets that are low in fiber and high in carbohydrates with a high glycemic index double their risk of diabetes, especially persons already predisposed to it. In this study, the foods that posed the greatest risks were white bread, white rice, potatoes, sugar, and soft drinks. People with the lowest incidence of diabetes had diets containing lots of whole grains, fiber-rich cereals, and other carbohydrates with a low glycemic index. It seems that high-glycemic, carbohydrate-rich foods put pressure on the pancreas to produce more insulin, causing the pancreas to eventually wear out. The inability to produce enough insulin results in diabetes.

HOW SUGAR HARMS

The complex carbohydrates found in vegetables, grains, and fruits are good for you; the simple sugars found in sodas, candies, frostings, and packaged treats can do harm, at least when eaten in excess. It's as simple as that. Here's why:

Excess sugar depresses immunity. Studies have shown that downing 75 to 100 grams of a simple sugar solution (about 20 teaspoons of sugar, or the amount that is contained in two average 12-ounce sodas) can suppress the body's immune responses. Simple sugars, including glucose, sucrose (table sugar), and fructose, caused a 50-percent drop in the ability of white blood cells to engulf bacteria. In contrast, ingesting a complex carbohydrate solution (starch) did not lower the ability of these

GLYCEMIC INDEX RATINGS*

(lowest to highest)

1. soybeans (15)	11. spaghetti (42)	21. soft drinks (68)
2. fructose (20)	12. grapes (45)	22. bread, white (69)
3. cherries (23)	13. oranges (46)	23. potatoes (70)
4. grapefruit (26)	14. sweet potatoes (48)	24. candy bar (70)
5. kidney beans (29)	15. All-Bran (51)	25. bread, whole wheat (72)
6. lentils (29)	16. oatmeal (54)	26. white rice (72)
7. milk (34)	17. corn (59)	27. refined cereals (80)
8. yogurt (36)	18. table sugar (sucrose) (59)	28. honey (87)
9. chickpeas (36)	19. bananas (62)	29. carrots (92)
10. apples (39)	20. raisins (64)	30. glucose (100)

The glycemic index is the relative rate of blood sugar rising when a given food is compared with glucose, which has a glycemic index of 100. While the GI provides some useful information, you should take these sugar ratings with a grain of salt. Many of these numbers were based on studies of only five or six middle-aged persons, and there are wide individual variations in the glycemic indexes. Also, these values were based upon eating the carbohydrate alone, yet consuming carbohydrates along with other foods (especially those high in fiber) could change the rate of absorption of the sugar and therefore the glycemic index. So, as with many nutritional concepts, let your body be your guide. How you feel and act following a high-carb meal is more important than someone else's numbers. This would be your personal glycemic index.

white blood cells to engulf bacteria. The immune suppression was most noticeable two hours after ingestion, but the effect was still evident five hours after ingestion. This research has practical implications, especially for teens and college students who tend to overdose on sodas containing caffeine and sugar while studying for exams or during periods of stress. Stress also suppresses immunity, so these sugar users are setting themselves up to get sick at a time when they need to be well.

Sugar sours behavior, attention, and learning. Studies of the effects of sugar on children's behavior are wildly contradictory, but the general consensus is that some children and adults are sugar sensitive, meaning their behavior, attention span, and learning ability deteriorate in proportion to the amount of junk sugar they consume.

Sugar promotes sugar highs. Some persons are more sugar sensitive than others, and children may be more sensitive to sugar than adults are. A study comparing the sugar response in children and adults showed that the adrenaline levels in children remained ten times higher than normal for up to five hours after a test dose of sugar. Studies have also shown that some children with Attention Deficit Hyperactivity Disorder (A.D.H.D.) react to glucose-tolerance tests with a dip to low blood-sugar levels. High adrenaline levels or low blood-sugar levels produce abnormal behavior. (See the discussion of sugars on page 302 in Chapter 31, "Feeding the Brain." For more on the connection between food and A.D.D., see "A.D.D. — A Nutritional Deficiency?," page 300, and "A.D.H.D. Foods," page 302.)

Sugar promotes cravings. The more sugar you eat, the more sugar you want. A high-sugar meal raises the blood-glucose level, which triggers the outpouring of insulin. This excess insulin lingers in the system, triggering a craving for more

SWEET NOTHINGS

Certain sugars belong in the same category as fake fats. They not only provide no essential nutrients to the body (in fact, your body can live better without them), but they actually may do harm.

Soft drinks. Many soft drinks provide a double-whammy of sugar and caffeine, a combination that sends most bodies (and minds) on an uncomfortable biochemical roller-coaster ride. Since caffeine is a diuretic, caffeine-containing sodas not only don't quench thirst, they can leave you feeling more thirsty. A 12-ounce can of cola contains about 10 teaspoons of sugar in addition to artificial flavors and caffeine. Here's what's going on in your body: The quick rise in blood sugar causes an insulin burst, which makes the liver respond by turning the excess sugar into fats. Caffeine exaggerates the roller-coaster effect of sugars in the bloodstream by triggering the release of hormones that release stored sugar in the liver. That can of cola will produce a sugar high, but a sugar low is sure to follow.

The junk sugars in soft drinks also take good things out of the body. High doses of sugar and artificial sweeteners increase the urinary excretion of calcium, leading to weaker bones, or osteoporosis, and to deposits of calcium in the kidneys (i.e., kidney stones). The phosphoric acid present in many soft drinks further robs the body of calcium by increasing the loss of magnesium and calcium in the urine.

Then there are the good things that junk sugars take the place of. Junk sugars fill children up, so they tend to eat less of more nutritious foods. Many children drink cola with a meal instead of milk. Or they reach for high-fat junk food to go with the empty calories in their soda. Unfortunately, television advertising has made junk soda along with a junk sandwich the American nutritional norm.

Packaged bakery goods. The combination of white sugar, white flour, and hydrogenated shortening makes packaged bakery goods a nutritionally empty package. Most sweet snacks, such as cupcakes and doughnuts, contain all three of these factory-made foods. Look for baked goods that are made with whole grains, contain no hydrogenated oils, and are sweetened with fruit concentrates.

NUTRITIP
Three "Sweet" Beans

If you are a sugar-sensitive person (you feel uncomfortable after a high-sugar meal), try a three-bean salad. Kidney beans, chickpeas, and pinto beans all have low glycemic indexes. No sugar rush — just good, steady nutrition.

sugar, thus adding another hill to the roller-coaster ride.

Sugar promotes obesity. People tend to eat and drink too many foods and beverages that are sweetened with refined sugar. Foods with a high glycemic index stimulate the production of LPL (lipoprotein lipase), the enzyme that encourages the body to store food in fat cells. Thus, low-fat diets that contain carbohydrates with a high glycemic

FROM SWEET TO SOUR CHILDREN

Research suggests that children are more sugar sensitive than adults, and, according to Dr. C. Keith Conners, author of *Feeding the Brain,* the effects are more pronounced in younger children. This could be related to the fact that the brain grows rapidly in the preschool years, exaggerating the effects of sugar on behavior and learning.

In an interesting study, researchers fed normal preschoolers a high-sugar drink, containing the amount of sugar in the average can of soda, and compared them with children who received a nonsugar drink. The sugar group experienced decreased learning performance and more hyperactivity than the nonsugar group.

Some children are sugar junkies. We've noted that some of our eight children have more of a sweet tooth than others. Whenever I bring home food gifts from patients and lay them on the kitchen table, within minutes the highly sugared ones are "missing," found later in someone's secret stash.

Children tagged with the A.D.H.D. label are often sugar sensitive. There may be several reasons for this. Hyperactive kids are impulsive and need instant gratification. They need more energy and they need it now! Unable to curb their appetite, they overdose on junk foods. Some studies of hyperactive children show a higher blood-sugar rise following a high-sugar meal than one finds in normally active children. Hyperactive children seem to metabolize sugar differently. In response to a high-sugar meal, hyperactive kids increase their output of the stress hormone cortisol, which plays an important role in regulating blood-sugar levels. Based on his own research, Dr. Conners concludes that while the neurotransmitters in the brains of normally active children signal the hormones to regulate blood sugar, brains of hyperactive children do not seem to send the same signals. (For related information, see "Breakfasts for Growing Brains," page 310, and "A.D.H.D. Foods," page 302.)

While studies show that activity levels go up in both hyperactive and normal children on high-sugar diets, the hyperactive children also become more aggressive. Adding protein to a high-sugar meal mellows out the behavioral and learning deterioration. Chalk up another point for eating a balanced breakfast.

index can actually cause weight gain. It's much easier to binge on chocolate chip cookies than fresh peaches or apples, which are more filling and pack a lot of fiber in the stomach. All those extra calories have to go somewhere. Your body says, "Ah, extra energy. I'll pack that away as fat and save it in case there's ever a famine!" Refined starches, such as white flour, white rice, white pasta, and cornstarch, are more likely to turn into body fat than natural starches, such as whole grains, which, because they contain more fiber, are digested more slowly and raise the blood sugar less drastically. Yes, fat will make you fat, but so will sugar. Put them together in soda and chips or high-fat baked goods, and you can expect to put on some pounds. So, even though fat has gotten the reputation as the unhealthful food, excess sugar deserves an equal reputation.

TART TOOTH

Instead of a sweet tooth, develop a tart tooth. As you explore new ways of eating, you will notice a difference in sweetness between traditional American desserts and those from some other cultures. Many American desserts are sickeningly sweet, a taste we have become accustomed to. Many European desserts tend to be less sweet, a taste that once you get used to it becomes quite enjoyable. Without providing an after-dessert blood-sugar plunge, these delicacies are also better for your mood. When you're making desserts, experiment with different amounts and different kinds of sweetness according to the tartness you desire and the natural tartness of the food. For example, some apples are sweeter than others, so, if you're baking an apple pie, keep in mind that they require varying amounts of sweeteners.

Sugar promotes diabetes. While the risk of developing diabetes lies more in the genes than in the diet, the old grandmothers' tale that too much sugar causes diabetes does have scientific support (see "Glycemic Index," above).

Sugar promotes heart disease. When bears are storing up body fat for their long winter hibernation, they consume lots and lots of carbohydrates. When you eat excess carbohydrates, your body turns these sugars into fat. The body stores excesses of most nutrients as a safeguard against starvation. If you eat more carbohydrates than you can burn off, the excess is stored as fats. People who eat too much sugar tend to have higher blood triglycerides, and this increases the risk of cardiovascular disease.

A SWEETER GUT FEELING

Change your sweet tooth to a tart tooth and after a few months of less added sugar in your diet, your intestines, your body, and your mood get used to the more comfortable after-meal feeling of complex carbohydrates. Eventually you will shun frostings, candy bars, and sugar-sweetened cereals and will be put off by how you feel if you eat a packaged sweet treat, especially one that is in the junk-food category. Once your tongue gets used to a tarter taste, you're well on your way to enjoying a healthier relationship with the sugars in your life.

CURBING YOUR CRAVINGS

The good news about the link between body chemistry and cravings is that there are other ways to stimulate the release of your well-being hormones and to keep them at steady levels. Here are some suggestions:

Exercise regularly. One of the healthiest ways to experience better living through better brain

NUTRITIP
No Sweet Rewards

How many parents, desperate to get some broccoli into their preschooler, promise candy for dessert if the vegetables get eaten? This is an unwise nutritional bargain. It teaches children to dislike their veggies and value their sweet treats. Besides, when your child gets older, there will be no one standing over her to encourage her to eat the good food first.

A SPOONFUL OF HONEY

Honey has been renowned as a source of energy and nutrition since humans discovered bees. The Romans regarded honey as "nectar of the gods," and Greek athletes energized themselves with honey before entering the arena. Egyptians put honey in tombs as food for the afterlife. In fact, honey was used as a sweetener centuries before humans learned how to extract sugar from sugarcane or beet. The biblical Promised Land "flowed with milk and honey," and Hippocrates, in his writings on the care and cure of the patient, extolled the nutritional virtues of honey. In short, history regards honey as man's original and most natural sweetener.

Is honey more nutritious than table sugar? Possibly. One reason that honey is touted over table sugar is the "extra nutrition" in the form of proteins, minerals, and vitamins that honey is supposed to contain. The fact is that the trace amount of these nutrients in honey is so insignificant that honey is not superior.

Whether or not the sugars in honey are more nutritious than those in table sugar is controversial. Nutritionists say no. Honey lovers say yes. The sugars in honey and ordinary table sugar (or sucrose) are both primarily a mixture of fructose and glucose, yet honey contains a small amount of other sugars. The composition of sugars in honey can vary from beehive to beehive, according to the source of the nectar. Because of its slower rate of absorption through the intestines and a stopover at the liver before being used by the body, fructose triggers less insulin and therefore less swings in blood sugar. For this reason, honey that contains more fructose than the equivalent amount of table sugar would be metabolically easier on the body. Yet, the glycemic index of honey is about the same as table sugar.

Many people prefer the taste of honey over that of table sugar as a sweetener. Since honey is sweeter than table sugar, when substituting honey for sugar in recipes, use half the amount of honey and decrease the liquid called for in the recipe by the volume of honey that you add. (The American Academy of Pediatrics recommends that honey not be given to infants under one year of age because of the rare possibility of their being infected with the germ that causes botulism.)

---

chemistry is to exercise vigorously, an average of twenty minutes a day. I never realized to what degree endorphins can be stimulated by exercise until I experienced this phenomenon. During the planning of this book, I was being treated for colon cancer. One day, at the peak of my double-whammy dose of chemotherapy and radiation, I experienced a common side effect of these treatments: extreme fatigue. It was the most awful feeling I have ever had, yet I was determined not to let the fatigue lure me into inertia. I wanted to do something about it. I forced myself to do a vigorous twenty-minute workout on my home treadmill. At the end of the twenty minutes, I felt like a new person. The endorphin rush was obvious. The wonderful thing about the brain's natural narcotics is that they give you the feeling of well-being without the unpleasant side effects. So, when you feel a carbo craving coming on, go take a brisk walk outside instead of running to the

SWEET TEETH

One of the ploys we use to get our children to brush their teeth is, "Don't forget to brush off the sugar bugs." Believe it or not, this dental-health marketing image is scientifically correct. The decay-causing bacteria that live in the mouth love sugar, and bacterial action on the sugars is what produces decay-forming plaque. Some sugars are more tooth-friendly than others. Believe it or not, the much maligned white stuff on the table is less likely to damage the teeth than the sweetener with a healthier reputation — honey. The stickier the sugar or the food it's in, the greater the chance of tooth decay. Table sugar dissolved in a hot cup of coffee is less likely to stick to the teeth than honey, raisins, and caramels. So, don't feed those sugar bugs in your mouth!

NUTRITIP
A Sweeter Feeling

If you have an overexcited and foggy feeling following a high-sugar meal or snack, you are a sugar-sensitive person. To avoid that unfocused feeling, concentrate on eating complex carbohydrates and avoid pure carbohydrate foods. Try combination foods, those containing not only carbohydrates but protein and fat, such as yogurt. The fat slows the rate of stomach-emptying and delays absorption of sugar into the blood. Eating raw foods rather than cooked ones also slows the absorption of sugar from the food and leaves you with a more comfortable feeling.

refrigerator. Do this often enough and you'll find yourself craving the exercise rather than the sweet snack. Really.

Graze on good foods. Instead of bingeing on three high-carbohydrate meals a day and snacking on junk-sugar foods in between, eat smaller, more frequent meals. Concentrate on eating complex carbohydrates throughout the day. Keeping your stomach satisfied, but not too full, reduces cravings. When you overeat, the feeling of fullness is usually followed four to six hours later by a feeling of emptiness, just in time for another round of overindulgence. If you're just a little bit full (i.e., satisfied) throughout the day, you're less likely to crave a sugar jolt. The key to weight control is to graze on foods that keep you full without being fattening.

Drink, drink, drink. Not alcohol, but water. Your stomach doesn't have to be full of food to suppress cravings. Water will do the trick. Drinking at least eight 8-ounce glasses of water throughout the day will trick your body into thinking it is satisfied. Carry around a bottle of water to sip. Herbal teas are also good.

Eat a healthy breakfast. Give your brain the best start by beginning each day with a balanced breakfast of complex carbohydrates and proteins, the biochemical partners that not only enhance learning and behavior for school and work but also stimulate the brain neurotransmitters that contribute to a feeling of lasting well-being. People who start the day with a healthy breakfast are less likely to experience a blood-sugar dip and carbo craving later in the morning. People who skip breakfast are more likely to overeat the rest of the day. (See the related discussions "Foods for Thought," page 299, and "Breakfasts for Growing Brains," page 310.)

Cut back on caffeine. Caffeine can trigger a drop in blood sugar. That morning doughnut with

THE CHEMISTRY OF CRAVINGS

Do you have a hard time putting your body on crave control? You are not alone, as many of us crave certain foods. The "wisdom of the body" principle says you'll crave the nutrients you need. But years of unwise eating and a lot of cultural conditioning have taught our bodies to crave foods they don't need.

New research suggests there is a physiological connection between carbs and cravings. Sweets trigger an increase in serotonin — a mood-elevating hormone. The body and brain get used to this higher level of serotonin and even depend on it for a sense of well-being. So, when the serotonin level dips, the craver dips into the chocolate to "correct" the situation. The cycle continues, and in time the sweets eater makes the association between food and mood and believes that sweets ensure well-being.

Another group of hormones, called "endorphins," are also implicated in food cravings. Sweets trigger the release of endorphins (named for *end*ogenous m*orphines*), the brain's natural narcotics, helping you to relax when stressed. So it seems there is a biochemical basis for the good feelings you have after munching on a morsel of chocolate. Endorphins are another part of the biochemical explanation for feelings of well-being. Exercise and sex also trigger endorphin release, and one or the other of these may be a better choice than another slice of cheesecake.

Besides serotonin and endorphins, many other neurochemicals affect cravings. One such is neuropeptide Y (NPY), whose job is seeing that your body (especially your brain) gets enough carbohydrates for energy. As your sugar stores are used up, the blood-sugar dip triggers the release of NPY, which prompts the brain to crave more carbs. This is the neurochemical explanation for why most people prefer a high-carbohydrate breakfast after using up their carbohydrate stores during a ten- to twelve-hour overnight fast. When your fat stores are being depleted, a fat-craving neurochemical called "galanin" is released. Crash dieting and stress can also trigger the release of these neurochemicals that urge you to heed your body's demand for fuel.

As you might expect, given the wisdom of the body, levels of food-craving neurochemicals fluctuate throughout the day. The carbohydrate-craving chemicals (e.g., NPY) are highest in the morning, stimulating you to eat a high-carbohydrate breakfast. Fat-craving neurochemicals are highest in the evening, when the body needs to store fat for the overnight fast.

Nutrient-craving hormones can also play tricks on adolescents. Besides the mood changes associated with hormonal shifts during puberty, hormones also may explain some bizarre adolescent eating habits. Rising estrogen levels prompt females to crave sweet and creamy foods, such as chocolate and ice cream. Males may lose their childish preferences for sweets and come to prefer protein-rich foods, which may account for how a fifteen-year-old boy can wolf down three beef sandwiches at one meal. Girls tend to put on more fat during adolescence in preparation for childbearing, and males tend to build more muscle.

ARTIFICIAL SWEETENERS

Feed your child artificial sweeteners and you may see an increase in artificial reactions. There is reason to believe that artificial sweeteners have no place in the diets of growing children, especially ones who already have problems behaving and learning. The many studies that have tried to show a connection between artificial sweeteners and behavior have produced confusing and conflicting results, so common sense has to take over. Artificial sweeteners (e.g., aspartame and saccharine) were originally developed as a sugar substitute for diabetics, but then the manufacturer discovered a huge market in a calorie-conscious society, one that has also been fed a lot of hype about the hazardous effects of sugar. Artificial sweeteners do not usually satisfy a body that is craving sweets or carbohydrates. In fact, they may so accustom the taste buds to sweet flavors that sweetener users want more sugar rather than less. The more sweets you eat, the more your taste buds get used to the sweet taste, so the more sweetness you need in order to satisfy your sweet tooth. The widespread use of artificial sweeteners or "low-calorie" drinks hasn't been able to stop the increasing incidence of childhood obesity, and, by fostering unhealthy eating habits,

may even contribute to it. As you ease more tartness into your diet, your taste buds regain their sensitivity to sweetness and are more satisfied with less sugar.

Also, some scientists are concerned about the biochemical quirks of artificial sweeteners. The sweetener aspartame is basically a combination of two amino acids, aspartic acid and phenylalanine. Amino acids have different effects on the brain than sugars do. In natural foods these amino acids enter the brain in company with other naturally occurring nutrients. Theoretically, it is also possible that the amino acids in the artificial sweeteners could compete with the natural amino acids in the foods, throwing the neurotransmitters out of balance. In reality, this is unlikely since the amount is so small. Another problem with artificially sweetened drinks is that people tend to drink a lot of them, whereas the calories in a sugar-containing soda will satisfy the appetite. Common sense says that feeding the brain an unnatural substance may cause it to perform in an unnatural way. Our advice for any artificial substance: WHEN IN DOUBT, LEAVE IT OUT.

---

coffee can leave you feeling desperate for another doughnut an hour later. Substitute fruit juice or herbal tea for the coffee, and the doughnuts won't look so tempting.

If your sweet tooth still craves sweets, switch from junk sugars to fruit sugars, preferably in the form of whole fruit, such as an apple or orange. Fructose sugars do not cause the blood levels of sugar and insulin to bounce around, and the fiber in the fruit will satisfy your stomach.

Try non-food substitutes. The best way to break any habit, including a food craving, is to substitute an alternative pleasure. Write down what conditions trigger your cravings, such as boredom, loneliness, anxiety, depression, and develop other ways to perk yourself up. Try exercise, a hobby, music, or just close your eyes for a few minutes and visualize something that relaxes you before going back to your everyday tasks.

NUTRITIP
Best Fruit Snacks

Fruits that contain higher amounts of fructose relative to glucose and sucrose are the most blood-sugar-friendly snacks. The primary sugar in pears and apples is fructose, which, combined with the high fiber content of these fruits, should produce steady sugar absorption with no sugar jolt during snack time. Some fruits, such as oranges, pineapples, peaches, and grapes, contain more glucose than fructose, so the sugar in them will be absorbed slightly faster.

Compromise a bit. It's okay to give in to your cravings occasionally. Your body is forgiving — within limits. If you continually resent giving up a food, you will eventually give in and eat it. You don't have to have a perfect diet. If you believe you can't live without ice cream, you can't. Just cut down on how often and how much you eat and try some alternatives, such as lower-fat ice cream or frozen yogurt. Eventually, as your body becomes wiser, you will crave what's better for you and the high-fat premium ice cream will taste far too rich.

Food cravings, like other habits, don't change overnight. It may take several weeks before these crave-curbing techniques feel natural and satisfying. Choose the ones that you think will work for you and try others as needed.

4

Powerful Proteins

LIKE THE STRUCTURAL steel of buildings, proteins provide the framework for every cell of the body. Just as workers at a construction site need a steady supply of building materials, tissues undergoing repair and those that are growing need a steady supply of protein to build and rebuild organs, muscles, antibodies, hormones, and enzymes — every kind of cell in the body. At eight months or eighty years, bodies need protein.

Protein is a reasonably worry-free food. Unlike with fat or sugar, it's nearly impossible to overdose on proteins, especially in children's diets. And for most Americans, getting enough protein is not a problem. Also, unlike with fats and carbs, there's no such food as an unhealthy protein.

PROTEIN LANGUAGE

Like the first two members of the nutritional Big Three, fats and carbohydrates, proteins have their own language. Here are some nutritional terms you should know.

- *Protein* comes from the Greek word *prōtos,* meaning "first." These nutrients are the basic elements of living cells, of first importance. Like carbohydrates and fats, proteins contain carbon, hydrogen, and oxygen, but they contain one more element that sets them apart from the other two — nitrogen.

- *Amino acids* are the molecules that make up the proteins. There are twenty different amino acids in the human body, but there are many possible combinations of these amino acids. Think of it this way: Amino acids are like letters, and proteins are like words. There are many ways to put letters together to make words, and each word has a different function, a different place in a sentence. The protein you eat is broken down into individual amino acids in the digestive system, and then different cells take the ones they need and recombine these amino acids into the proteins that make up your body. Picture a Scrabble board full of words. Then imagine the tiles getting dumped, mixed up, and reassembled into new words.

- *Essential* and *nonessential* describe the two kinds of amino acids. Of the twenty amino acids in the human protein "alphabet," eleven are nonessential amino acids, meaning your body can make them; you don't have to eat them. Nine are essential amino acids, meaning your body can't make them, so it's essential that you

GROWTH SPURTS

Growing children need more "grow foods" (i.e., proteins). During the first two months of life, 50 percent of the protein in a baby's diet is used for growth, and the other 50 percent is used for continued maintenance of the tissues. By three years of age, only 11 percent of dietary protein is used for growth, and the rest is used for repair and maintenance of healthy tissues. During the periodic growth spurts of infancy, childhood, and adolescence, you may need to perk up the proteins in your child's diet anywhere from 5 to 15 grams more a day.

Animal proteins are better tailored to meet the needs of infants and growing children than are plant proteins, which is why nature provides human milk for babies. The complete proteins in breast milk are more suited to a growing infant's needs than is plant protein, which is found in some formulas. Even babies in vegan families get an animal-based food if they are breastfed.

Essential Amino Acids	Nonessential Amino Acids
histidine	alanine
isoleucine	arginine*
leucine	asparagine
lysine	aspartic acid
methionine	cysteine*
phenylalanine	glutamic acid
threonine	glutamine
tryptophan	glycine
valine	proline
	serine
	tyrosine*

get them from foods. (See the related discussion of how proteins are broken down into amino acids through the process of digestion, page 99.)

COMPLETE AND INCOMPLETE PROTEINS

Getting the right kinds of protein is similar to shopping for clothes. Some clothing comes in complete sets. The jacket is sold with the skirt or pants, and together they make a complete outfit. Other clothing you mix and match: jeans from one rack, a shirt from another, maybe a sweater from a different store across town. Proteins, too, come in complete sets or as incomplete parts that work together. A *complete protein* contains all nine of the essential amino acids; a protein missing one or more of these is an *incomplete protein*. Foods that come from animal sources contain complete proteins, since animal tissues have an amino acid composition similar to our own. Both grains and legumes contain significant amounts of protein, but these proteins do not contain all of the essential amino acids. Except for soybeans, plant proteins do not contain all the essential amino acids, so they are called "incomplete proteins."

Another way to evaluate proteins is to consider the *biological value (BV)* of a protein, meaning, not only how rich it is in essential amino acids but also how well it can be digested by the intestines. Animal proteins are around 95 percent digestible, and plant proteins range between 80 and 90 percent digestible.

---

* These amino acids fall into the "semi-essential" category, meaning, they are essential for growth, but not for maintenance of the tissues. Therefore, children need them in their diet. Adults can make enough for maintenance of the tissues, but children cannot make enough of these amino acids for growth.

Complementing and combining proteins.
While it may seem that animal proteins are better nutritionally, the differences in quality between animal and plant proteins are of more theoretical interest than practical significance. People can grow just as well on plant proteins. (Plant-protein eaters may even be healthier, since they avoid the fat that comes with animal protein.) One plant food can supply the amino acids missing in another. Proteins from different kinds of plants complement each other and, in fact, many common and traditional foods are based on complementary proteins.

Don't be misled into thinking that you must eat meat twice a day or even once a day to get the protein you need. Even though plant proteins are not complete proteins, you can make up for what any one food lacks by eating a wide variety of plant and animal foods. A hefty salad with a sprinkling of parmesan cheese and a topping of sunflower seeds is a healthy protein lunch.

COMPLEMENTARY PROTEINS

whole grains	+	legumes
whole wheat bread	+	peanut butter
brown rice	+	beans
whole grain crackers	+	lentil soup
whole wheat pita	+	hummus

Plant proteins can also be combined with animal proteins to make complete proteins, but the animal proteins don't have to come from meat. There are many possible combinations of grains and legumes with dairy products:

whole grains	+	dairy products
cereal	+	milk
pizza	+	cheese
granola	+	yogurt
pasta	+	cheese
vegetables	+	**dairy products**
broccoli	+	cheese sauce

QUESTIONS YOU MAY HAVE ABOUT PROTEINS

How much protein do I need daily?

The amount of protein you need depends primarily on the size of your body and how fast it is growing, and, to a lesser extent, on your gender and how much you exercise. Babies need more protein per pound than moms, moms more than grandmothers, and dads more than moms. As a general guide, this is the amount of protein that the average person needs at various ages:

Age	Protein Per Pound	Minimum Daily Protein Needs
birth–6 months	1 gram	13 grams
6 months–1 year	.75 gram	14 grams
1–6 years	.6 gram	16–24 grams
7–15 years	.5 gram	28–75 grams
adults	.36 gram	50–60 grams

THE MOST POWERFUL PROTEINS

Some proteins are more powerful than others. What makes one protein more powerful than another is not only whether it contains all the essential amino acids, but how efficiently these amino acids are metabolized. That's why nutritional scientists use the biological value (BV) ratings of proteins, which measure how well the body utilizes amino acids in a protein. Here's how the main proteins rate (from highest to lowest) according to how well they are utilized in the body.

- whey protein (the lactalbumin extract from dairy proteins that is found in protein supplements; also the predominant protein in human milk)
- egg white
- fish
- dairy products
- beef
- soy
- legumes (e.g., beans, lentils)

Notes:

- These amounts are *average* recommended dietary allowances (RDA's). Practically speaking, most people eat different amounts of protein each day.

- Vegans (eating plant proteins only) should add 25 percent to these values. Because the body metabolizes animal protein more easily than plant protein, eating more plant protein makes up for this difference.

- Pregnant and lactating women should add 15 to 25 grams a day.

- During growth spurts in infancy, childhood, and adolescence, add 5 to 15 grams.

- During periods of increased tissue repair (illness, injury, or strenuous athletic training), add 10 to 20 grams.

- Male adolescents and adults usually need 10 to 20 grams more protein daily than females do.

- As a rough and very general guide, if you shoot for a gram of protein per pound per day for infants and children, three-quarters of a gram for adolescents, and half a gram per pound per day for adults, you're in the right nutritional ballpark, and getting even more than the RDA for protein.

What happens if I eat too much protein?

Too much protein is not a problem, unless you really overdose, which would mean eating twice the amount your body needs for a long time. When your body has more protein than necessary, it simply disassembles the excess protein, uses the amino acids it needs, and discards the leftover nitrogen through the kidneys. The body can't store excess dietary protein the way it stores excess fat. When someone eats too much protein over a long time, the body will either break down the protein and use it as an energy source or deposit it as fat. You virtually never have to worry about children getting too much protein; in fact, parents usually worry about picky eaters not getting enough. Excess protein is not usually a worry for adults either, unless they are suffering from kidney disease.

Are high-protein weight-loss diets safe?

Be careful with these. It is generally unwise to use a high-protein diet to lose weight. The protein overdose sends the kidneys into overtime. As the kidneys work to eliminate the excess protein, they also dump a lot of water out of your system. On

JUST HOW MUCH PROTEIN DO YOU REALLY NEED?

The usual figures that are thrown around concerning protein needs are "15 to 20 percent of total daily calories." For most individuals this is much too high. The average infant, child, and adult can get all the protein they need without having daily calories from protein exceed 10 percent of their total calories. For example, if you eat an average of 2,000 calories a day, about 200 calories of this should be protein. Protein contains 4 calories per gram, so this would be about 50 grams of protein (200 grams ÷ 4 calories = 50 grams). Most children and adults get at least 10 percent of their total daily calories as protein without even trying. In times of increased protein needs (such as pregnancy, lactation, adolescent growth spurts, or high-endurance exercise), this figure may increase to 15 percent.

the bathroom scale, this looks like a dramatic weight loss, but it is not a real weight loss. (What you really want to lose is fat.) If you lose too much water weight too fast, you could harm your health. It is wise to consume extra amounts of water if eating extra protein. High-protein diets are potentially harmful for people with kidney or liver disease. Before trying this type of diet, be sure to consult your doctor and a registered dietitian.

The reason that high-protein diets "work" is the same reason that other weight-loss diets work: They are lower in calories. High-protein diet plans substitute fish and vegetable protein for meat and dairy protein, and this reduces the amount of fat in the diet. Basically, high-protein diets are weight-loss gimmicks. Use common

sense. Any diet in which you eat fewer calories than you burn will result in loss of body fat, regardless of whether the diet contains primarily fat, carbohydrates, or proteins. Eat a balanced diet and don't eat more calories than you burn. That's the secret of weight control.

I'm exercising vigorously to stay lean and doing weight training to build muscle mass. Do I need to eat extra protein?

Just eating more muscle will not make you gain muscle. But, if you're trying to build your muscles through exercise, you may need more protein. How much depends upon how hard you're working out. An average person working out to stay healthy, but not on a vigorous exercise and weight-training program, will need around half a gram of protein per pound per day. Studies have shown that athletes undergoing vigorous exercise for two hours per day need double that amount of protein, around a gram of protein per pound per day. Serious weight lifters may even need to go up to a gram and a half of protein per pound per day. For most teens and adults on vigorous exercise programs, increasing their daily protein by one-third (roughly 16 to 20 grams — 2 to 3 ounces of meat or fish) is sufficient.

I've heard that in order to reap the benefits of complementary proteins, I need to eat them at the same meal. Is this true?

No. It used to be believed that for two incomplete plant proteins to complement each other and give the body all the essential amino acids, they had to be eaten at the same meal. Being a vegetarian seemed complicated, even risky. Now we know that this is not only nutritionally incorrect, it is an insult to the wisdom of the body. When you eat a protein, your body disassembles it into amino acids and then reassembles these amino acids into

FOODS THAT PACK THE MOST PROTEIN

Perhaps the fairest and most practical way of rating protein foods is to look at the amount of protein in relation to the total calories in a food. The following chart will show you how to get enough protein without overdosing on fat.

Protein Food	Grams of Protein per Serving	Percentage of Calories as Protein
Fish, tuna (4 ounces)	25–30	83%
Egg white (1)	3.5	82%
Cottage cheese, nonfat (½ cup)	15	75%
Poultry, breast, no skin (4 ounces)	25	75%
Kidney beans (½ cup)	7	60%
Tofu, firm (3 ounces)	13	45%
Yogurt, plain nonfat (1 cup)	12	40%
Beef, lean (4 ounces)	30	40%
Egg, whole (1)	6	33%
Milk, 1% (8 ounces)	8	32%
Peanut butter (2 tbsp.)	8	17%
Cereal (1 cup) with ½ cup milk	6–8	17%
Nuts or sunflower seeds (1 ounce)	7	16%
Pasta (1 cup)	7	15%
Whole wheat bread (1 slice)	3	15%

the types of proteins needed by different cells. New studies show that incomplete proteins (plant proteins) eaten as much as twenty-four hours apart combine in the body to provide all the essential amino acids. So, you could eat grains at breakfast and legumes at dinner, and the body will still be able to mix them all together and make what it needs. As long as you eat a variety of protein foods from a variety of sources, you don't have to constantly worry whether they are "com-

plete" or "incomplete" proteins. Your body will do the thinking for you.

I'm worried that my three-year-old daughter is not eating enough protein. How can I be sure?

You'll be surprised how easy it is for your child to get enough protein. In fact, most Americans, children included, eat more than the RDA for protein. If she is at an average weight for three-year-olds, around 30 pounds, she needs an average of 18 grams of protein. She can get this amount from any *one* of the following:

- 8 ounces of yogurt in a cup of cereal

- a tuna fish sandwich using 2 ounces of tuna

- ½ cup cottage cheese and a piece of toast

- a peanut butter sandwich using two slices of whole wheat bread and 2 tablespoons of peanut butter, plus ½ cup milk

- two scrambled eggs with cheese

- a 2-ounce hamburger on a whole wheat bun

- 1 cup chili con carne with beans, plus ½ cup milk

5

Care About Your Calcium

"DOCTOR, I'M WORRIED my child isn't getting enough calcium. He just won't drink his milk!" Nutritionists as well as parents fear that many preschool children do not get their recommended dietary allowance (RDA) of calcium. Getting enough calcium is also a concern for many adults, especially women during pregnancy, lactation, and around menopause. The good news is that calcium is found in most of the foods that everyone normally eats. Here's what you should know about getting enough calcium in your own diet and in your child's diet.

WHY DO YOU NEED CALCIUM?

We all know that calcium is necessary for strong bones and teeth. What you may not know is that calcium is required for every cell of the body to function in a healthy way. Besides acting as a cellular cement for bones, calcium is used by nerves and muscles, and it also contributes to proper blood clotting. Here's an overview of the good things calcium does for your body.

Calcium promotes healthy bones. Just as lime is necessary for strong concrete, calcium is needed for strong bones. Calcium is continually deposited into multiplying bone cells, like the cement that holds together the particles of stone and sand in a chunk of concrete. The stronger the bone development during childhood, the healthier those bones will be in the adult. That is, the stronger the foundation, the sturdier the eventual building.

During adolescence, bones grow rapidly, so teens need a lot of calcium in their diet. Once a person reaches full growth, his or her calcium needs stabilize, but there are periods when calcium needs increase, such as during pregnancy, lactation, and healing from injuries. In old age, the bones begin to lose some of their sturdiness (this is called "osteoporosis," or "fragile bones"). There are several reasons for this, some hormonal and some related to the fact that calcium absorption lessens in elderly intestines. Also, certain medications decrease the body's ability to absorb calcium, including antacids. Senior citizens need to be particularly conscious about the level of calcium in their diet and about which medications interfere with calcium absorption.

It's best not to wait until you're fiftysomething to start preventing osteoporosis. Building stronger bones with a calcium-rich diet and weight-bearing exercise in your twenties and thirties is more likely to prevent osteoporosis than using some preventive measures in your fifties.

Other functions of calcium. Besides promoting healthy tooth enamel, calcium helps muscles. Muscles can cramp, and in the case of heart muscles even fail, if they are not supplied with just the right amount of calcium. Nerve impulses, the transmission of information between nerve fibers, will not function properly without just the right amount of calcium, since calcium is a part of neurotransmitters, such as serotonin and norepinephrine. For example, muscles twitch (a condition called "tetany") when the calcium supply to neuromuscular cells is insufficient. Calcium is one of the most vital minerals for optimal functioning of your entire body.

HOW MUCH CALCIUM DO YOU NEED?

While the body at any age needs calcium, there are stages in a person's life when calcium requirements increase. Here are the daily requirements in milligrams of elemental calcium:

- Pregnancy: 1,500 to 2,000 mg.
- Lactation: 1,200 to 1,500 mg.
- Infants (birth to 1 year): 400 to 600 mg.
- Children (1 to 10 years): 800 mg.
- Preteens and teens: 1,200 to 1,500 mg.
- Adults: 1,200 mg.
- Seniors: 1,500 mg.

HOW DOES CALCIUM WORK?

As with other minerals, the body has a marvelous system for keeping the concentration of calcium in the blood and tissues just right. This is necessary because if calcium concentrations fall too low or get too high, certain organs will fail to function. The intestines regulate calcium entry. Children can absorb around 75 percent of the calcium from their diet, whereas adults may absorb as little as 15 percent. If you eat too much calcium or already have enough calcium in your blood, the intestines simply absorb less of the calcium in the food you eat. If your body needs calcium, the intestines absorb more. Bones are the second regulator. If you don't get enough calcium in your diet, your body may borrow what it needs from your bones. This works for a time, yet continued withdrawals of calcium from the bone bank can lead to osteoporosis. A hormone called "parathyroid" oversees all this calcium activity like a vigilant bank manager, keeping the calcium concentration just right. When calcium levels fall, this hormone stimulates vitamin D to increase absorption of calcium from the intestines and to release calcium from the bone bank until a proper balance is restored.

MAKING THE MOST OF YOUR CALCIUM

Various factors affect how much of the calcium you ingest really gets into your blood. Here are the facts you should know to make the most of the calcium in your diet or any calcium supplements you take:

- Stress from tension and worry can decrease calcium absorption. The calcium in the diet is excreted rather than used.

- Labels on calcium supplements can be misleading. The figure that is important is the amount of *elemental* calcium provided by the supplement. This is the actual amount of usable calcium. The rest of the calcium in the tablet is coupled with a salt that makes it unavailable to the body. For example, calcium glutamate is only 9 percent elemental calcium. A 500-milligram tablet of calcium glutamate contains only 45 milligrams of elemental calcium, even though you may have been led to believe that you are taking 500 milligrams of calcium. Calcium carbonate, on the other hand, is 40 per-

BEST SOURCES OF CALCIUM

Best Dairy Sources	milligrams
Yogurt, nonfat, plain (1 cup)	450
Yogurt, low-fat, plain (1 cup)	400
Yogurt, nonfat, fruit (1 cup)	300
Parmesan cheese (1 ounce)	336
Milk, low-fat (1 cup)	300
Romano cheese (1 ounce)	302
Cheddar cheese (1 ounce)	200
Cottage cheese (1 cup)	155

Best Nondairy Sources	milligrams
Sardines (3 ounces)	371
Orange juice, calcium-fortified (1 cup)	300
Rhubarb (½ cup)	174
Tofu (3 ounces)	190
Salmon (3 ounces, canned)	180
Blackstrap molasses (1 tbsp.)	172
Figs (5)	135
Amaranth flour (½ cup)	150
Artichoke (1 medium)	135
Beans (½ cup, baked)	75
Broccoli (½ cup, chopped)	47
Collards (½ cup, chopped)	180
Soybean nuts (¼ cup)	116
Kale (½ cup, chopped)	90
Okra (½ cup)	77
Tempeh (½ cup)	77
Spinach (½ cup, canned)	136
Turnip greens (½ cup, chopped)	100
Beet greens (½ cup, boiled)	82
Almonds (1 ounce)	80
Almond butter (2 tbsp.)	86
Cereal, calcium-fortified (½ cup)	100–200
Bok choy (Chinese cabbage) (½ cup)	79
Orange (1 medium)	50
Papaya (1 medium)	73
Sesame seeds (1 ounce)	280

cent elemental calcium; a 500-milligram tablet of calcium carbonate provides 200 milligrams of usable calcium. Labels on some supplements make this distinction, listing both the type of calcium compound in the supplement and the amount of elemental calcium provided. Other products are not as carefully labeled. Read labels carefully and compare several brands when you shop.

- Calcium is best absorbed when taken in smaller amounts more frequently and with meals. For example, your body absorbs more calcium if you take one 250-milligram tablet twice a day rather than one 500-milligram tablet once a day. If a higher-dose calcium tablet is a better buy, break it in half.

- Dairy products are a rich source of calcium, and lactose, the sugar contained in milk, facilitates calcium absorption. However, chocolate milk is not such a good source of calcium; because chocolate contains calcium-binding oxalates, it can interfere with calcium absorption.

- Soft drinks that contain citric or phosphoric acid can decrease the absorption of calcium. A 12-ounce cola can rob the body of 100 milligrams of calcium.

- Vitamin C improves the absorption of calcium, which is why drinking calcium-fortified orange juice makes sense.

- High-fiber diets can interfere with calcium absorption, so it's best not to mix a high-fiber food with a high-calcium one. If you do mix them, boost your calcium as you increase your fiber.

- The calcium-to-phosphorus ratio of a food or supplement determines how much of the calcium is absorbed. The ideal calcium-to-phosphorus ratio is 2 to 1, close to the proportion found in human milk, which has an almost perfect calcium-to-phosphorus ratio of 2.3 to 1. The ratio in cow's milk is 1.3 to 1. The higher the phosphorus content of the food, the more calcium is excreted in the urine, leading to a loss of calcium. Foods high in phosphorus (e.g., meat, poultry, corn, potatoes, beer, and buckwheat) can interfere with calcium absorption.

- The presence of estrogen facilitates calcium absorption, so women after menopause are at increased risk of calcium deficiency and therefore need to increase their daily intake of calcium.

- You may read that vegans run the risk of calcium deficiency because the calcium in vegetables, like iron, is bound by the fibers and phytates (mineral-binding chemicals in plants) in the vegetables which may interfere with calcium absorption. This theoretical worry may be balanced out by the lower phosphate content of vegetables, which improves calcium absorption, and by the fact that most people have the enzyme phytase, which breaks down the phytic acid in vegetables. Also, vegans can simply eat more veggies.

- Couch-potatoism, or lack of exercise, may contribute as much, or more, to osteoporosis than a lack of calcium does. Weight-bearing exercise (just about any exercise except swimming or cycling) not only builds muscle, it builds bone.

- Ignore what you may read about losing bone mass while breastfeeding. After weaning, breastfeeding mothers regain the bone mass they may have lost, and some even get a perk by developing more.

6

Pumping Up Your Iron

YOU HEAR ABOUT bodybuilders pumping iron. You have to do more than lift a lot of iron to build strong muscles — you have to eat sufficient iron as well. Here's how to perk up your body with enough iron.

WHY DO YOU NEED IRON?

Iron is necessary to make hemoglobin, the substance that carries oxygen through your blood to all the cells in your body. Hemoglobin is what makes red blood cells red. With insufficient iron, and therefore not enough hemoglobin, red blood cells become small and pale and don't carry enough oxygen. You may have heard the expression "tired blood." This refers to blood that is low in iron and that can't carry enough oxygen to vital organs and muscles. "Tired blood" results in a tired body.

Iron is needed not only for blood but also for brains. Neurotransmitters, the neurochemicals that carry messages from one nerve to another, require sufficient iron to function properly. A person with an iron deficiency may have a tired mind as well as a tired body.

WHERE DO YOU GET IRON?

How much iron is absorbed from food depends on the food itself and the body's needs. Animal sources of food contain more iron than plant sources, and they are a more efficient source of iron.

Animal iron. Iron from animal tissue is called "heme iron." This is the iron that the animal has used to make hemoglobin — just like humans. It is found in animal tissues (muscles and organs) that have blood in them. Even though milk and egg yolk are from animal sources, the iron in these foods is not heme iron. As a general rule, the redder the meat, the greater the quantity of heme iron. Dark meat, such as the drumstick or thigh of the chicken or turkey, contains more heme iron than the white breast meat. Very red organ meats, such as liver, are the richest sources of heme iron. Depending on various other factors, anywhere from 15 to 35 percent of heme iron is absorbed by the body.

Plant iron. Plant iron is chemically different and is known as "non-heme iron." Plant foods may contain more iron than some animal sources, but only 2 to 20 percent of non-heme iron gets absorbed by the body.

Recycling used iron. Red blood cells wear out naturally, and the bone marrow replaces them every three to four months. But the body is efficient: Much of the iron from the worn-out red blood cells is stored and reused in new blood cells.

Improving Iron Absorption

Just adding up the milligrams in the box on page 64 will not tell you how much iron your body is getting from the food you eat. Iron absorption is influenced by a number of factors. For example, if the body is deficient in iron, the intestines will absorb a higher percentage of the iron in the diet. (The body's ability to vary the efficiency of mineral absorption is a safeguard against the toxic effects of iron excess.) The U.S. Department of Agriculture takes these factors into account when recommending dietary allowances of iron at different life stages. Knowing more about the percentage of iron that is absorbed form certain foods in certain conditions can help you get more usable iron out of the food you eat.

Plants contain substances that bind non-heme iron, making it hard to absorb through the human intestines. But combining certain foods can increase iron absorption. Fruits and vegetables rich in vitamin C enhance iron absorption from both meat and plant sources. Remember Popeye's spinach? He ate whole cans of spinach alone to boost his strength. But, we know now that he should have combined his spinach with a food rich in vitamin C. This is because spinach contains oxalic acid, which lessens the amount of iron that is absorbed.

In grains and legumes, substances called "phytates" bind with the iron and make it less available to the body. Eating foods rich in vitamin C along with plant sources of iron helps to unbind phytates and the oxalic acid and increase iron absorption. Vitamin C can double the amount of iron absorbed from a food. Meat, poultry, and fish also enhance the absorption of iron from plant sources. They contain a compound called "meat-protein factor," which improves the absorption of plant iron eaten at the same time. Grandmother's plateful of meat *and* vegetables was nutritionally correct. Meat can double the amount of iron absorbed from veggies. The best partners for getting the maximum amount of iron out of food are meat and foods high in vitamin C eaten together at the same meal.

HOW MUCH IRON DO YOU NEED?

Children and adults need different amounts of iron at different times in their lives. Rapid growth increases iron needs. So does iron loss. Here are some facts on iron needs at different ages and stages:

- Babies store iron from their mothers' blood while they are in the womb. Babies born prematurely need extra iron because they have not had enough time in the womb to develop sufficient iron stores.

- Term babies are born with a large reserve of iron, which should last for a few months. If baby does not receive any extra dietary iron, these iron stores get used up. This is why formula-fed babies should receive an iron-fortified formula, beginning at birth or at least within the first few months afterward and continued throughout the first year. Human milk contains relatively small amounts of iron, but it is very well absorbed. Breastfed babies rarely need iron supplements.

- Between six months and one year, babies' mother-provided iron stores may run out. This is the reason your doctor will check your infant's hemoglobin levels around the nine- and twelve-month checkup, especially if your doctor suspects anemia because of baby's dietary history or because baby appears pale.

IRON BINDERS

The following foods hinder iron absorption:

- tea and coffee (drink these beverages an hour before or after meals)
- high-fiber foods, such as bran (some high-fiber foods contain phytic acid, which binds iron, making it less absorbable; if getting enough iron is a concern for you, it's best to eat your high-fiber foods at a different meal than your iron-rich foods)
- soy proteins
- antacid medicines
- milk or dairy products consumed with a meal
- solids consumed right after breastfeeding (space breastfeedings and solid foods an hour apart if you're concerned about your baby's iron intake)

- Toddlers, ages one to three, with their finicky eating habits may also be prone to iron-deficiency anemia.

- Preschoolers and school-age children, ages three to eleven, are not likely to become iron deficient for two reasons: They are not growing as

rapidly as they did in infancy, and they tend to eat more iron-rich foods, such as hamburgers.

- Adolescents need more iron because they are going through a period of rapid growth, increasing their need for all nutrients.

- Teenage girls and women of child-bearing age need approximately 5 milligrams a day more of dietary iron than men because of blood loss through menstruation.

- Pregnancy increases the need for iron in order to supply two growing bodies. Also, the woman's blood volume increases during pregnancy, calling for more iron.

- Athletes require increased amounts of iron to perform well during high-endurance sports. Athletes engaged in endurance training may become iron deficient due to increased elimination of iron during prolonged vigorous exercise.

HOW MUCH IRON DO YOU NEED EACH DAY?*

- Children, 1 to 10 years   10 mg.
- Teen males   12 mg.
- Adult males   10 mg.
- Teen and adult females   18 mg.
- Pregnant women   30 mg.

Average RDA for iron in milligrams

NUTRITIP
Women Need More Iron.

An active, menstruating woman should eat at least 18 milligrams of iron daily. This is easier advised than done. A well-balanced diet supplies around 6 milligrams of iron for every 1,000 calories. Yet most women eat about 2,000 calories per day, which amounts to only around 12 milligrams of iron a day. Add to this diminished iron intake the fact that women eat more fruits and vegetables (which contain poorly absorbed iron) and are generally not big meat eaters. This is why many women are anemic or borderline anemic. It would be wise for women to have not only a hemoglobin-level check done yearly but also a serum ferritin test to check their total iron stores.

- Vegans (vegetarians who eat only plant products) may be at risk for iron deficiency, since plant foods are a less efficient source of iron than animal foods. (For more on vegetarians and iron deficiency, see page 170.)

- People on crash diets are prone to iron deficiency since they tend to eat fewer iron-rich foods.

- Iron deficiency among meat eaters is unusual. Most Americans eat too much meat.

- Iron-deficiency anemia may be a hidden cause of poor school performance, since iron deficiency has been shown to be linked to reduced ability to concentrate, decreased performance on school and intelligence tests, and a general overall decrease in academic and work performance. Some studies indicate that when anemia is corrected, academic performance is improved.

PREVENTING IRON-DEFICIENCY ANEMIA FROM BIRTH TO ADULTHOOD

Iron deficiency can cause anemia, which is a shortage of hemoglobin in the blood. This can lead to weakness, fatigue, a pale face and earlobes, and brittle, spoon-shaped nails. There are other causes of anemia besides nutritional deficiencies, including massive or chronic blood loss.

The best way to tell if you have enough iron in your body is to find out if you have enough iron in your blood. A finger-stick hemoglobin check can be done in your doctor's office. The test requires only one tiny drop of blood, and the results are available within a few minutes. Many pediatricians use this test to check hemoglobin levels in infants and toddlers. Your doctor may check hemoglobin levels at other ages of increased iron needs, too, such as during female adolescence

---

IRON DEFICIENCY AND DEVELOPING BRAINS

It is very important for growing infants to get enough iron in their diet. Infants between one and two years of age who have iron-deficiency anemia have been found to have lower scores on mental- and motor-functioning tests; their scores are lower also at five years of age. The late Frank Oski, who was a professor at the Johns Hopkins University School of Medicine and was one of the country's leading pediatric hematologists, summarized the importance of preventing iron-deficiency anemia: "Three studies . . . have now suggested that iron-deficiency anemia occurring at an apparently crucial time in infancy results in irreparable cognitive damage. Attention must be directed to prevention of iron deficiency. Breastfeeding, or the use of iron-fortified formulas until one year, can achieve this desired goal."

---

or pregnancy. Here are normal hemoglobin values:

- infants and children: 11 to 13 grams per 100 milliliters.
- women: 12 to 16 grams per 100 milliliters.
- men: 14 to 18 grams per 100 milliliters.

You can prevent iron-deficiency anemia by making wise food choices for yourself and your family. Getting your daily iron from food is preferable to taking iron supplements, which sometimes cause abdominal discomfort and constipation. Here are some ways to ensure there is enough iron in your family's diet.

CORRECTING YOUR CHILD'S ANEMIA

Borderline anemia can usually be corrected just by increasing your dietary supply of iron, without taking iron supplements. If your child is anemic, here's how to restock the iron-deficient body's stores and elevate the hemoglobin level to normal:

Step 1: Using diet to correct anemia in infants requires about 1 milligram of dietary iron per pound per day. So a 20-pound infant would need a minimum of 20 milligrams of iron per day or about twice the usual RDA. Depending on your infant's willingness to eat a lot of iron-rich foods, it can be difficult to correct anemia with dietary measures alone. The good news is that the intestines compensate for iron deficiency by increasing the percentage of iron absorbed from foods, and you can further improve iron absorption by combining good food iron sources with vitamin sources. You'll usually need even more dietary iron than 1 milligram per pound to correct anemia, but if your infant is only slightly anemic, it is worth trying the dietary increase for a couple of weeks. Then have your doctor recheck your baby's hemoglobin.

Step 2: If dietary iron does not produce a significant improvement in your infant's hemoglobin and/or serum ferritin level, it would be wise to begin giving your child iron supplements in the form of drops or pills. (Consult your doctor for dosage and timing.) The usual oral dose is 2 milligrams per pound given three times a day, between meals to enhance absorption. The iron syrup that is usually recommended for children is ferrous sulfate or ferrous succinate. During the first three weeks of treatment, the hemoglobin increases at a rate of 0.15 to 0.25 grams per day, so if your infant has a hemoglobin level of 9 and it should be 11, expect it to take around three weeks to reach the desired level. In order to replenish the depleted iron stores, it's best to continue oral iron supplements for at least two months after the hemoglobin becomes normal.

Step 3: If your baby's hemoglobin is not increasing by at least 1 gram after two to four weeks of treatment, your doctor may either want to increase the dosage of iron supplement or do some further blood tests to determine if the anemia has other causes besides iron deficiency.

Breastfeed your baby as long as possible. Once upon a time it was believed that breastfed babies needed iron supplements because human milk was low in iron. But studies indicate that breastfed babies at four to six months of age have a higher hemoglobin level than infants who are fed an iron-fortified formula. Breastfed babies have been found to have sufficient iron stores for six months or longer. Human milk remains an im-

portant part of baby's diet even after the introduction of solids.

Use an iron-fortified formula. If bottlefeeding, use an iron-fortified formula, preferably beginning at birth, but at least starting by three months of age. Continue using an iron-fortified formula for at least one year or as long as your baby's doctor recommends, which is usually until your in-

SIGNS OF IRON-DEFICIENCY ANEMIA

- paleness (especially noticeable in the face and earlobes of infants and children; in the palms and nail beds of adults)
- weakness
- fatigue
- shortness of breath
- irritability
- difficulty concentrating
- increased susceptibility to infections
- intolerance of cold temperatures
- constipation
- brittle, thin, spoon-shaped nails

fant is eating adequate amounts of other dietary sources of iron. Do not use low-iron formulas, which do not contain sufficient iron for a growing baby's needs.

Delay feeding cow's milk to infants; limit it for toddlers. The Committee on Nutrition of the American Academy of Pediatrics recommends that parents delay using cow's milk as a beverage until a baby is at least one year of age. There are

NUTRITIP
Don't Skin the Iron.

Leave the skin on the potatoes when making homemade fries. This way you'll get more nutrition into a french fry–loving picky eater. The potato skin is rich in nutrients and contains five times the amount of iron as the whole rest of the potato. And don't forget to eat the skin on your baked potato.

two iron-related reasons for this: Cow's milk is low in iron, and cow's milk can irritate the intestinal lining, causing bleeding and the loss of iron. This is a tiny amount of blood loss, but over a long period of time it can be significant. The combination of poor iron intake and increased iron loss sets a baby up for iron-deficiency anemia, and excessive milk consumption is a common cause of iron-deficiency anemia in toddlers. An eighteen-month-old who consumes 40 ounces of milk a day may be plump but is probably very pale. Unless advised otherwise by your baby's doctor, limit your toddler's cow's-milk intake to no more than 24 ounces a day.

Combine foods wisely. Eating a food rich in vitamin C along with a good iron source will help your body use the iron. Here are some classic examples:

- spaghetti with meat and tomato sauce
- meat and potatoes
- chicken fajitas with broccoli, sweet peppers, and tomatoes
- hamburger and coleslaw
- nitrate-free hot dogs and orange juice
- fresh fruit, iron-fortified cereal
- fresh fruit with raisins (for fruits that are high in vitamin C, see Chapter 7)

Try prune juice as a regular beverage. Prune juice is one of the few juices that are high in iron (3 milligrams of iron per cup). The process involved in making prune juice retains more of the fruit's original nutrients than the juicing of other fruits.

Cook in iron pots. The acid in foods seems to pull some of the iron out of the cast-iron pots. Simmering acidic foods, such as tomato sauce, in an iron pot can increase the iron content of the brew more than tenfold. Cooking foods contain-

BEST IRON-RICH FOODS

	Iron (in milligrams)		Iron (in milligrams)
Meat and Poultry		**Vegetables (continued)**	
Beef (4 ounces)	3.5	Tomato paste (4 ounces)	3.9
Ground beef (4 ounces)	2.5	Tomato puree (4 ounces)	1.1
Lamb (4 ounces)	2.5	Tomato sauce (4 ounces)	0.8
Pork (4 ounces)	1.0	**Grains and Cereals**	
Veal (4 ounces)	1.5		
Lunch meat (2 slices)	0.9	Pasta (4 ounces)	1.0–2.0
Hot dog (1)	0.5	Bagel (1 ounce)	1.8
Chicken liver (4 ounces)	10.0	Bread (white, 1 slice)	0.6
Liver (beef, 4 ounces)	6.5	Bread (whole wheat, 1 slice)	1.0
Liver (calf, 4 ounces)	16.0	Cream of Wheat (4 ounces)	5.0
Chicken (light meat, 4 ounces)	1.0	Breakfast cereal (iron-fortified, 1 ounce)	4.0–8.0
Chicken (dark meat, 4 ounces)	1.6	Grains for baking (amaranth and quinoa flour, ½ cup)	8.0–9.0
Turkey (light meat, 4 ounces)	1.6		
Turkey (dark meat, 4 ounces)	2.5		
Seafood		**Fruits and Juices**	
Clams (4 ounces)	3.0	Apricots, dried (10 halves)	1.6
Oysters (½ cup)	8.0	Figs (5)	2.0
Shrimp (4 ounces)	2.0	Peaches, dried (6 halves)	3.1
Tuna (3 ounces)	1.0	Prune juice (8 ounces)	3.0
Vegetables		Raisins (4 ounces)	1.5
Beans (½ cup)	2.0	**Others**	
Chickpeas (½ cup)	2.0	Nuts (1 ounce almonds, peanuts)	1.0
Artichokes (½ cup), raw	2.0	Tofu, firm (3 ounces)	2.0–7.0
Beet greens (1 cup)	2.7	Brewer's yeast (1 tbsp.)	1.4
Potato (with skin, 1)	2.5	Infant formula (iron fortified, 8 ounces)	3.0
Potato (without skin, 1)	0.6	Blackstrap molasses (1 tbsp.)	3.5
Pumpkin (4 ounces)	1.7	Chili con carne with beans (1 cup)	4.0
Sauerkraut (4 ounces)	1.7	Sunflower seeds (1 ounce)	1.9
Peas (4 ounces)	1.0	Pumpkin seeds (1 ounce)	4.0
Spirulina (1 tsp.)	5.0		
Lentils (4 ounces)	3.0		
Barley (4 ounces)	2.0		
Jerusalem artichokes (4 ounces)	2.5		
Sweet potatoes (4 ounces)	1.7		

NUTRITIP
Labels Can Be Misleading.

The percentage of iron listed on the package label is certainly not the amount of iron that gets into your bloodstream. This is especially true of iron-fortified cereals, in which only 4 to 10 percent of the iron listed actually gets absorbed. The amount of iron absorbed from any food depends on the type of iron in the food, the body's need for iron, and the company of other foods eaten at the same meal.

ing other acids, such as vinegar, red wine, and lemon or lime juice, in an iron pot can also increase the iron content of the final mixture.

Bake with iron-rich grains. The usual wheat used to make bread and pastries is relatively low in iron (around 1 milligram of iron per half cup). Lesser-known grains, such as amaranth (8 mil-

SIDE EFFECTS OF IRON SUPPLEMENTS

Adults who are iron deficient can take ferrous sulfate tablets, 60 milligrams, two or three times a day. Children usually take 2 milligrams per pound three times a day. Expect the stools to become green or dark black. This is harmless. Liquid iron may cause a temporary black stain on the teeth, so brush your child's teeth immediately after giving him iron and have the child swish his mouth with water. Some children and adults may experience constipation or abdominal upset from the iron, necessitating a change in form or dosage of the iron preparation.

ligrams per half cup) and quinoa (9 milligrams per half cup) are much richer in iron. Barley grains contain 4 milligrams of iron per half cup. Mixing these grains into the wheat flour you use when you bake will increase the iron content of the finished product.

IRON DEFICIENCY WITHOUT ANEMIA

A normal hemoglobin level indicates that you are not anemic, meaning, your blood is not low in iron. Yet, the hemoglobin level obtained in your doctor's office does not reflect the total body stores of iron. It's possible to have a normal hemoglobin, that is, a normal amount of iron in the blood, yet have vital tissues throughout your body be deficient in iron. Some people have symptoms of iron-deficiency anemia, even with a normal hemoglobin. To really be sure you have enough iron in your body, your doctor may send you to the laboratory to measure what is called your "serum ferritin," the level of iron in your blood that accurately reflects your iron stores. Based on the lab results, your doctor will advise you whether or not your child needs iron supplements. If your serum ferritin level is normal, you can rest assured that you have adequate iron stores throughout your body.

Serum ferritin levels detect iron deficiency in the early stages: a low hemoglobin level reflects a much later stage of iron deficiency. This is an important consideration, since with a normal hemoglobin and low ferritin levels, the iron stores can be restocked by simply increasing the amount of iron in your diet. By the time the hemoglobin is low, iron supplements are usually needed. Symptoms of iron-deficiency anemia, such as being tired, irritable, and having difficulty concentrating, may be present long before anemia is reflected by the hemoglobin tests. A serum ferritin is an earlier and more sensitive indicator of iron deficiency.

7

Value Your Vitamins

MOTHER IS RIGHT when she says, "Get your vitamins." These substances, indeed, are vital to life. In the early 1900s these nutrients in foods were thought to be *amines,* or organic compounds. Since they also appear to be *vital* to life, they were termed "vit-amines." Unlike the Big Three nutrients (fats, proteins, and carbohydrates), vitamins contain no calories and are not sources of energy, yet they work at the cellular level to help metabolize the nutrients from food. Vitamins are important to the health and well-being of every family member. To be your family's nutritionist, you must know how to value your vitamins.

VITAMIN FACTS YOU SHOULD KNOW

There are thirteen vitamins that are essential to humans. Vitamins are divided into two categories, according to the way the body absorbs them. Fat-soluble vitamins (A, D, E, and K) are absorbed with the help of fats in the diet and are stored in the fats of the body. Because your body can store these vitamins for a long time, unless your diet is chronically lacking one of these it is unusual to have a deficiency of a fat-soluble vitamin. The other vitamins — vitamin C and the B-complex vitamins — are water-soluble vitamins, meaning,

they do not need fat for absorption, and they are not stored very long in the body. If there's an excess of water-soluble vitamins, either from food or from a supplement, they are flushed through the body rapidly and are eliminated quickly in the urine.

Except for vitamin D, and a bit of vitamin K, your body cannot make vitamins. You must get them from foods. So, if your diet is deficient in one or more vitamins, your body will feel the effects of these missing essentials.

NUTRITIP
Getting Nutrients the Old-Fashioned Way

Popping a pill may not be the best way to fortify your diet. A better way is to get the nutrients you need directly from food. Nutrients in food take advantage of the valuable nutritional principle of "synergy": Some nutrients work better in the body when grouped with other nutrients, the 1 + 1 = 3 effect. This is especially true of antioxidants. A bowl of fresh assorted fruits may produce healthier effects than a bunch of synthetic powder in a pill.

It's best to get your vitamins from foods and not from supplements, since one nutrient in a food may help another one be better absorbed. Except for vitamin A, it's impossible to overdose on vitamins in food (and to overdose on vitamin A, you'd have to eat a lot of carrots). Vitamin supplements are drugs, which have both benefits and risks. Taken in just the right amount, they can help the body; overdosing, as on any drug, has side effects and may harm the body. Although there are situations in which your body might need a boost from supplements, if you and your family eat a balanced diet you don't need to worry that you or your children aren't getting enough vitamins. What is lacking in one food will be found in another. This is particularly true in fruits and vegetables. Many of the vitamins that are found in vegetables, which children may shun, are also found in fruits, which most kids enjoy.

The following is the most important information you need to know about the most significant vitamins. Even though beta carotene is not usually regarded as a vitamin, because the body converts it to vitamin A we have included it. Because the two vitamins pantothenic acid and biotin are found in so many foods that deficiencies of them are rare, we have omitted them from the following list.

Please note that the RDA of some of the nutrients on the following pages has been updated as a daily value (DV) in the appendix (see page 401).

Vitamin	How Much You Need (RDA)	What It Does
A	*Children* Birth to 1 year: 375 RE (retinol equivalents) 1 to 3 years: 400 4 to 6 years: 500 7 to 10 years: 700 *Teens and Adults* Females: 800 RE Males: 800	Promotes healthy vision by making retinol, a pigment necessary for retina of eye, to accommodate to night vision; promotes healthy skin and teeth; boosts immune system
Beta carotene	no RDA established	Beta carotene is a precursor to vitamin A, meaning the body converts it to vitamin A according to its need. The intestines extract from foods the amount of beta carotene the body needs to make the vitamin A it needs (no more, no less). So the intestines protect the body from excess vitamin A in case you habitually eat too much food rich in preformed vitamin A.
B-1 (Thiamin)	*Children* Birth to 1 year: 0.3 to 0.4 mg 1 to 3 years: 0.7 4 to 6 years: 0.9 7 to 10 years: 1.0 *Teens and Adults* Females 1.1 mg. Males 1.5	Helps cells convert sugars to energy, especially high-energy-utilizing cells in heart and brain
B-2 (Riboflavin)	*Children* Birth to 1 year: 0.4 to 0.5 mg. 1 to 3 years: 0.8 4 to 6 years: 1.1 7 to 10 years: 1.2 *Teens and Adults* Females: 1.3 mg. Males: 1.7	Like B-1, acts like a co-enzyme, helping to convert carbohydrates to energy; also essential for red blood cell production

Deficiency Signs	Best Food Sources	What Else You Should Know
Night blindness, dry eyes, dry, scaly skin, increased susceptibility to infections Deficiency unlikely since so many foods are rich in either preformed vitamin A or its precursor, beta carotene	Liver, carrots, sweet potatoes, pumpkin, apricots, green, leafy vegetables, mango, cantaloupe, tuna	Measured in retinol equivalents (RE); may also see international units (IU), a less precise measurement. One IU is a little more than 3 RE. Is the only vitamin you can get too much of from food; excess (ten times the RDA) potentially harmful, causing scaly skin, liver damage, gastrointestinal upset, and birth defects
Deficiency signs are the same as listed those under vitamin A.	Yellow-orange fruits and vegetables and dark green vegetables: dried apricots, sweet potatoes, carrots, cantaloupe, peaches, pumpkin, kale, winter squash, mango	Best to get your vitamin A from beta carotene, which, in addition to making vitamin A, is an antioxidant, which protects against heart disease and cancer. Excess may cause *carotenemia,* yellowish orange skin, especially in palms and soles (but not the eyeballs); this harmless curiosity disappears if you cut back on carotenoids.
Weakness, nervous-system malfunction, heart failure Deficiency rare in America, except in alcoholics, since alcohol excess impairs absorption of thiamin	Whole grains, seeds, nuts, wheat germ, sunflower seeds, pork, oats, tuna, salmon, avocados, pasta and cereals (whole grain or fortified), beans, legumes, tofu, artichokes	Discovered after Japanese sailors (eating a diet high in refined white rice) died from heart failure, due to a vitamin B-1 deficiency known as beriberi; when white rice was replaced with whole-grain rice, condition disappeared.
Dry, scaly, cracked skin; eyes ultrasensitive to bright light; sore red tongue Deficiency rare in America	Organ meats, dairy products, seafood, eggs, meat, fortified breads and cereals, almonds, tofu, artichokes, beet greens, spinach, sweet potatoes	While less familiar grains (quinoa and amaranth) are moderately good sources of riboflavin, the popular grains (wheat, barley, rice, oats, corn, and rye) are not, which is why milk or yogurt is a riboflavin-rich partner to cereal. Enriched grains contain varying amounts of riboflavin.

Vitamin	How Much You Need (RDA)		What It Does
B-3 (Niacin)	*Children* Birth to 1 year: 1 to 3 years: 4 to 6 years: 7 to 10 years:	5 to 6 mg. 9 12 13	Like B-1 and B-2, a co-enzyme in cellular conversion of sugars into energy, especially in digestive and nervous systems
	Teens and Adults Females: 15 mg. Males: 19		
B-6 (Pyridoxine)	*Children* Birth to 1 year: 1 to 3 years: 4 to 6 years: 7 to 10 years:	0.3 to 0.6 mg. 1.0 1.1 1.4	Acts like a co-enzyme in protein metabolism, specifically, helping the cells assemble amino acids into protein parts. Also needed to help the cells convert proteins and liver glycogen to energy in case extra energy is needed. Also boosts immune system, and is helpful in building brain's neurotransmitters
	Teens and Adults Females: 1.6 mg. Males: 2.0		
B-12	*Children* Birth to 1 year: 1 to 3 years: 4 to 6 years: 7 to 10 years:	0.7 micrograms 1.0 1.4	Helps build a strong myelin sheath to insulate nerves; necessary component in healthy red blood cells
	Teens and Adults 2 micrograms		
C (Ascorbic acid)	*Children* Birth to 1 year: 1 to 3 years: 4 to 6 years: 7 to 10 years:	30 to 35 mg. 40 45 45	Builds strong connective tissue that stabilizes muscles and bones; antioxidant; enhances iron absorption; promotes wound healing; maintains integrity of capillaries; boosts immune system; important in production of neurotransmitters
	Teens and Adults 60 mg.		

Deficiency Signs	Best Food Sources	What Else You Should Know
Dry, cracked, inflamed skin; digestive and nervous systems malfunction Deficiency rare in developed countries since it's added to lots of fortified foods, and the body can manufacture niacin from tryptophan, an amino acid found in many protein foods	Tuna, swordfish, salmon, meat, peanuts and peanut butter, wheat germ, wheat bran, fortified cereals and pasta, barley, rye, buckwheat, wild rice, sunflower seeds, potatoes, avocados, mushrooms	Excessive doses in *supplements* may cause flushing of face, tingling of skin, and headache; these harmless but annoying symptoms quickly wear off.
Convulsions, nervous system malfunction; inflamed skin Deficiency rare, since B-6 is found in most protein foods, and typical American diet is high in protein	Tuna, salmon, avocados, potatoes, meat, bananas, chickpeas, prune juice, sunflower seeds, sweet potatoes, artichokes, rice bran	Megadoses (100 times the RDA) taken for months can cause nervous-system damage.
Anemia, nerve damage Deficiency rare, since liver can store many years' supply of B-12	Seafood, meat, yogurt, milk, cheese, eggs	Because B-12 is found in animal sources, vegans need special precautions (see page 171)
Bleeding gums, reduced wound healing, easy bruising, depressed immune function	Guava, papaya, cantaloupe, kiwi, strawberries, orange juice, chili peppers, sweet yellow peppers, broccoli	Adult RDA of 60 mg. considered low by many nutritionists; 200 to 500 mg. a day may be better for optimal health; long-term excess doses of 1 to 2 grams could cause kidney stones.

Vitamin	How Much You Need (RDA)	What It Does
D	*Children* Birth to 6 months: 300 international units 6 months to 24 years: 400 *Adults* 200 international units	Promotes absorption of calcium and phosphorus for strong bones
E	*Children* Birth to 1 year: 3 to 4 mg. 1 to 3 years: 6 4 to 6 years: 7 7 to 10 years: 7 *Teens and Adults* Females: 8 mg. Males: 10	One of the big three antioxidants, along with vitamin C and beta carotene; protects cell membranes against damage (see "All About Antioxidants," page 362)
F (Folic acid)	*Children* Birth to 1 year: 25 to 35 micrograms 1 to 3 years: 50 4 to 6 years: 75 7 to 10 years: 100 *Teens and Adults* 400 micrograms	Acts like a co-enzyme that aids in the production of DNA, the blueprint for cell reproduction; necessary in red-blood-cell production and in formation of spinal bones in fetus
K	*Children* Birth to 1 year: 5 to 10 mg. 1 to 3 years: 15 4 to 6 years: 20 7 to 10 years: 30 *Teens and Adults* Females: 65 mg. Males: 70	A vital substance in the blood-clotting mechanism

Deficiency Signs	Best Food Sources	What Else You Should Know
Fragile, easily fractured bones and weak muscles — a condition called "rickets"	Sunshine stimulates a cholesterol-like substance in the skin to make vitamin D; dietary sources not necessary as long as skin is exposed to as little as 15 minutes of sunshine three times a week; vitamin D–fortified milk	Persons living in cloudy winter climates, indoor-bound persons, or those with little sun exposure should have vitamin D–fortified foods. Because of growing bones, children need more vitamin D than adults (the only vitamin a baby needs more of than an adult).
Anemia, neurological damage; effects of deficiency less clear than with other vitamins	Polyunsaturated oils and seeds (sunflower, safflower, canola, corn), almonds, peanut butter, wheat germ, tomato puree, avocados, peaches, oat bran, fortified cereals Top source: sunflower seeds	May have heart-healthy and anti-cancer benefits (see page 391)
Anemia; spina bifida in fetus, delayed growth	Asparagus, pinto beans, lentils, chickpeas, artichokes, spinach, kidney beans, avocados, papaya, wheat germ, fortified cereals	Called "folic acid" from *folium,* Latin for "leaf," since first discovered in spinach leaves. To prevent spina bifida in fetus, pregnant women should get 800 micrograms of folic acid daily.
Bleeding, diminished blood clotting Deficiency rare, since normal resident intestinal bacteria make vitamin K for the body	Green, leafy vegetables, kale, broccoli, onions, lettuce, cabbage, spinach	Routinely given to newborns who may be born deficient in vitamin K, either by injection or in a new oral preparation

8

Becoming Water Wise

YOU'VE HEARD OF vitamin deficiencies and iron deficiencies. Ever heard of someone having a water deficiency? Probably not, but the dry truth is that most children and adults don't drink enough water. And while you're thinking about getting enough water into your body, consider also the quality of the water you drink.

WATER — THE BEST HEALTH "ADE"

Why Does Your Body Need Water?

Over 50 percent of an adult's body is water; that figure goes as high as 72 percent in an infant. Blood is 80 percent water, and even muscles are 70 percent water. The waterway flows through your body, delivering nutrients to cells and carrying away waste. Water acts as your body's cooling system, moving heat to the skin surface, where it evaporates in sweat and breath. Water lubricates joints, softens skin, makes muscles work more smoothly, and prevents constipation. If your body is temporarily short of water — a condition called "dehydration"— every organ in your body is affected.

How Much Water Do You Need?

Infants need around 1½ ounces of water per pound per day. So, each day a 20-pound baby needs around 30 ounces of fluids, most in the form of milk. Breastfed babies don't need any extra water, but a small amount of water is necessary for formula-fed infants. In fact, some pediatricians feel that offering excessive water to infants under one year of age may actually be nutritionally unwise because excess water may fill up baby and replace needed calories.

Adults need half as much water as infants do — between ½ and ¾ ounce of water per pound per day, depending on the amount of exercise, heat loss, illness, and so on. A 120-pound woman should drink at least eight 8-ounce glasses of fluid per day.

You need to drink more water if:

You're exercising. Prehydrate yourself by drinking at least two glasses (16 ounces) of water an hour or so before you work out. As you work up a sweat, take frequent sips of water, as dehydration makes muscles tire more easily. After exercising, top off with two more glasses of water to rehydrate yourself.

HEALTH WATER

Water, the original health drink, is underrated and overshadowed by commercial substitutes. Consider these health uses of plain water.

Drown the cold. You've heard the expression "Starve a fever, feed a cold!" This bit of medical folklore is only half true. Best is to drown the fever *and* the cold with water. Fever makes you perspire and lose water, which dehydrates not only your body but also your brain, causing you to think and feel even worse from dehydration. During a cold, the mucous membranes of your nose and breathing passages lose water and dry out. Drinking water keeps these mucous membranes moist, which allows the inflamed lining of your nose and breathing passages to heal more quickly. Dehydration also thickens the mucus, making it difficult for the tiny hair filaments in your nose (called "cilia") to oscillate back and forth and move the mucus and the germs along. As a result, the mucous plugs collect in the nose, sinuses, and airways and serve as a culture medium for bacteria. Keeping the mucus and the membranes moist and waterlogged keeps mucous plugs from forming and even getting stuck in the lower airways, where they are difficult to cough up. In fact, among pediatricians, water has often been dubbed the "best and most readily available cough syrup."

Drink to go. Not drinking enough fluids is also a subtle contributor to problems with constipation, especially in the very young and very old. The colon is your body's fluid regulator. If you're not drinking enough, your colon steals water from the waste material and gives it to the body, causing the stools to be water deprived or hard. People eating high-fiber diets actually increase their risk of constipation if they don't drink extra water along with fiber-rich foods, since fiber needs water to do its intestinal sweeping job. More fluids in your diet put more fluids in your bowels, lessening constipation.

Drink to think. Water even contributes to healthier brains. The brain is a water-loving organ. If it doesn't get enough, it doesn't work right. Dehydration can impair concentration, which is most apparent following sweaty exercise or doing brain work in hot weather. So, drink to help you think.

You're sick. Bodies lose a lot of water through illnesses that cause fever, vomiting, or diarrhea. Becoming dehydrated makes you feel doubly sick.

You're pregnant. Blood volume increases by 40 percent during pregnancy, and extra fluids are also needed for the ongoing manufacturing of amniotic fluid. Water also helps maintain overall well-being during pregnancy. Drinking lots of water helps move along and dilute the body's waste products, lessening problems with constipation and reducing the risk of urinary tract infections. Pregnant women need to drink more than the usual eight 8-ounce glasses of fluid a day to keep body and baby well hydrated. If you don't like to drink that much plain water but are worried about weight gain from drinking extra juice, flavor your water with just a teaspoon of frozen juice concentrate. Space this fluid intake evenly throughout the day, consuming larger, more frequent drinks along with smaller, more frequent meals. The swelling of ankles, feet, and hands during pregnancy is not a signal to cut back on water. Some of this is the normal swelling that occurs with pregnancy, or it may be a sign that your body is retaining too much salt, in which case drinking more water will actually help decrease the swelling.

You're breastfeeding. Enjoy an extra glass of water before each nursing. Milk is the baby's water source, as well as his source of nutrition.

You're hot. During hot weather or while working in the hot sun, bodies perspire more. Drink several glasses of water before going outside and drink more water afterward.

You're thirsty. Obviously, you should drink water when you're thirsty. Thirst means your body already has a water shortage. It's best to drink enough water so you don't get thirsty. If you get thirsty, quench your thirst and then drink two more glasses of water. This is especially important for seniors, since the thirst signal declines with age.

Are You Drinking Enough Water?

Don't rely on thirst to judge if your body is adequately hydrated. Waiting till you're thirsty to take a drink of water is waiting too long. If you're drinking around ½ ounce of water per pound per day, plus an additional two or three glasses during times of increased water need, chances are you're drinking enough. (This amount includes *all* fluid sources: soups, fruits, milk, etc.) Also, your kidneys can give you a clue. Notice the color of your urine. If your body is low on water, your kidneys try to conserve it by concentrating the urine. If

you have enough or too much water in your body, the kidneys excrete more water in the urine. So, if your urine is almost colorless or slightly yellow, you are probably drinking enough liquids; if your urine is darker than usual, like apple juice, you need to drink more water.

WHAT ABOUT WATER QUALITY?

Over a lifetime you will put more water into your body than any other kind of food or drink. So, paying attention to the water you drink is at least as important, if not more so, than inspecting the food that you eat.

The Safe Drinking Water Act, passed in 1974 and amended in 1986 and again in 1996 with more rigorous standards, required the U.S. Environmental Protection Agency (EPA) to set maximum allowable levels of contaminants in municipal water supplies and to periodically monitor compliance with these standards. Under these laws, the EPA issues maximum contaminant levels (MCLs) for eighty-three contaminants (e.g., pesticides, radioactive materials, chemicals, and bacte-

---

WATER-ADE VS. SPORTS-ADE

For ordinary mortals who exercise, water will do just fine to hydrate the body and lessen muscle fatigue. If you exercise moderately for less than an hour a day, water is as good as a sports drink. However, athletes doing heavy training or playing in competition, especially for longer than an hour, will perform better with a sports drink, which replenishes lost water, electrolytes, and carbohydrates. Otherwise, the body steals these needed nutrients from muscles, which protest this robbery by tiring out. (See "Sports Drinks," page 368.)

ria). As part of the law, the EPA must continually update its monitoring to include many more contaminants. The law also makes the EPA responsible for setting up criteria for safe purification procedures and for monitoring water purification in the United States. It sounds on the surface like the government has taken tap water in tow, and the water drinker can imbibe without worry.

Not exactly. Even though U.S. water is touted to be the safest in the world, and water-borne disease is less common in the United States, there are still concerns about contaminants in the public water supply. Here are some of the reasons:

- Many municipal water-purification plants are too old or the city is too poor to totally comply with EPA standards.
- There may be contaminants that enter the water supply that are not on the EPA's hit list, and thus they escape detection.
- Current testing and purification technology may miss some contaminants, which get past filtering systems and enter the water supply.
- Some germs, such as cryptosporidium, may be resistant to current disinfecting methods. Cryptosporidium is the chlorine-resistant parasite that was implicated in the 1993 Milwaukee water-contamination episode in which forty thousand people suffered gastrointestinal illnesses and more than one hundred immunocompromised people died. Even so, this germ is still not on the EPA's "most wanted" list for monitoring and detection. Other germs, such as

E. coli and *Giardia,* are tiny enough to slip through some filtration systems.
- The long-term effects of drinking a gallon of chlorinated water every day for seventy years have not been determined.

Contaminants of Concern

Here are the specific contaminants to be concerned about:

Chlorine. While chlorine (a chemical also found in household bleach) is a disinfectant that kills germs, it may also pose health hazards. Chlorine reacts with the leftover organic waste products in water to form a possible carcinogen, trihalomethane, which may increase the risk of bladder and rectal cancers. Chlorine vapors can be inhaled through shower steam (so ventilate your shower well) and even absorbed through the skin during showering with chlorinated water. (You can eliminate this risk by placing an inexpensive, replaceable, activated carbon filter in the showerhead and by using a chlorine-free ozone-filtration system in your pool or spa.) There is also the possibility that chlorine used to kill germs in water might upset the balance between harmful and useful bacteria in the human intestines, perhaps even killing the weaker bacteria and allowing the stronger, and sometimes more harmful, ones to multiply unchecked. While chlorination of the water supply has eliminated certain public health problems, such as water-borne outbreaks of cholera and hepatitis, the questions about the overall safety of chlorination are still unanswered.

Agricultural chemicals. Pesticides and herbicides have been implicated as possible carcinogens, and these substances get into the water supply in many parts of the country. If you live in an agricultural area, it is best to drink bottled water during "run-off months," that is, the peak periods of

WATERED-DOWN SAFETY

You drink a glass of water that looks safe and tastes okay, and you don't feel any the worse afterward. So what's the worry about the water? The problem is that disease doesn't develop all of a sudden. Contaminants damage cells little by little, yet it may take years, or even decades, for the whole organ to fail or for tests to find cancer. This is why safe water is of such importance. You drink water every day, but you may not know for fifty years whether the water you drank was good or bad for you. Actually, you'll never know if it was the water, the food, the air, or other factors. Here are some alarming statistics:

- The Natural Resources Defense Council (a nonprofit, public environmental-watchdog agency) reports that more than two-thirds of the nation's water-treatment plants are obsolete and perhaps unsafe.

- Despite the Safe Drinking Water Act in 1986, which banned lead in plumbing, in a 1993 report the EPA admitted that 819 water-treatment plants in the United States produce water containing above-safe levels of lead.

- The government's Office of Technology Assessment reported that the water in one-third of 954 American cities tested was seriously contaminated.

surface-water contamination that follow harvesting. In 1995, an alarming study of tap water samples from many agricultural areas revealed that thousands of infants were drinking infant formula mixed with pesticide-contaminated water.

Bugs in the water supply. Bacteria sometimes found in water supplies include cryptosporidium, *E. coli,* and *Giardia.* There are plenty of other sources for these germs in the environment, and most healthy people can fight them off with no problem. But for people whose immune systems don't work as well — those already ill, the very young and the very old, people receiving cancer treatment, or those with AIDS — bacteria in the water supply can be life-threatening.

Toxic metals. The main metal menace in water is lead, which seeps into water from old pipes and plumbing solder. Lead plumbing materials were not banned until 1986, so many homes and mu-

nicipal water systems still have pipes held together with lead solder.

Radioactive material. Another concern is the seepage of radioactive material into groundwater and surface water. This problem is of particular concern if you live near old radioactive dumping sites or downstream from them. Theoretically, these potential toxins are monitored by EPA testing.

WHAT YOU CAN DO ABOUT YOUR WATER

In a rich and technologically advanced country like the United States, parents should not have to worry about the purity of the water that flows from the tap. Yet, the fact is that many municipalities do not deliver the pure water they promise. If consumers were more aware of the problems, perhaps there would be more pressure on the government to improve the water supply. Here's how to find out whether or not you're drinking safe water.

Check Out the Source

Call your local water-utility officials and inquire about the source and safety of your water. Don't know who to call? Look for a phone number on your water bill. Or, call your local government offices for more information. Here are the questions to ask:

- What is the source of the water — groundwater or surface water? Groundwater is water found deep beneath the ground, such as huge reservoirs naturally formed deep in the earth's surface. Theoretically, this water is cleaner, since the ground acts as a natural filter. Because of the natural soil filtration, groundwater is more likely to be free of cryptosporidium than surface water is. Surface water, that which flows from rivers, lakes, streams, and man-made reservoirs, is more likely to pick up pollutants from the earth's surface.

- When was the last time the water was tested by the EPA?

- What were the results of the last EPA tests? Ask for a copy of the most recent laboratory testing results. Utility companies are required by law to provide consumers with information on contaminants in water.

- Is chlorine the main disinfectant used?

- What other disinfectant procedures are employed besides chlorination?

- Is fluoride added to the water?

If you don't get a favorable response or are unclear about the test results, contact your local health department for clarification or the EPA Safe Drinking Water Hotline at 800-426-4791 or hotline-sdwa@epamail.epa.gov and ask for information about EPA standards (see also their web site, http://www.epa.gov/OGWDW/index.html). The Safe Drinking Water Act requires periodic updating of EPA monitoring standards, but there has been no update since October 1996. When calling the EPA, ask for a complimentary copy of the booklet "Water on Tap: A Consumer's Guide to the Nation's Drinking Water."

The EPA has delegated the task of monitoring the safety of drinking water to each state's government, and while states must at least comply with the EPA's standards, some states may set higher standards. Check with your state government offices to find out more about your state's regulations. *The EPA does not monitor drinking water unless it receives a complaint.*

Test the waters. If your water comes from your own well or if you're unsatisfied with your community's water testing, do it yourself. Be sure you use a state- and EPA-certified testing laboratory. You can obtain a list of EPA- and state-certified water-testing laboratories by calling the EPA hotline (see above). Costs of testing range from $25 to $100, depending on how extensively you want your water examined.

Some tap water may be high enough in sodium to be of concern to people who are on a low-sodium diet for medical reasons. If you consume a lot of tap water, and your doctor has put you on a low-sodium diet, have your water tested for sodium content.

Filter Your Water

If you're uneasy about drinking the water coming out of your tap, there are many steps you can take to improve the water quality. Some families choose to purchase some kind of filtration system.

With filters, like so many other commodities, you get what you pay for. The more chemicals and contaminants you want removed from your

FLUORIDE IN YOUR WATER

The benefits of fluoride were discovered in one of nature's own experiments: The incidence of tooth decay was found to be 50 percent less in areas with naturally fluoridated water, while the incidence of major diseases in these areas was the same as in the general population. Studies of large numbers of people over many generations have attested to the value of fluoride as a safe and effective nutritional supplement for the prevention of tooth decay. Fluoride has been added to drinking water for almost fifty years now, and follow-up studies have validated the cavity-lowering effects of fluoride supplementation and failed to show any increase in diseases due to this public-health measure. There are many myths that persist about fluoride, but these have been disproven. Fluoride does not cause weaker bones or cancer.

According to public-health officials, fluoride supplementation ranks along with water purification and vaccines as one of the top public-health measures of the twentieth century. The American Academy of Pediatrics, the U.S. Department of Public Health, and the American Dental Association have all recommended that from six months to sixteen years, children with growing teeth should receive fluoride supplements either in their diet or in the water they drink.

Fluoride that your child ingests either in food or water enters the bloodstream and becomes incorporated in the tooth enamel even before the teeth erupt, making them strong and more resistant to decay. Fluoride applied topically through toothpaste or by your dentist also makes the teeth more resistant to decay and strengthens the enamel as it repairs itself from normal wear. Fluoride is a naturally occurring trace mineral, and, like calcium, iron, and other minerals, it is often found naturally in water. Unlike other minerals, it has a narrow risk-to-benefit ratio. This means that just the right amount of fluoride helps the teeth, but too much harms the teeth, causing a condition called "fluorosis." While most cases of fluorosis are mild, causing a few white spots or patches on the teeth, more severe cases can cause a brownish mottling and weaken tooth enamel. Because it's important to give infants and children just the right amount of fluoride, the drops are available only by prescription and should be given to your infant or children in only the exact dosage your doctor prescribes.

To be sure your children get the right amount of fluoride — not too much and not too little — follow these recommendations:

- If your child drinks several glasses of water a day, and the local water supply has a fluoride concentration of at least 0.3 parts per million, your child does not need fluoride supplements in the form of tablets or drops. Check with your family doctor or dentist as to your child's individual fluoride needs. You can check the fluoride content of your water by calling your local water department.

- Even if your local tap water is fluoridated, your infant or child may not drink enough tap water to receive sufficient fluoride. In this situation, consult your doctor about giving your child fluoride supplements. If you drink bottled water, it will not be fluoridated unless you specifically request it.

FLUORIDE IN YOUR WATER (CONTINUED)

- Don't use fluoride-containing toothpastes and mouthwashes in children under the age of two, since toddlers tend to swallow toothpaste.

- If your child uses a fluoridated toothpaste, allow only a pea-sized dab a day. *This will provide the recommended daily dose of fluoride without risking overdose.* Don't allow your children to use the generous amounts of toothpaste they see in TV commercials.

- Ready-to-feed infant formulas are not made with fluoride-supplemented water. Ask your child's doctor if fluoride supplements are needed.

- Breastfeeding babies do not need additional supplies of fluoride. The American Academy of Pediatrics recommends that fluoride supplements not be given to any infants younger than six months of age because of the concern about fluorosis in this age group.

- Depending on your child's age and the fluoride concentration in your local water supply, the American Academy of Pediatrics recommends the following fluoride supplementation schedule.

Age of Child	Fluoride Concentration in Local Water Supply (Parts Per Million)		
	< 0.3 ppm	0.3–0.6 ppm	> 0.6 ppm
6 months to 3 years	0.25 mg fluoride daily	0.00	0.00
3 to 6 years	0.50 mg	0.25 mg	0.00
6 years to at least 16 years	1.00 mg	0.50 mg	0.00

water, the more expensive the filter is likely to be.* But if you think of food and water as medicine, pure water, even at the price of a filtration system, is still one of the least expensive pills you can swallow. Remember, too, that it's not enough just

to filter your water and forget about it. Be sure you change cartridges frequently and according to the manufacturer's instructions.

If you are investing in an expensive water-purification system, before you sign on the dotted line, arrange for before-and-after tests of the water. Tell the filter company that you expect to have your money refunded if your filtered, tested water contains more contaminants than the manufacturer claims. You may have to pay for the testing, but it may save you from paying for a high-priced but less effective system.

---

* No matter what kind of filter you have, it won't purify all the water in the house. Most families attach the filter to the kitchen tap. But what about the bathroom taps and the glass of water your children drink before going to bed? Also, consider the many public water fountains (parks, school, movie theaters) that your child drinks from while away from home. For this reason, it would be better if municipal water were made purer at its source.

Here are the most common types of filters, what they remove, and what they don't:

Carafe filter. Like a coffee pot filter, a carafe filter fits on top of a water pitcher and filters the water as you pour it through.

- Removes lead, chlorine, and some sediments.
- Doesn't remove bacteria, pesticides, and other agricultural chemicals.
- Care: Replace filter every month or two.
- Cost: Under $30 initially. Replacement filters cost $7 to $8 each. Even though the start-up cost is low, by the time you factor in the cost of replacement filters, at least $1 per week, and the inconvenience of having to remember to buy new filters, this type may not be the best buy.

Faucet filter. These filters are also called "point-of-use carbon filters." The water passes through a carbon bed that absorbs the contaminants. These filters are designed to fit directly onto your faucet or to a hose attached to the faucet, or they are connected directly to the cold-water line under the sink. You can install the faucet and hose types yourself; the under-the-sink type may require a plumber. This type can also fit on showerheads.

- Removes chlorine, lead, some pesticides and industrial chemicals, radon, and some bacteria, such as cryptosporidium.
- Consult the packaging of different models to see what contaminants are not removed.
- Care: Replace filter every six months to a year (otherwise they become so clogged with contaminants that the water coming out the filter may be less pure than the water going in).
- Cost: $30 to $300, plus the cost of replacement cartridges. Over the long run, these may be cheaper than the carafe filters on a per-gallon-of-water basis.

Whole-house activated carbon filters. This system attaches to your central water supply line and has the advantage of filtering the water that comes through all the taps.

- Removes chlorine and most industrial chemicals.
- Doesn't remove bacteria or nitrates.
- Care: Change filter as needed.
- Cost: Up to $500.

Reverse-osmosis purification system. This bulky large-tank system attaches to the cold-water pipe under your sink and flushes the water through carbon filters and a membrane that separates out most of the contaminants. Be aware that the system wastes several gallons of water for every one gallon it purifies. Check the model for how much water it wastes.

- Removes nearly all contaminants, including bacteria and industrial chemicals. (*Note:* This type of system also removes most of the fluoride in your water.) Check different models for exactly what they remove — some systems can remove 95 percent of contaminants.
- May not remove all industrial chemicals, depending on the power of the system.
- Care: Replace filter parts once a year. Replace the membrane less often according to manufacturer's instructions.
- Cost: $700 to $1,000 initially, but the overall filtering cost may be as little as 10 cents a gallon.

Other Ways to Improve Your Water Quality

Distill it. In some ways, a distillation system provides the purest water, and in other ways it doesn't. In this type of system, the water is boiled and the vapor collected, with most of the contaminants and bacteria left behind. The problem with this system is that there are still gases, such as chlorine, and some pesticides in the remaining water. Nevertheless, steamed, distilled water is about the purest you can get. Some home-distillation systems can remove 98 percent of the contaminants, which leaves you with water that is more pure than with filters.

Run it. Run your water for a full minute in the morning before taking a drink from the tap or making the coffee. First-draw water is likely to contain more lead from sitting in the pipes overnight.

Cool it. Drink water only from the cold tap. Lead more easily leaches from the pipes or faucet into hot water.

Boil it. Boiling water allows the chlorine to escape, which could improve the taste of some heavily chlorinated waters. (Note, however, that taste is not an accurate indicator of the purity or safety of drinking water.)

Buy bottled water. Many families choose to buy bottled water for drinking and cooking. Bottled water must be stored in a cool, dark place, such as in the pantry. Once it is opened, it must be recapped and refrigerated. For details on the different kinds of bottled water (e.g., spring water, mineral water, etc.), see the box "Bottled vs. Tap Water."

IMPROVING YOUR HYDRATION HABITS

To get the most health, enjoyment, and safety out of your water, here are some additional family water tips:

Drink water-rich foods. Don't like to drink plain water? No problem. Many foods, such as juice, soups, fruits, vegetables, and milk are 80 to 90 percent water. While it's healthier to get in the habit of drinking a lot of plain water (and model this wet taste for your children), if you absolutely

must have some sweet-tasting water, try water-logged fruits, such as (you guessed it) watermelon, juice Popsicles, fruit-rich smoothies, and plain water flavored with juice.

Watch out for water robbers. Shun caffeine-containing coffee, teas, and colas, along with alcoholic beverages, as these have a diuretic effect, causing your body to eliminate more water. This precaution is especially important if your hydration is already marginal, such as while you are exercising or if you are sick. Sugared drinks can also rob you of water, since sugar may lessen the absorption of water by the intestines. Drinking large amounts of juices that are high in sorbitol (such as prune and pear juice) or even overdosing on apple juice can produce diarrhea-like stools and increase water loss from the intestines.

Find fluid companions. Get in the habit of taking along a bottle of water when you ride your bike, drive in the car, and especially when you go on outings with active, thirsty toddlers. When water is close at hand in your purse, diaper bag, or front seat, you're likely to drink more of it. Keep a glass of water or water bottle on your nightstand and imbibe as soon as you get up.

Provide plane water. While traveling in airplanes, you may notice that your nose and mouth become dry and your breathing harder. Next you may notice you are feeling tired and thinking less clearly. What is happening is that you are getting dehydrated. The dry cabin air has only around 7 percent humidity, which dries out your breathing passages and sucks water out of your body as it tries to moisturize them. As a frequent flier, I fill up with at least two glasses of plain water or juice around half an hour before boarding the plane. I tote along some bottled water in my carry-on bag and bring a squirt bottle of salt water (available over the counter at pharmacies as saline nasal spray, but you can make your own) so that I can

BOTTLED VS. TAP WATER

There are several factors to consider when deciding whether commercially bottled or your own tap water is best for your family. When you look at the labels on the various bottles of water in the grocery store, here are the terms you are likely to see and what they mean:

- **spring water:** natural underground water that comes up to the surface
- **mineral water:** water containing only the natural minerals from its underground source, but not less than 250 parts per million of dissolved solid material
- **sparkling water:** water that has natural or added carbonation
- **purified water:** water with all the contaminants filtered out (A word of caution to mothers mixing this water with formula: "Purified" does not mean "sterile." For newborns it still should be boiled.)
- **drinking water:** ordinary tap water
- **artesian water:** water from an underground, natural reservoir

Now, which one do you choose?

Consider the source. This is one of the main facts you want to know: Where does the water come from? Does the bottle really contain that pure-as-snow, fresh mountain spring water that the label's picture seems to portray? Or is it simply municipal water that has been ultrafiltered or purified? If the bottle doesn't list a source, the stuff inside may be little better than what comes from the tap. If you're not sure, don't be afraid to call the 800 number listed on the bottle and ask. Members of the International Bottled Water Association (IBWA) must list the source of the water (e.g., spring). If the bottler doesn't list the source, the contents are probably municipal water.

Consider the tester. Bottled water is regulated by the Food and Drug Administration (FDA) because it's considered a food, and according to FDA guidelines the label must identify the source of the water. However, it does not have to specify what's in the water. Tap water, on the other hand, is regulated by the Environmental Protection Agency (EPA) and by state governments. Would you rather have your state or local government or the FDA test your water? The International Bottled Water Association includes 85 percent of bottled-water processors, and the organization claims to have a stricter code than the EPA. Members must submit to an annual, unannounced inspection by an independent third-party tester. So, at least in theory, bottled water seems to have a slight safety edge over tap water. One thing you can be certain of in nearly all bottled waters, though: The water is chlorine-free. And, bottled, distilled water is the cleanest water you can buy. For general information about bottled water, call the International Bottled Water Association (800-WATER-11).

JUNK WATER

Sure, fruit drinks are cheaper than pure juices when it's your turn to furnish snacks for the soccer team. The supermarket shelves are running over with colored sugar water, sold in the guise of "fruit drinks." These are little more than high-priced water with corn syrup and a touch of juice for color and flavor. Many of these drinks or punches contain chemical colorings that have never been proven safe. Moreover, they foster unhealthy drinking habits in children, who become so accustomed to the sweet taste of fluids that they refuse to drink plain water.

spritz a few drops into my nose every hour. I order double-fluid drinks, such as water and juice, and periodically order a cup of hot water to treat my dried-out nose with a little steam bath. I avoid alcoholic and caffeinated drinks while flying, since as diuretics they contribute to dehydration. Sure, waterlogging your body during plane travel stimulates frequent treks to the bathroom, but even these trips down the aisle are good for your body.

Watch out for water diets. Beware of crash diets and their unhealthy claims that you can lose a lot of weight fast. Especially suspect are the "high-something" diets, such as high-carb, high-protein, high-grapefruit, and so on, which tend to be not only nutritionally unbalanced but possibly downright dangerous. These diets often cause you to lose a lot of water. Yes, you may weigh less, but it's usually temporary. You don't lose fat, which is your real goal. Essentially what happens is you urinate out the weight rather than burn off the fat, and soon your body decides it wants that water back.

Try waterless meals. It's best not to consume too much fluid with meals. The body normally produces its own fluids to help digest food, beginning with saliva in the mouth and digestive juices in the stomach and small intestine. Drinking too much fluid with a meal can dilute these natural digestive juices, contributing to indigestion. Better to drink most of your fluids between meals. An exception to this is alcoholic beverages, such as wine, which are best consumed with food, since the food in the stomach and intestines slows the absorption of alcohol, minimizing blood-sugar swings and reducing the risk of intoxication. If you do like drinking water with meals, it's best to drink a little room-temperature water, since ice water slows digestion.

Try water a bit before breakfast. Beginning your day with several glasses of water rehydrates you after the night and helps your body begin the day in better biochemical balance.

Love that lemon-ade. If your tap water tastes of chlorine, adding a squirt of lemon juice to each glass of water can make it more palatable.

Forget fizzy water. Carbonated water does nothing more for your body than make you belch. In fact, the gas from carbonation makes you feel fuller sooner, so you drink less. If you enjoy the fizz, add a little seltzer to plain water.

Try water for weight loss. Can you drink more and weigh less? Yes, thanks to a biological quirk that is friendly to fat reducers. Your body is a natural water heater. When you drink water, which is nearly always a lower temperature than your body, the body expends energy (and therefore calories) to bring the water up to its own temperature. So you're not only drinking a noncaloric beverage, you're burning calories! That's a darn good drinking deal. Your body can burn around 100 calories a day using energy to heat a gallon of cool water that you drink. That translates into nearly a pound of fat loss in a month. Beware of any weight-loss programs that advise drinking less water. Water contributes to health by helping the kidneys flush toxins out of the body. When the kidneys are working optimally, other organs of the body, especially the liver, are more in balance.

WHAT ABOUT WATER SOFTENERS?

Water softeners have little to do with purification. Instead, they make the water more pleasant to wash with. Hard water contains a lot of calcium and magnesium. Water softeners replace the calcium and magnesium with sodium to soften the water. Whether you soften your water depends upon whether you like to wash in hard or soft water. However, there is one health implication: If you are on a low-salt diet but drink lots of tap water, you should find out exactly how much sodium is in your softened water.

Your family deserves pure-water swimming. If there are health concerns about showering in chlorinated water (from either inhaling water-chlorine vapor or from absorbing chlorine through the skin), what about being immersed for hours in a heavily chlorinated public pool or inhaling the steam as you sit meditatively in a chlorinated spa or even your own heated pool? There is a better way. European pool-filtration technology is way ahead of American, since in Europe many pools are indoors and the concentration of chlorine gases in the pool room can be nauseatingly uncomfortable. (Take a deep breath next time you walk into the hotel indoor pool.) To solve this problem, Europeans invented an ozone-filtration system in which the water is zapped with bacteria-killing ozone as it goes through the filter, and then the ozone self-destructs as the water reenters the pool. This is the system that we have installed on our pool and spa, and it is probably the healthiest $500 we have ever spent. Actually, by the time you factor in the savings of having a chemical-free pool and the lower maintenance cost, it's probably the most cost-effective way to filter your pool water, too.

9

Fantastic Fiber

GRANDMA ALWAYS TOLD you that "roughage" was good for you, and now research is proving that fiber in foods is important to health. Fiber is the part of fruits, vegetables, and grains that is neither digested nor absorbed. Why should fiber matter to good nutrition, since it doesn't provide any calories or nutrients? Fiber helps keep your intestines working comfortably and helps prevent many diseases. This chapter tells you why fiber is so fantastic.

Fiber comes in two forms, insoluble and soluble. Each acts differently in the intestines and benefits the body in different ways. Soluble fiber acts like a *sponge;* insoluble fiber acts like a *broom.*

Soluble fiber. Found in dried beans and peas, oat bran, rice bran, barley, and even fruit pectin (the substance used to thicken jams and jellies), soluble fiber absorbs water in the intestines, mixes the food into a gel, and thereby slows the rate of glucose digestion and consequent absorption into the bloodstream.

Insoluble fiber. This is the stringy stuff that holds plants together. It's called "insoluble" because it doesn't dissolve in water. It can be found mainly in plant leaves, peels, skins, and the coverings of whole grains (e.g., wheat bran). Like a disposable diaper, fiber can absorb many times its own weight in water. This water adds bulk and softness to the stools and keeps them moving along more comfortably. Think of eating fiber as similar to brushing your teeth — it cleans out your intestines daily.

FIBER FOR YOUR HEALTH

Fiber is an important part of a healthy diet. It can help you control your weight and your cholesterol level, and it does other good things for your body, too. Here are some reasons for eating a diet high in fiber:

Fiber curbs overeating. Fibers are filling without being fattening. High-fiber foods require more chewing, and the prolonged chewing, besides predigesting the food, satisfies the appetite, so you eat less. Fiber stays in the stomach longer, absorbs water, swells, and helps you feel full. Because of this feeling of fullness, people on high-fiber diets tend to eat more slowly and eat less, especially less fat. Best fibers for weight control are bran and the pectin from fruits.

Fiber steadies your blood-sugar level. Fiber, especially the soluble type, found in psyllium, bran, citrus fruits, and legumes, mixes the food into a

HOW MUCH FIBER DO YOU NEED?

To get the full health benefits of dietary fiber, adults should eat from 25 to 35 grams of fiber each day. Most American adults eat only around 11 grams. To calculate how much daily fiber your child needs, follow this formula: *age of child in years + 5.* For example, a five-year-old would need 10 grams of fiber a day.

How much fiber is too much? Your intestines will tell you. Gradually build up the amount and variety of your daily fiber intake. Signs of insufficient fiber in a diet are:

- constipation
- infrequent stools
- hard stools
- abdominal pain
- a general feeling of "sluggish bowels"

Signs of too much fiber are:

- excessive gas
- bloating
- abdominal pain
- stools uncomfortably frequent and large in overall volume

---

gel, thereby slowing the absorption of sugar from the intestines. This steadies the blood-sugar level and lessens the ups and downs of insulin secretion. So a breakfast and lunch containing moderate amounts of soluble fibers, such as bran, fruit, and oats, can be especially valuable to a child who shows behavior and learning difficulties from blood-sugar swings. Keeping insulin levels low and stable also helps the body store less fat, another perk for people trying to control their weight.

NUTRITIP
Fiber Tips for Kids

The skins of fruits are rich sources of fiber, so don't peel apples and pears. Cut these fruits up into easy-to-eat wedges, but leave the skins on. Serve your child nectar (which contains pulp) rather than fiberless plain juice. Better yet, serve the whole fruit rather than its juice.

Fiber slows fat absorption. Fiber slows down the absorption of fat (and therefore calories) from the foods you eat. This is another weight-control perk offered by a high-fiber diet. The stools of people eating high-fiber diets have a higher fat content than stools from those eating low-fiber meals.

Fiber reduces cholesterol. A diet high in soluble fiber, such as that found in oat bran, whole oats, psyllium, legumes, barley, fruit, and prunes, lowers blood levels of the harmful type of cholesterol (LDL) without lowering the good cholesterol (HDL) levels. As it travels through the intestines, soluble fiber absorbs water and forms a gluey gel that picks up cholesterol and carries it out of the body. Yet, doctors caution, adding more soluble fiber to your diet is not a license to eat high-cholesterol foods. High-fiber diets are usually low in fat, too, and the cholesterol-lowering effects may be related to less fat in the diet as well as to fiber. Recent studies show that eating an extra 10 grams of fiber daily (the average American adult eats only 11 grams of fiber a day) decreases the risk of dying from heart disease by 17 to 29 percent.

Fiber promotes regularity. Insoluble fibers, mainly the cellulose in skins of fruits and vegetables and the husks of grains, help prevent constipation; their sponge effect absorbs much water into the stools, making them soft and bulky. This type of stool stimulates the intestines to contract in an undulating way, called "peristalsis," which sweeps stools along. In cultures that typically eat higher-fiber diets, people tend to produce stools that are softer, larger, and more frequent, unlike the smaller, harder, and less frequent stools associated with the typical Western diet.

Fiber reduces cancer risk. While soluble fiber helps protect against cardiovascular diseases, insoluble fiber protects against colon cancer. The incidence of colon cancer is significantly lower in cultures where people eat lots of high-fiber foods. Increasing your consumption of insoluble fiber, such as that found in whole grains, especially wheat bran (e.g., All-Bran), is one of the most effective dietary changes you can make to decrease your risk of colon cancer. Here's how fiber decreases the risk of colon cancer:

- *Fiber increases peristalsis.* One of the theories explaining the relationship between a high-fiber diet and a lower risk of colon cancer suggests that the longer the potential toxins are in contact with the lining of the colon, the greater the chance that these lining cells will become cancerous. So anything that decreases the contact time between the stools and intestinal walls will lower the risk of cancer. The bulkier, softer stools that result from a high-fiber diet stimulate peristalsis, the involuntary muscular contractions that keep food moving through the intestines. So fiber acts like a biological broom, sweeping potentially toxic waste products through the intestines more quickly. A high-fiber diet can cut the transit time in half, thereby reducing the time that the lining of the bowel walls is exposed to potential cancer-causing substances.

- *Fiber binds carcinogens.* Besides moving carcinogens (toxins that can transform normal cells into cancerous ones) through the bowels faster, fiber binds them, further lessening their contact time with the intestinal wall. The water and bulk of the stools also dilute carcinogens, decreasing their potential to do harm. In addition, fiber absorbs bile acids and other potential irritants that may predispose the intestinal lining to cancer. Studies of persons at high risk for colorectal cancer showed that those eating a high-fiber diet (primarily wheat bran) had a much lower chance of going on to develop colon cancer than those on a low-fiber diet. While more and more studies confirm the link between high-fiber diets and lowered risk of colon cancer, the effect of fiber on other cancers is less clear. Preliminary studies have shown that high-fiber diets may decrease the risk of stomach and breast cancer. There are several possible explanations for this. Fiber binds estrogen in the intestines, thereby reducing the chance of breast cancer. Fiber also binds toxins, keeping them away from vulnerable tissues.

  A recent article in *The New England Journal of Medicine* received a lot of publicity by reporting on the results of a study in which the eating habits of eighty-eight thousand nurses were tracked over sixteen years. The study found that there was no difference in the incidence of colorectal cancer between those who ate a low-

---

NUTRITIP
Children's Fiber

A child's age plus 5 grams is about the minimum amount for a child over two. So, a six-year-old should eat at least 11 grams of fiber; a fifteen-year-old should eat at least 20 grams.

TEN EASY WAYS TO BOOST YOUR DAILY FIBER

1. Consume whole fruits and vegetables instead of juice. The peel on apples and the white pith on oranges are rich sources of fiber, as are potato skins.

2. Cut back on refined foods. "Enriched flour" means the fiber-containing parts have been removed.

3. Try a daily yogurt smoothie made in the blender with a couple of handfuls of fresh fruits, such as strawberries, bananas, papaya, blueberries, and pears. Blend in a heaping tablespoon of psyllium husks. Drink it quickly before it gels.

4. Snack on dried fruits, such as apricots, figs, prunes, and raisins.

5. Use whole grains instead of white. White bread and white rice have had the fiber processed out of them. (This is why white bread and white rice are constipating.) Instead use whole grains: bread made with whole wheat flour, whole-grain cereals that contain wheat bran or oat bran, whole-grain cornmeal, wheat germ, and barley. Instead of white rice, use brown or wild rice.

6. Be a bean freak. Nearly all varieties of beans are a rich source of fiber, especially kidney beans, which can be served in many forms, such as in salads, soups, burritos, or chili.

7. Dip it. A chickpea dip (i.e., hummus) is nutritious and fiber rich.

8. Choose a high-fiber cereal. If you find that high-fiber cereals are not the most palatable, try mixing a couple of tablespoons of All-Bran or psyllium husks into your favorite cereal to boost the fiber content. Add lots of milk, rice beverage, or juice and enjoy.

9. Choose your lettuce wisely. Iceberg lettuce is useless as a source of fiber or any other nutrients. Spinach and romaine lettuce are healthier choices.

10. Fresh fruits have more fiber than canned fruits because much of the fiber is in the peel, which is usually removed in processing.

Simply emphasizing grains, fresh fruits, and vegetables in your diet will automatically get you enough fiber. A diet that revolves around meat, eggs, and dairy products will not contain enough fiber.

---

fiber diet and those who ate a high-fiber diet. In my opinion, the conclusions of this study are questionable. The study is purely a statistical analysis, and it contradicts the findings of other studies. In addition, it makes good physiological sense that a high-fiber diet could reduce the risk of many cancers, including colorectal cancer. As a physician, whenever I read the results of any study that doesn't agree with common sense and sound physiological principles, I question its relevance. As is the case with many

"conclusions" in medicine, tune in for the results of similar studies soon to come.

- *Fiber promotes healthy intestinal bacteria.* Fiber promotes overall colon health by discouraging the growth of harmful bacteria in the intestines and encouraging the growth of beneficial bacteria. This is thought to contribute to the lowered risk of colorectal cancer associated with a high-fiber diet. Fiber also contributes to a friendlier intestinal environment — the friendly bacteria in the colon ferment fiber into short-chain fatty

NUTRITIP
Fiber Soaks Up Fat

Eat high-fiber foods with high-fat foods to decrease the absorption of fat. Increase your daily fiber and you'll absorb fewer calories a day.

SILLY PSYLLIUM

This super fiber is made from the husks of psyllium seeds. It has more water-absorbing capability (called "stool-bulking capacity") than any other fiber. Yet stronger is not necessarily better. Because of its high water-absorbing capacity, if not used wisely, psyllium can actually gum up the stools, resulting in constipation, the very problem it was meant to cure. This is known as the "psyllium syndrome." If using psyllium, take two precautions: Begin with only 1 teaspoon, then gradually increase the amount until your stools are soft and you have no bloating or intestinal discomfort. And drink at least eight 8-ounce glasses of water a day when using psyllium.

acids (SCFA's), healthy nutrients that can be used by the body. The friendly bacteria in the intestines seem to prefer rice bran and barley bran, balanced sources of soluble and insoluble fiber, to make these nutritious fatty acids. These foods are also rich in vitamin E compounds called "tocotrienols," which are natural cholesterol-lowering substances.

FIBER-EATING TIPS

Getting enough fiber is really quite simple. If you follow the recommendations of the Food Guide Pyramid on page 112 and include the amounts of healthy grains, fruits, legumes, and vegetables it suggests, you will automatically get enough fiber in your diet. Here are some tips on eating your fiber:

- *Increase the amount of fiber in your diet gradually.* Your intestines will be more comfortable with this approach than with a sudden onslaught of high-fiber foods. Too much fiber too soon is likely to catch your intestines off guard, leading to bloating and gas. Each week increase the amount of fiber in your diet by about 5 grams a day for adults and 1 to 2 grams a day for children until you reach your individual intestines-friendly daily amount. This is usually somewhere between 25 and 35 grams a day for adults, and half that for children. Keep experimenting with the amount and type of fiber that give you a comfortable "gut feeling."

- *It's important to eat fiber from a variety of sources.* By eating many types of high-fiber foods, you are more likely to balance out the right amount of soluble and insoluble fibers. The more soluble the fiber, the more it ferments, and therefore the more gas it produces.

NUTRIMINDER
The 3 B's of Fiber

Remember the three B's of fiber: bran, beans, and berries. One serving of bran plus one serving of beans each day will give you more than half of your total daily fiber needs. And remember: Bran and berries blend very well into yogurt smoothies.

BEST FIBER FOODS*

Food	Serving Size	Total Fiber (grams)[†]
All-Bran cereal	½ cup	10–13
Psyllium husks	2 tbsp. (1 ounce)	16
Wheat bran	¼ cup	7
High-fiber cereals	1 ounce (½ cup)	10–14
Flax meal	¼ cup	8
Apple (with skin)	1 medium	3.5
Oat bran	¼ cup	4
Prunes	3 medium	3
Kidney beans	½ cup	7.3
Lima beans	½ cup	4.5
Navy beans	½ cup	6
Lentils	½ cup	3.7
Peas	½ cup	3.6
Spaghetti (whole wheat)	1 cup	3.9
Apricots (dried)	5 halves	1.4
Banana	1 medium	2.4
Blueberries	½ cup	2.0
Grapefruit (with membrane)	half	1.6
Pear	1 medium	3.2
Bread (whole wheat)	1 slice	1.4
Figs (dried)	3 medium	5.3
Chickpeas (garbanzo beans)	½ cup	7
Potato (with skin)	1 medium	2.5
Broccoli	½ cup	2.3
Sweet potato	½ cup	3
Orange (with membrane)	1	2.6
Spinach	½ cup	2.1
Pita bread (whole wheat)	1 piece	5
Corn	1 ear	5
Barley	½ cup	8

Best Sources of Soluble Fiber

    oat bran
    kidney beans
    lentils
    sweet potatoes
    oranges
    broccoli
    pears
    apples
    barley
    peas

Best Sources of Insoluble Fiber

    wheat bran
    legumes
    skin of fruit
    seeds and nuts: sunflower seeds, soybean nuts, almonds

* Journal of the American Dietetic Association *86 (1986): 732.*
† *The RDA for fiber is 25 grams for adults; for children it is child's age in years + 5.*

NUTRIMINDER
The 4 A's of Fiber

Remember the four A's of fiber: apples, artichokes, apricots, and avocados.

- *Spread out your dietary fiber throughout the day.* Overdosing on fiber at any one meal is liable to produce bloating and gas.

- *Drink a lot of water with your fiber.* For fiber to do an adequate sweeping and sponging job, there has to be an adequate amount of water for it to absorb. Otherwise, fiber may actually contribute to constipation rather than prevent it, or it may soak up water and other nutrients needed elsewhere by the body.

- *Get your fiber from food, not from pills.* The fiber in the pill may not work the same way biologically as the fiber in food. For fiber to do its job, it needs to be eaten in the company of other foods and with a lot of fluids.

- *Avoid fiber-induced nutritional deficiencies.* Overdosing on fiber can interfere with the ab-

---

NUTRITIP
Fiber — A Family Food

In addition to being friendly to aging bowels, fiber is also valuable for school-age children, mainly because it delays the absorption of sugars in the food into the bloodstream, making the blood sugars more stable — and, consequently, making the children more likely to behave and learn better. Send your child off to school with a breakfast containing at least 5 grams of fiber, the amount contained in a medium-fiber cereal and one serving of fruit.

---

sorption of valuable nutrients. Fiber can push food through the intestines so fast that some nutrients, such as calcium, zinc, vitamins, and iron, don't have a chance to be fully absorbed. Trying to avoid eating high-fiber foods at the same time you eat foods containing these nutrients is impractical. If you're on a diet that includes more than 35 grams of fiber a day, you should consider taking vitamin and mineral supplements.

10

Food Digestion: Taking a Trip Through the Intestinal Tract

HOP ON THE intestinal train for a food-informative ride. From mouth to anus, your intestinal tract is a twenty-five-foot-long *dis*assembly line. Whole food is taken in at one end, and waste is expelled from the other. En route, nutrients are taken out of the food and absorbed into the bloodstream according to the body's needs. The whole process is called "digestion." (When things go wrong, it's called "*in*digestion.")

WHAT IS DIGESTION?

Digestion is basically a process of breaking down big food particles into individual molecules, tiny enough to squeeze through the intestinal lining into the bloodstream. Your body uses mechanical and chemical means to do this. By understanding the way the digestive process works — and how you can make it work better — you can improve your own "gut feeling." Let's follow a representative food — say, a peanut butter and jelly sandwich — from top to bottom and study the stops along the way.

Digestion Begins in the Brain

Before you eat, you imagine how good the food is going to taste. You get an eyeful when you walk past the buffet table at the beginning of the party. Or the aroma of freshly baked bread draws you into the bakery. Your eyes and your nose get your body and mind in the mood for food, and just the thought of food gets your digestive juices flowing. Your mouth waters, and your stomach churns at the very thought of what is soon to grace your palate. Even before the first bite, you think, sniff, and drool your digestion machine into action. Just anticipating eating gets the intestinal tract ready for the job coming its way.

Chew! Chew!

Mom's admonition to chew your food is good advice. When the sandwich enters your mouth, the first step in food breakdown begins. Your teeth break the bread down into smaller particles, increasing the surface area through which the chemical food processors — enzymes — can penetrate the food. Chewing breaks up the fiber that holds the food together and unwraps the food package so that the digestive enzymes have easier access to the contents inside. The saliva, which is already flowing in anticipation of eating, bathes the broken-down bread and peanut butter and jelly with the first digestive enzyme, called "salivary amylase." Amylase breaks the chemical bonds between the carbohydrate molecules, changing them into smaller sugar molecules. Uncoupled from their friends, these are now free to be broken down even further, if necessary. Even the fat in the food gets a head start on digestion while it's in the mouth by receiving a tiny squirt of a fat-digesting enzyme called "lingual lipase." (Note that the names of most of the enzymes are a combination of the suffix -*ase* and the nutrient they work on, such as lipase digesting lipids, proteinase digesting proteins, and lactase dissolving lactose.) Saliva also lubricates the food, making that sticky peanut butter slip and slide down the ten-inch-long esophagus, the tube that connects the mouth and the stomach. Saliva is the body's own health juice; besides helping with digestion, it contains a recently discovered substance called "epidermal growth factor" (EGF), which facilitates the growth and repair of injured or inflamed intestinal tissue. Perhaps this is why animals lick their wounds.

Taking small bites, chewing the food well, and swallowing slowly are things you can do to better prepare the food package for the next part of its journey. Also, taking time to chew foods well slows down your eating. You'll swallow less air (so you'll have less burping), and you can be more aware of signals that tell your stomach it's getting full. When each step along the disassembly line is done well, the next job is easier. If the food is hurried to the next stop, the "workers" there rebel because they have to work harder, and they cry "indigestion." By taking small bites, chewing your food well, and swallowing it slowly, you help the food particles go down the tube without discomfort. Mom not only chewed you out for "swallowing your food whole," but you also probably got many mealtime sermons on "eating slowly." Again, mother-nutritionist was right.

Churn! Churn!

When it enters the stomach, the mush from your mouth gets mixed together further. The stomach is your body's mechanical and chemical food processor. It's a pouch composed of sheets of muscle that encircle the stomach in different directions. When they contract, they twist and churn the food the way you would knead bread dough. The lining of the stomach secretes gastric juices, including hydrochloric acid, which dissolves the food, a protein-splitting enzyme called "pepsin," and a fat-digesting enzyme called "lipase." Like fruits or vegetables pureed in a blender, the food is churned and mixed with the digestive juices until it resembles thick soup. This glob is called "chyme." The circular muscles of the stomach also have the job of keeping the food in the stomach long enough to be broken down from a solid to liquid. Sometimes these muscles can malfunction. The muscle at the lower end of the stomach (called the "pylorus") can become too thick and tight in the first few weeks or months of infancy, keeping the stomach contents from emptying. When this happens, the food comes back up forcefully. This condition is known as "pyloric stenosis" and is manifested by vomiting of increasing frequency and severity. The muscle at the top end of the stomach, called the "gastroesophageal sphincter," can become too loose, so the stomach contents don't stay in during churning. This leads to a condition called "gastroesophageal reflux," or GER (see the box on page 96).

Hydrochloric acid is strong enough to eat through meat and potent enough to kill most of the harmful bacteria that may be in food. So the stomach not only digests, it disinfects. It is the body's food processor and the body's food purifier. Yet it does not destroy all the bacteria we ingest. Some of the bacteria that are able to survive the harsh conditions in the stomach eventually take up residence in the intestine where, in return for

GER — THE GREAT MASQUERADER

Once upon a time a fussy baby was labeled with "colic," which is really a five-letter word short for "the doctor doesn't know why." New insights into the cause of colicky behavior and frequent, painful night-waking episodes reveal that oftentimes babies hurt because of some underlying medical problem. In fact, in our practice we have replaced the term "colicky baby" with "hurting baby," which motivates the parents and the doctor to keep searching for the cause. One of the most common hidden medical causes of colic is a condition known as "gastroesophageal reflux" (GER), in which irritating stomach acids are regurgitated into the esophagus, causing pains that adults would call "heartburn." GER is caused by a malfunction of the valvelike muscles between the stomach and the esophagus. Besides triggering colicky behavior, GER is a subtle cause of unexplained bouts of wheezing or asthma in infants and children.

Here are clues that your baby suffers from reflux:

- painful blasts of crying (more than the usual baby cries)
- frequent spitting up (but not always)
- inconsolable bouts of abdominal pain
- painful bursts of night waking
- fussiness particularly after eating
- arching or writhing as if in pain
- seems more comfortable when carried upright, sleeping on the stomach, or sleeping propped up at a 30-degree angle
- frequent, unexplained bouts of wheezing and chest infections and episodes of apnea
- sour breath; throaty noises

If you suspect GER, mention it to your doctor. The diagnosis is usually made based on the history given by the parents. A doctor can confirm the diagnosis by placing a stringlike tube into baby's esophagus (only minimally uncomfortable), leaving the tube in place overnight, and measuring the amount of stomach acids regurgitated into the esophagus. If the reflux is severe, your doctor will prescribe medicines that lower the amount of stomach acid produced and accelerate stomach emptying. Besides these medications, try these home remedies to ease your baby's discomfort:

- Keep baby upright and quiet for at least thirty minutes after feeding.
- Offer smaller, more frequent feedings.
- Wear your baby in a carrier as much as possible. Carried babies cry less. Babies reflux more while crying.
- Breastfeed. Studies show that GER occurs less frequently in breastfed babies.
- If you are bottlefeeding (and if recommended by your doctor), thicken baby's feedings with 1 or 2 tablespoons of rice cereal in each 8-ounce bottle.
- Discuss with your doctor the safest sleeping position for your baby. Babies with severe reflux sleep best on their stomachs and propped up at a 30-degree angle by elevating the head of the crib. (Babies without reflux should be put down to sleep on their backs.)

From one-third to one-half of all babies have some degree of reflux during the first three months. The good news is that most infants outgrow reflux at around seven to nine months of age.

NUTRITIP
Fast Absorbing Food

The mouth and stomach are mainly food processors. The small intestine is in charge of absorption. Yet, some substances, such as alcohol and caffeine, and some drugs, such as aspirin, can be absorbed through the lining of the stomach, accounting, for example, for the tipsy feeling or the buzz that can occur even before someone finishes an alcoholic drink or a cup of coffee. Consuming these mind-altering substances on an empty stomach increases the speed of their absorption.

---

all they can eat, they fulfill an important role in the health and digestive process.

For comfortable digestion to occur, the stomach lining should secrete just the right amount of acid at the right time — no more, no less. If the lining pours out acid when the stomach is empty (which can happen when you are under stress), the acid irritates the stomach lining, causing uncomfortable sensations, or indigestion. Also, if there is no food to absorb the acid, the excess acid enters the first part of the intestine, the duodenum, which is more sensitive. Since there is no food to digest, the acid digests the lining of the duodenum, causing what are called "duodenal ulcers." Substances such as alcohol or coffee on an empty stomach (accompanied by stress) can cause you to be "eaten up inside." Or, the excess acid can squirt up into the esophagus, which also has a sensitive lining, causing the heartburn, or reflux, mentioned above.

Belches, rumblings, and vomiting. When your stomach is empty and you are hungry or anticipating eating, the stomach contractions just squeeze air, making the noise experienced as rumblings. Belches, rumblings, vomiting, and retches are occupational hazards for the hardworking stomach. Most belches follow the swallowing of air, which occurs not only when you swallow food but also when you swallow saliva, or when you get hungry or tense. Since you swallow several thousand times a day, it's no wonder that the upper end of the intestines needs to kick back some air. Add to that the internal gases produced from fermentation in the lower intestines, and it's no wonder that the average human is a bit of a "windbag."

The vomiting reflex is designed to protect the intestines from unwanted material. It simply sends it back out the way it came in. The brain triggers the muscles of the diaphragm, abdomen, and stomach to contract suddenly, forcing the stomach contents up and out. While vomiting is not always desirable, often (e.g., after experiencing food poisoning) vomiting brings gut feelings of relief.

Grazing for good digestion. The size of a meal shouldn't be more than the size of your stomach. To help your eyes get a picture of the approximate size of your stomach, open your fist so that the tips of the thumb and forefinger touch. Your stomach is about the width of this open fist and twice as long. Next time you are about to binge, place your fist next to your heaping plate and notice the mismatch. (Compare the tiny fist of a tiny toddler next to a full plate. You can now see why tiny tummies can get upset easily.)

All parts of the intestinal tract — from top to bottom — were designed for grazing, that is, eating small, frequent mini meals rather than three big squares a day. The term "square meal" doesn't imply a complete balanced meal must be eaten at every sitting. In some ways children are smarter eaters than adults. Left to their own devices, they tend to nibble and graze throughout the day. Most adults would experience less indigestion if they ate five mini meals rather than three maxi meals a day.

Seep! Seep!

By the time the peanut butter and jelly sandwich is chewed and churned, it's ready to be pushed from the stomach into the small intestine, where the real digestive action is. Most of the sandwich's proteins and carbs empty from the stomach into the small intestine within a couple of hours, but the fats, since oil and water (i.e., digestive juices) don't easily mix, remain in the stomach a few hours longer. (This is why you feel fuller longer after a high-fat meal than you do after a high-carbohydrate or high-protein meal.)

As the chyme, the food mush, enters the small intestine, the most important part of digestion — absorption — begins. The first part of the small intestine is called the "duodenum" (from the

---

INDIGESTION

Do you suffer from indigestion? You don't have to. While heartburn and indigestion used to be discomforts that many adults just learned to live with, new insights have uncovered the medical reasons and effective treatment for these upsets.

While the terms "heartburn" and "indigestion" have no medical definition, if your "heart" burns or you "indigest," there is usually a medical reason. The most common medical reason for these symptoms is a condition known as "gastroesophageal reflux" (GER), sometimes called "gastroesophageal reflux disease" (GERD). Reflux happens when the muscle between the stomach and the esophagus fails to contract enough to keep food and digestive juices in the stomach. If you experience pain just below your breastbone shortly after eating, wake up with this pain during the night, or have periodic episodes of unexplained wheezing, suspect that you may have GER and discuss the diagnosis and treatment with your doctor. Besides medications that lessen the amount of stomach acid you produce and help the stomach empty faster, here are some self-help measures you can try to lessen the regurgitation of acid and foods back up into your esophagus after eating:

- Graze. Eat small, frequent meals, or mini meals, rather than three large meals a day.
- Take small bites and chew your food well. Smaller food particles empty faster from the stomach.
- Eat foods that pass through your stomach quickly, primarily proteins and carbohydrates, rather than foods that linger in the stomach for a while, such as high-fat foods.
- Remain upright and quiet for thirty minutes after eating. Moving around jostles the acid in your stomach, aggravating the condition.
- Don't go to bed with a full stomach. Eat dinner earlier in the evening and keep it low-fat. Remember: "Don't dine after nine."
- Relax. Stress produces stomach acid.
- Get friendly with your blender. Fruit-and-yogurt smoothies and blended vegetables are liquid enough to pass through the stomach quickly, minimizing the chance of reflux.

Despite what the advertisements tell you, it's best not to self-diagnose and self-medicate if you suspect you suffer from GER. Consult your doctor or gastroenterologist for proper diagnosis and the most up-to-date treatment for this most uncomfortable condition.

Latin for "twelve" — so called because the adult duodenum is around twelve finger breadths long). More digestive processes occur in the duodenum than in any other part of the intestinal tract.

In order for food to become muscle, it has to get through the intestinal lining, and here's where some exciting changes occur. First, because the more delicate lining of the small intestine doesn't like the irritating stomach acids, it secretes the body's own antacids — called "bicarbonates" — to neutralize the food. As the food moves down the intestinal disassembly line, it passes by stations where it gets squirts of digestive juices that further break down the proteins, carbohydrates, and fats into molecules small enough to seep into the bloodstream.

Each nutrient requires specific intestinal juices that work on its molecules in particular ways. Trypsin and peptidase are enzymes that disassemble the protein necklaces into individual amino acids, which enter the bloodstream through "doors" in the intestinal lining specially marked "for amino acid entry only." Carbohydrates are disassembled into individual sugar molecules by the enzymes lactase, sucrase, maltase, and pancreatic amylase, and the individual sugar molecules enter the bloodstream through doors marked "sugars only." (If the intestinal lining is injured, these doors are not so selective, allowing allergens to pass through that are potentially harmful to the body — a condition known as "leaky gut syndrome.") Behind each door runs a blood vessel that quickly ferries the nutrients throughout the body, where they can be burned for energy or reassembled into tissues.

Meanwhile, back at the stomach, the fats are finally getting ready to leave. As they enter the small intestine, the fats get a squirt of bile from the gallbladder and some lipase from the pancreas. The bile emulsifies the fat, the way soap breaks up grease. Like soap, bile does not really dissolve the fat but rather breaks it down into tiny particles, which are then more easily broken down by the pancreatic enzyme lipase for absorption into the bloodstream. The individual fatty-acid molecules exit the intestine through doors marked "fats only." However, unlike proteins and carbs, which go through their own doors and into the bloodstream quickly, fats go into microscopic holding rooms within special cells in the intestinal lining. Here they are stuffed into microscopic bags, which are then taken out the back door and loaded onto ferryboats in the bloodstream called "lipoproteins." (Two of these lipoprotein boats are the cholesterol-carrying HDL and LDL; see page 24.) These molecular ferries then circulate throughout the bloodstream, loading and unloading fat molecules at cell loading docks. Picture each cell of the body as having hundreds of loading docks on the membrane. If the cell doesn't need any more fat, it shuts down the docks, so that the lipoprotein ferryboats can't dock and are forced to circulate around the bloodstream until they find some other place to deposit the fat. The two places always receiving more fats are the liver and the fat cells. So the ferryboats either deposit the excess fat around the waist, the hips, *or wherever there are fat cells,* or transport the extra fat into the liver, where it is dissolved by bile and excreted out into the intestines as waste.

A supply-and-demand process. The enzymes involved in digestion work on a supply-and-demand basis. If the glands in the intestinal lining and the pancreas secrete enough enzymes to break down and absorb all the food that comes by, the intestines feel fine. But if there is more food than there are enzyme workers to process it, the doors close, and the excess travels down into the large intestine, where it is not very welcome. The result is indigestion. How to keep this supply-and-demand digestive process in balance? You guessed it. Give the enzymes a fighting chance by grazing or eating smaller meals. Overwhelming the intestines with too much food sets you up for indigestion.

The luxurious intestinal lining. The lining of the intestines is more like a plush carpet than a smooth sheet. Here's why. Trillions of microscopic projections, called "villi," grow out from the cells of the intestinal lining. This enlarges the cell's surface area, thus increasing the contact between the food and the cells. The more contact these cells (and their rich blood supply) have with the food, the more nutrients can be absorbed.

The intestinal lining is only one cell thick, which is a good news/bad news phenomenon. The good news is that because the lining is thin, nutrients are easily absorbed. They come in the front door of the cell and go out the back door into the bloodstream. The bad news is that this delicate lining is easily injured by irritants and infection. When this happens, food cannot be absorbed efficiently, leading to diarrhea, abdominal pain, gas, and bloating. When the cells are damaged, there may not be enough enzymes available to digest certain foods, such as lactose. Temporary lactase deficiency is common following intestinal irritation or infection. This is the reason that doctors advise smaller, more frequent feedings of more easily digestible foods during recovery from an intestinal infection, so as not to overload the healing intestines that may be undergoing a temporary enzyme deficiency. It may also be necessary to avoid milk and other lactose-containing foods. The cells of the intestinal lining do regenerate and heal, but complete healing may take several weeks. Diarrhea or looser stools may occur for four to six weeks following an intestinal infection.

Water and Waste

By the time the peanut butter and jelly sandwich has completed its twenty-foot-long, ten-hour journey through the small intestine, most of the nutrients have been absorbed. The leftovers enter the final five feet of the journey, called the large intestine, or "colon." Little digestion occurs in the colon, since it has few villi and low levels of intestinal enzymes. Food processing in the colon is often described as the calm after the storm. Yet the colon is not just a passive waste collector and eliminator. It plays an active and important role in the health and well-being of the whole body, accounting for the phrase, "Your body is only as healthy as your colon."

The first vital function of the colon is to regulate the body's water balance. As the waste from the food passes through the lower part of the intestine (called the "jejunum") and enters the colon, the colon absorbs excess water from the food and furnishes it to the water-thirsty body. If, however, the waste matter lacks water, the colon fills the stool with water to prevent constipation. Healthy water balance in the colon leads to healthy stool patterns. In fact, one of the most important changes a person will notice after following our L.E.A.N. program (see Chapter 35) is having several smaller, soft (but not diarrhea-like) stools a day rather than the usual American pattern of one huge bowel movement once a day or every other day. Passage of four to six soft, not uncomfortable, bowel movements a day suggests that your colon is in biochemical balance.

Bugs in the bowels. Billions of bacteria reside in the intestines, primarily in the large intestine. Called "intestinal flora," because they are like the plant life of the intestines, they contribute to the healthy life of the colon — and the whole body. These intestinal bacteria are also known as "probiotics" because they add health to life. (The term "probiotics" is also used for bacteria supplements in a bottle, either in powder or capsule form.)

The two main healthful bacteria in the colon are *Lactobacilli* and *bifidus* bacteria. They live symbiotically in the colon, meaning, in a mutual give-and-take relationship. These bugs give good stuff to the body in return for a warm place to

GOOD TASTES

Taste buds are located primarily on the tongue, but they are also found throughout the lining of the mouth, especially in babies. Four types of taste receptors are located around the tongue. Sweet and salty tastes are best perceived at the tip and front sides of the tongue. Sour receptors are located on the sides of the tongue, and bitter receptors toward the back. You can use this anatomical knowledge to your advantage when introducing solid foods to infants. Since taste buds for sweetness enjoy front-row seats on the tongue, and babies prefer sweet and/or salty foods, place these foods on the front of your infant's tongue. The prominent location of the taste buds for sweetness explains why babies prefer the sweeter taste of fruits rather than vegetables as first foods. If your baby is used to the sweet taste of breast milk or the bland taste of formula and rejects the different tastes of solid foods, place new foods toward the middle of the tongue where there are fewer taste receptors. After experimentation with various foods on various areas of the tongue, you will discover which combination works. The fact that the bitter taste buds are located at the back of the tongue may be an adaptive phenomenon for the primarily plant eating humans. Nutritious plants tend to be sweet, while poisonous plants tend to be bitter. When bitter plants touched the back of the tongue, they would trigger the gag reflex as a protective mechanism and be spit out.

Cold temperatures dampen taste buds, which is why frozen yogurt tastes much sweeter when

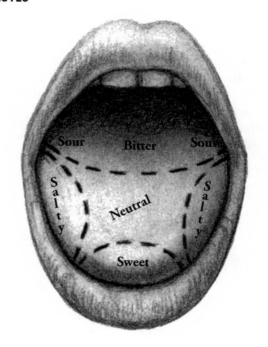

melted. To get your child to accept an unpleasant-tasting medicine, trick the taste buds by letting your child suck on a Popsicle, ice, or anything cold just before giving the medicine. Salt dilutes sour tastes, which is one reason why it is added to vinegar-containing dressings.

Taste buds change their preferences with age. While infants and young children prefer sweet foods in most cases, this young sweet tooth diminishes as a person ages.

---

live. The healthy bacteria keep the harmful bacteria in check. They also ferment the soluble fiber in food, forming short-chain fatty acids (SCFA's), which nourish the cells of the large intestine, stimulating healing and reducing the development of intestinal cancer. SCFA's are also absorbed from the intestines and travel to the liver, where they decrease the liver's production of cholesterol. In addition, SCFA's inhibit the growth of yeast and disease-causing bacteria.

NUTRITIP
Gut Feelings

Take your cues from your intestines. The intestinal lining and muscular walls are richly supplied with nerves, anatomically referred to as the "gut brain." They react to emotions as well as foods, which is why stress or nervousness can give you indigestion or abdominal pains.

More gut sounds. Air-swallowing produces belches. Gas at the other end is another matter. When the normal bacteria that live in the large intestine "eat" certain foods (such as the polysaccharides in beans), the byproduct of the bacteria's own digestive process is gas. While the colon absorbs some of this gas so it doesn't bother anybody, some causes bloating and the rest of the gas is expelled as flatus. The odorous gas is a combination of methane and hydrogen sulfite.

Most of the gas you hear, feel, or smell is a result of the intestinal bacteria digesting the sugars and fiber that manage to reach the large intestine.

THE WISDOM OF THE BODY

Once upon a time there was a popular nutritional principle called "the wisdom of the body," which meant that our bodies would tell us which foods we need — as long as we learn to listen. According to the "wisdom of the body" principle, if your body is deficient in a particular nutrient, your desire to eat food containing that nutrient increases.

In the 1920s pediatrician Clara Davis did a famous study to validate the concept of the wisdom of the body. In this study, infants who had been exclusively breastfed but were newly weaned were offered a dozen different foods at each meal. It's noteworthy that all these foods were in their natural state — unprocessed, unseasoned, and unsweetened. Over time and without coercion, these babies, making their own food choices, established eating patterns that provided them with the balanced nutrition they needed.

For most people, the body has become less wise because of stupid things done to it. The body can make wise choices only when programmed with the language of good nutrition. Otherwise, it's garbage in, garbage out. If all your body knows is high-fat junk food, that's all it can ask for.

The problem for many of us is that we have confused our bodies with years of poor eating, so much so that the body no longer knows what is good and what is bad. Even food cravings — the revered biological signal, the inner voice of a wise body saying what it needs — can't be trusted in a body that's biochemically out of tune. As you improve your nutrition, the wisdom of your body will return, though this may take several months. Eventually you will crave the foods that help you and shun those that harm you. When you go against your body's signals (and everyone does this occasionally), your body will remind you of why you normally choose to skip a particular food.

The wisdom of the body is related to the "gut feeling" that you have after eating. Certain foods, certain volumes, and certain combinations leave you feeling pleasantly satisfied; others leave you uncomfortably full and bloated. Excessive gas, flatulence, bloating, burping, headaches, lethargy, and sweats are all signals that you are not eating wisely.

Since these bacteria love starch, the prime gas producers are polysaccharides in starchy foods, such as beans, brussels sprouts, prune juice, and just about every type of grain, except rice, which seems to be the most socially acceptable starch. Galactose from milk and the soluble fiber pectin are also favored foods of the resident bacteria.

How much gas is produced and by what foods varies from person to person. To put your large intestine on emission control, keep your own food-gas diary and adjust your diet accordingly. Most of the time the volume of food you eat is more at fault than the type of food. Overwhelming the intestine with more starch than it can absorb sets you up for unwanted blasts.

The End

The rhythmic contractions of the colon move waste material (called "feces") into the last five inches of the large intestine, called the "rectum," where the final waste products are eliminated. Normal passage of feces or stools (called "defecation") occurs when the nerves lining the rectum sense the presence of feces that need to be evacuated. The presence of feces in the rectum stimulates a reflex (called the "defecation reflex"), which causes the muscles of the abdomen and upper rectum to contract and the muscle encircling the anus to relax, allowing easy passage of stools. This reflex is very efficient as long as people don't do something to mess it up. Eating too little fiber, not drinking enough fluids, eating too much fat (fat slows intestinal transit), and simply not paying attention to the evacuation warnings of the rectum will all cause the reflex to stop working. (Kids between five and ten, especially boys, are prone to ignore this reflex.) Feed your intestines properly and listen to their signals, and they will work well for you.

II

MAKING WISE FOOD CHOICES

With toddler in tow, you push your shopping cart through the supermarket aisles, bombarded on all sides by enticing packaging with unintelligible fine print. You may wonder, What do all these terms on the labels mean? What information can I trust? How can I make the best choices for my family? In this section we will help you become a wise shopper so that you can select from the overwhelming variety of foods in the store and put together menus that meet the nutritional needs of every member of your family. We'll take you through a buffet of top foods and point out how one food compares to another in nutritional content. Besides buying nutritious foods for your family, you need to be concerned about safety, so we'll tell you not only about which foods are the most nutritious, but also which foods are least likely to contain substances harmful to your family's health. Here's a guide to foods that give you the most nutritional bang for your buck.

11

Making Your Own Family Food Guide

Now that you've digested the nitty-gritty of nutrition, you're probably wondering, What should I eat? We know there's more to dinner than the biochemistry of proteins and carbohydrates. In this chapter we'll tell you about our top twelve foods — foods that provide a lot of good nutrition and are good to eat as well. These are family foods: What's good for the goose is good for the goslings. Kids will like most of these foods as much as adults do.

THE TOP TWELVE FAMILY FOODS

Admittedly, any "top foods" list will be a bit biased based on personal preferences, but we have tried to honor certain criteria in selecting our top twelve. We believe that the key to healthy eating is to fill your plate with foods that provide high-quality nutrition, those foods that are most *nutrient dense.* This means foods that pack a lot of nutrition alongside relatively few fats and calories. To be on our list, a food must do the following:

- supply a significant amount of nutrition per serving
- supply nutrients vital to bodily functions
- supply nutrients that keep you healthy

- be versatile (able to be prepared in a variety of tasty ways)
- be readily available at an affordable price
- contain minimal amounts of substances that may be harmful to your health (e.g., hydrogenated fats, saturated fats, added sugars)

So here's our answer to "What's for dinner?" Start with the foods on page 108, and you're on your way to serving nutritious meals to the whole family.

LEAST NUTRITIOUS FOODS

In the early days of medical school, aspiring young physicians are admonished, "First, do no harm." That sage advice also applies to food. On page 108, we serve you a list of our top twelve foods, nutrient-dense foods that pack a lot of nutrition and contribute to health. In contrast to those "top foods" is our hit list of worst foods (see page 110) — those that not only provide little nutrition but also can harm your health. Truthfully, these are foods to die for.

Hot Dogs

Grind up various parts of an animal that would otherwise have no commercial value, stuff them into an artificial casing, and serve them as a nutrient-poor food. What do you have? A hot dog.*
Hot dogs supply absolutely nothing of any nutritional value that can't be gotten more safely from many other foods. The typical hot dog packs more problems than nutrients. Specifically, most hot dogs are likely to contain all of the following:

- nitrates and nitrites, which are health-harming food additives
- high levels of saturated fat
- lots of sodium: one hot dog can contain a child's total recommended dietary allowance (around 500 mg.)
- who knows what in the casing, since ingredients are not listed on the label.

Pack a nutritionally poor hot dog in an impoverished (dubbed "enriched") white bun and you have a double junk food.

A healthier hot dog? Let's be frank: Parents depend on hot dogs. What else will a picky eater pick? To preserve their market share of American kids' cuisine, frankfurter makers have begun serving up improved alternatives: fat-free and low-fat franks, all-beef franks (which simply means the meat comes from somewhere on the cow), turkey franks, and even veggie dogs made with tofu and other soy products. Some hot dog alternatives are even free of nitrates, nitrites, preservatives, and food coloring.

Should you get the hot dog out of your house completely, or should you simply switch to one of the more healthful varieties? You can be pure or practical. A nutritional purist would ban all hot

dogs, believing that it's important for the child to make the connection between hot dogs and poor nutrition, so that he won't be tempted when the only available dog is the chemical-laden standard-issue variety. A more practical-minded parent (in search of convenience foods) might try some of the alternative hot dogs mentioned above, reasoning that those lower-fat alternatives will program a child to recognize what a healthy hot dog is supposed to feel like in the gut. Then when the child goes out to the ballpark and tastes an all-American high-fat hot dog, the uncomfortable sensations that follow become their own lesson. Model healthy hot dog habits. If your child sees you eating hot dogs or sausages, most of which are as high in fat as hot dogs, it's hard for her to understand why these foods are off-limits to her.

We define a junk food as "a food that is likely to do more harm than good to the body." We've used hot dogs as our, pardon the expression, "model" junk food. They're high in saturated fats, hydrogenated fats, added sugars, additives, food colorings, nitrates, and nitrites. The rest of our list of least nutritious foods, foods you should be cautious about, is on page 110.

COLOR YOUR CUISINE

Modern food science confirms what grandmother taught: "As long as you have lots of color on your plate, you're eating healthy." The stuff that gives color to your food is the same stuff that provides nutrients to your body. Those color-rich biochemicals are called "phytonutrients" (meaning, plant nutrients), or "phytos" for short. In general, the darker the food, the more nutritious it is, such as the deep blue of blueberries, the dark red of tomatoes, the deep red of grapes, the deep orange of a sweet potato, and the dark green of broccoli, kale, and peppers. Choose colorful foods over less colored ones: red grapes over green, pink over lighter grapefruit, dark, leafy green vegetables over paler

---

* Hot dogs can even be dangerous: The diameter of a chunk of hot dog is about the same as that of a child's windpipe. Even a low-fat, no-nitrate hot dog should be cut into tiny pieces for a child under three.

TOP TWELVE FOODS*

Food	Important Nutrients
Avocado	B vitamins, vitamin A, vitamin E
Chickpeas (especially tasty when made into hummus)	protein, fiber, folic acid, vitamin B-6, calcium, zinc, iron
Eggs	protein, vitamin A, riboflavin, vitamin B-12, folic acid
Fish (salmon, tuna)	protein, niacin, vitamin B-12, zinc, iron, omega-3 fatty acids
Flax seeds and flax oil	omega-3 fatty acids; seeds also rich in protein, fiber, thiamin, riboflavin, niacin
Kidney beans	protein, fiber, thiamin, folic acid, calcium, zinc, iron
Lentils	protein, fiber, riboflavin, vitamin B-6, folic acid, iron; most intestines-friendly legume
Sweet potatoes	fiber, vitamin A, beta carotene, vitamin C, riboflavin, carotenoids
Tofu (firm)	protein, fiber, vitamin A, thiamin, folic acid, calcium, zinc, iron, unsaturated fats, anti-cancer phytonutrients
Tomatoes	vitamin A, vitamin C, health-promoting carotenoids, especially lycopene
Whole grains	protein, fiber, vitamin A, thiamin, riboflavin, niacin, vitamin B-12, folic acid, zinc, iron
Yogurt (plain, nonfat)	protein, calcium, zinc, folic acid, riboflavin, *Lactobacilli* for colon health

* *These foods are listed in* alphabetical order, *not ranked according to which are the most nutritious.*

Honorable Mention

Almonds	protein, fiber, riboflavin, calcium, zinc, iron, vitamin E, unsaturated fats
Artichokes	protein, fiber, vitamin A, vitamin C, thiamin, riboflavin, niacin, folic acid, calcium, zinc, iron
Broccoli	vitamin A, vitamin C, folic acid, beta carotene, anti-cancer phytonutrients
Cantaloupe	carotenoids, vitamin A, vitamin C, beta carotene
Garlic	heart-healthy and anti-cancer phytonutrients
Orange	fiber, calcium, vitamin A, folic acid, vitamin C, carotenoids
Papaya	fiber, vitamin C, folic acid, carotenoids
Peanut butter	protein, fiber, niacin, zinc, vitamin E
Peppers (sweet and hot)	vitamin A, vitamin C, vitamin B-6, health-promoting phytonutrients, folic acid
Pink grapefruit	vitamin C, fiber, carotenoids
Sunflower seeds	protein, unsaturated fats, fiber, niacin, folic acid, zinc, iron, vitamin E, selenium
Turkey	protein, niacin, vitamin B-12, zinc, iron

ones, red onions over white, and spinach instead of lettuce. On page 111 is a list of foods that display a lot of color and information on what those colors do for you. Enjoy your colorful plate!

UNDERSTANDING THE FOOD GUIDE PYRAMID

In 1992 the U.S. Department of Agriculture replaced the popular concept of four food groups with the Food Guide Pyramid. The new pyramid gave greater prominence to plant foods, stressing that grains, fruits, and vegetables are the basis of a healthy diet. Meat and dairy products were placed further up in the pyramid, to show that people should eat less of these foods.

The pyramid is a guide to filling your plate with the right food proportions. It can help parents set these food priorities for their family:

- *mostly* grains, fruits, and vegetables
- *adequate* legumes, dairy, fish, poultry, and meat
- *fewer* fats and sweets

There are problems with the pyramid. With so many special-interest groups to please — beef and dairy farmers, food manufacturers, consumer groups — compromises are inevitable. While the

TERRIBLE TEN JUNK FOODS

Junk Food	The Unnutritious, Potentially Harmful Stuff That's In It
Beef jerky	high sodium, high percentage of saturated fat, high in nitrates and nitrites, added food colorings (Healthy alternatives are available.)
Colored, sweetened cereals	hydrogenated oils, dyes: yellow #6, red #40, blue #2, blue #1 (Most don't contain whole-grain flour yet may display the American Heart Association's heart-healthy seal of approval.)
Doughnuts	white flour, hydrogenated oils, icing, lots of sugar
Potato chips	hydrogenated oils, high in salt
Gelatin desserts	dyes, high sugar
Candies	hydrogenated oils, high sugar
Punch	dyes, high sugar
Sodas	high sugar, caffeine, dyes, carbonation
Juice drinks or "cocktails"	very little juice, mostly corn syrup and other sweeteners
Marshmallows	mostly sugar, sticky for teeth

food guide pyramid helps the consumer make wise choices about the *quantity* of food to eat, it does not address the *quality* of the food within each group. Fats are all lumped together, whether they're saturated, hydrogenated, or not. White bread with minimal fiber holds the same place as the more nutritious whole wheat bread. Oils are omitted even though nutritious oils like flax, olive, and canola provide omega-3 fatty acids and monounsaturated fats so necessary for growing children and for keeping adults healthy. Meat, poultry, fish, legumes, eggs, and nuts end up in the same box, though their effects on your body are vastly different — as you will discover in later chapters of this book.

The USDA Food Guide Pyramid (see the illustration page 112) stacks up the five food groups in their relative proportions. In our "Food Guide Wheel" (see page 114) we have improved the food pyramid by making several changes:

HEALTHY COLORS

Color	Food Sources	Nutrients	Health Benefits
Red	tomatoes tomato sauce ketchup watermelon pink grapefruit guava juice red peppers	lycopene beta carotene vitamin C	Lycopene is a potent antioxidant and one of the top ten anti-cancer carotenoids; it has been linked to reductions in the risk of prostate cancer. Anthocyanins have anti-cancer properties. Red peppers contain much more beta carotene (and more vitamin C) than green peppers.
Pink	pink grapefruit	lycopene, beta carotene	Like lycopene, beta carotene is an antioxidant, good for the eyes. It also reduces the risk of cancers and cardiovascular disease.
Orange or deep yellow	apricots and peaches (especially dried) sweet potato carrots pumpkin winter squash mango yellow peppers	beta carotene vitamin C	Some orange/yellow vegetables, such as pumpkin and summer squash, contain the phytonutrient lutein, which helps protect against degeneration of eye structure with aging. Carotenoids are the phytos that protect plants from sun damage. Perhaps they do the same for humans.
Dark green	kale, other "greens" asparagus watercress spinach broccoli parsley, fresh dill, fresh romaine lettuce zucchini green peppers	beta carotene	Dark green foods are rich in antioxidants.
Blue or dark purple	blueberries bilberries cherries grapes red wine plums purple cabbage	anthocyanin	The pigment anthocyanin has anti-cancer properties.
Black or dark red	black beans kidney beans	calcium iron	Black beans are higher in fiber and calcium; red beans contain slightly more iron.

THE FOOD GUIDE PYRAMID

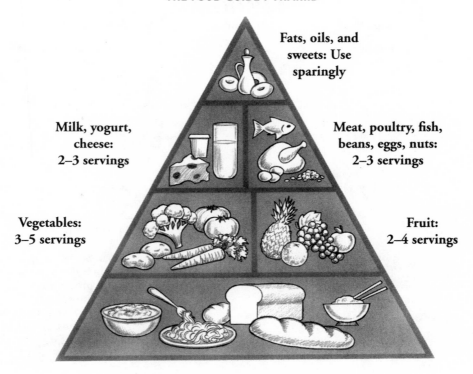

Fats, oils, and sweets: Use sparingly

Milk, yogurt, cheese: 2–3 servings

Meat, poultry, fish, beans, eggs, nuts: 2–3 servings

Vegetables: 3–5 servings

Fruit: 2–4 servings

Bread, cereal, rice, and pasta: 6–11 servings

- We not only suggest how much to eat of each food group but also note which foods within each group are better choices (e.g., "lean meat" rather than "meat" and "whole grains" rather than "grains").
- We describe not only which foods to eat but which ones to avoid.
- We give legumes and seafood a place of their own, since they merit ranking near vegetables and fruits.
- We include information on how often to eat certain foods. Grains, vegetables, legumes, dairy products, vegetable oils, and fruits are foods to eat daily; seafood, poultry, and eggs are eaten three times a week; meat is eaten once a week; wine should be consumed in moderation, sweet treats in moderation.
- We include nutritious oils, which contain essential fatty acids, instead of just stating "use oils sparingly."
- We make soy foods a separate group because of their health-building properties and because they are a healthier protein source than meat and poultry.
- We include only low-fat or nonfat dairy products.

Children can follow the same food wheel guidelines as adults, but with smaller servings. Kid-sized servings are one-third to one-half the

WHITE IS WRONG

Even though white is a symbol of purity, even of health, when it comes to the nutritional value of foods, white has been blacklisted. This is especially true of foods that have been man-made white by processing, such as *white flour* and *white rice*. In these two foods, the most nutritious brown part of the food (the bran; and in wheat, the germ) has been factory-removed by processing or bleaching, and the colorless stuff that remains is nutrient poor. Even a naturally white potato, though nutritious, is less so than its yellow friend, the sweet potato (which botanically is a root, not a potato). So, leave the white bread for the birds. Think brown.

size of adult servings. For example, kids should eat half a slice of bread instead of one slice, ¼ cup of vegetables instead of ½ cup, ½ ounce of cheese instead of 1 ounce, 2 to 3 ounces of meat or fish instead of 3 to 4 ounces, and one egg instead of two eggs.

RDA: WHAT DOES IT REALLY SAY?

The recommended dietary allowances (RDA's) were originally set up by the National Academy of Sciences during World War II as general guidelines for feeding the country's soldiers. These recommendations have grown to be guidelines for the general public and were last revised in 1997 and given a new name. RDA's are now known as "daily values" (DV's). Another term you may see is "DRV's" (daily reference value), which are dietary guidelines for protein, carbohydrates, fat, saturated fat, cholesterol, fiber, sodium, and potassium. Yet another new term is "RDI's" (reference daily intake), which are guidelines for essential vitamins and minerals. Daily values (DV's) are made up of both DRV's and RDI's. The current DV's for adults and children are listed in the Appendix, page 401.

The DV estimates the amount of a nutrient needed by an average, healthy person to avoid showing signs of deficiency. The recommendations have built-in safety margins, so in many cases the DV far exceeds the minimum amount of a nutrient necessary to avoid severe health consequences. Most children and adults can thrive on 50 percent of some of the recommendations. The minimum level of vitamin C needed to prevent scurvy, for example, is around 10 milligrams, yet the DV is set at 60 milligrams to allow for individuals with certain health problems, such as cancer and cardiovascular disease, who may require more vitamin C.

The DV specifies the minimum of a nutrient needed to stay healthy. This concept is not to be confused with the amount of nutrients the body actually uses, since we typically absorb much less of a nutrient than is actually in the food. The DV allows for low absorption rates for calcium and iron, for example. Practically speaking, you don't have to get every milligram of every DV every day, since everyone's diet varies widely from one day to the next. What you don't get one day you make up for the next.

The DV numbers represent *averages* only. You as an individual may have a different nutritional need from someone else. Realistically, it is not possible for the committees that calculate the DV's to present optimal values for every person and every situation. The DV has been likened to the minimum wage — enough to stay well, but perhaps not enough for some people, at least, to thrive. The DV numbers are based upon the amount a person needs to keep from getting sick, plus a margin of error. This may be less than the

THE FOOD GUIDE WHEEL

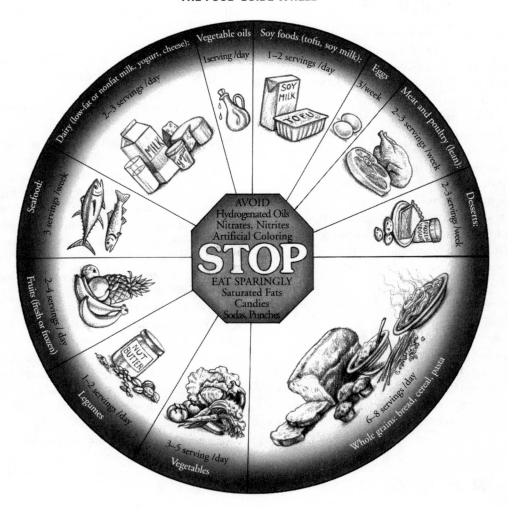

amount needed to achieve *optimum* health. Of course, optimum health is more difficult to evaluate and quantify than deficiencies are.

Some nutritionists believe that the DV has not kept pace with the latest nutritional research and that some of the recommendations may be thirty years out of date. The DV's have come under fire particularly regarding the recommended level of antioxidant nutrients, such as vitamin C, E, and beta carotene. For some people, the DV's for these

health-promoting nutrients should be at least two to five times the current values. On the other hand, the DV's may be too high for some individuals. They were initially figured for young, active, military males, which means they may be less appropriate for the very young, very old, or for women. A valid, but unavoidable, criticism of the concept behind the DV is that it does not respect the biochemical individuality of each person.

Comparing the proportions of the different spokes of the wheel, you will see immediately the relative importance of the various foods that make up a healthy diet for an average adult or child. For an adult, these proportions are based on a 2,400-calorie diet.

Whole grains. *The grain group, a prime source of energy, supplies about one-quarter of the daily calories for most children and adults (more or less, depending on energy expenditure). 1 serving=1 slice of bread, ¾ cup of dry cereal, ½ cup of cooked cereal, ½ cup of rice or pasta*

Vegetables, legumes, and fruits. *Together these groups comprise another quarter of a total daily healthy diet.*

Vegetables: 1 serving = 1 cup of raw or ½ cup of cooked vegetables, ¾ cup of vegetable juice

Fruits: 1 serving = ¾ cup of fruit juice, 1 medium apple, orange, or banana, ½ cup of fruit

Legumes: 1 servings = ½ cup of canned beans, 2 tbsp. of nut butter, 1 cup of cooked lentils or beans, 1 ounce (3–4 tbsp.) of seeds or nuts

Seafood. *1 serving = 4 ounces*

Dairy. *1 serving = 1 cup of milk, 1 cup of yogurt, ½ cup of cottage cheese, 1 ounce of cheese*

Soy foods. *1 serving = 3 ounces of tofu, 8 ounces of soy milk*

Vegetable oils. *Flax, canola, and soy, plus nut oils. 1 serving = 1 tbsp.*

Eggs. *3 per week.*

Meat and poultry. *1 serving = 4 ounces*

Desserts and treats. *Keep sweet treats a minor part of your diet and gradually make them less sweet and less fatty. 1 serving = 200-calorie equivalent of pie, cake, cookies, or ice cream*

NUTRITIP
Kids and Colors

To get your children to appreciate the nutrient value of foods, teach them that colors mean healthy foods, or, in kid-language, "grow foods." Remind them: "Did you get your reds today?"

The DV's are based upon measures of physical health only, not mental or psychological health. This is important in view of the growing suspicion that some emotional and behavioral difficulties of schoolchildren could be the result of nutritional deficiencies.

The DV's, like the Food Guide Pyramid, recommend quantities of nutrients without being specific about the quality. A particularly glaring oversight is in the lack of recommendations for sufficient essential fatty acids in growing children.

Despite their shortcomings, the DV's are still reasonable for most individuals. Think of the DV's as a guide, not a goal, and then work out your own nutritional needs and those of your family. As you learn more about nutrition, you can determine your own FDA (family dietary advice), IDA (individual daily averages), or even set up an IRA (individual recommended average). Whatever you call it, be sure to get your ODA (optimal daily average). You can become your own nutritional expert.

12

Learning About Labels

I F ONLY WE LIVED and shopped in a pure world where labels told the whole truth and nothing but the truth. But while consumers rely on labels to make wise nutritional choices, food processors use labels to sell their products. Sometimes these two functions of a label — providing accurate information and enticing someone to buy the product — are in conflict. Labels can be misleading, especially if you don't learn to read between the lines and examine the fine print. Knowing what the words on the label really mean is a big step in learning to make nutritious choices at the supermarket.

FRONT-OF-PACKAGE COME-ONS

Ignore the hype on the front of the package. This part of the label is designed by the food processor's marketing and advertising departments. It will contain whatever trendy words will help sell the product. While the meanings of many of these terms are regulated by law, it's still easy to be deceived by them. The food itself may not be as good for you as these large and colorful words lead you to believe. Manufacturers cannot legally lie on a food label, but they can stretch the truth a bit. Be wary of these tricky terms:

- Consider the word "pure." Everyone wants to eat food that's pure. You would not want to put contaminated food into your body. But "pure" has no regulated, agreed-upon meaning in food labeling. It tells you nothing about what's in the package that perhaps should not be there.

- "Natural" is probably the least trustworthy of all the label terms. While the term "natural" sounds appealing, it really says little about the nutritional quality of the food or even its safety. In reality, "natural" is empty of nutritional meaning. Consumers believe that "natural" means the food is pretty much as Mother Nature grew it, but this is seldom the case. And even then, "natural" is not the same as "nutritious," or even "good for you." The fat marbling in a New York strip steak is "natural," but it's not good for your arteries.

- "Made from" simply means the food started with this product. For example, the claim "made from 100 percent corn oil" may be technically correct but also misleading. Consumers are led to believe they are eating 100 percent corn oil. They think of fields of corn under a clear blue Iowa sky. But a lot can happen to that corn oil before it gets to the grocery store. The label really means the processor started with

LABEL TERMS YOU SHOULD KNOW

These front-of-the-box claims have specific meanings, defined by government regulation. Read the definitions carefully. Some promise less than you might think.

- *"Calorie free"* means the food contains less than 5 calories per serving.
- *"Low calorie"* means the food contains 40 calories or less per serving. (For serving size, check the "Nutrition Facts" box on the back of the package.)
- *"Reduced calorie"* means the food contains at least 25 percent fewer calories than regular versions of the product.
- *"Lite"* or *"light"* means the food contains one-third fewer calories or no more than one-half the fat of the regular version of the product.
- *"Fat free"* means the food contains less than 0.5 grams of fat per serving.
- *"Free"* means the food contains none or trivial amounts of a substance, such as sodium, fat, cholesterol, calories, or sugars.
- *"Low fat"* means 3 grams of fat (or less) per serving.
- *"Reduced fat"* means at least 25 percent less fat than regular versions of the food. (Note that a "reduced-fat" mayonnaise or margarine will still contain plenty of fat. "Reduced fat" may be many calories away from "low fat.")
- *"Cholesterol free"* means the food has no more than 2 milligrams of cholesterol and 2 grams or less of saturated fat per serving.
- *"Low cholesterol"* means the food has no more than 20 milligrams of cholesterol (or less) and 2 grams or less of saturated fat per serving.
- *"Low saturated fat"* means the food has 1 gram or less of saturated fat per serving.
- *"Lean"* means fewer than 10 grams of fat, 4 grams of saturated fat, and 95 milligrams of cholesterol per serving or per 100 grams of a food. "Extra lean" means the food has less than 2 grams of saturated fat and less than 5 grams of total fat.
- *"Fresh"* means unprocessed, uncooked, unfrozen (e.g., freshly squeezed orange juice). Washing and coating of fruits and vegetables are allowed. If a food has been quickly frozen, it can be described as "fresh-frozen," which is commonly done with fresh fish.
- *"Healthy"* means the food may contain no more than 3 grams of fat (including 1 gram of saturated fat) and 60 milligrams of cholesterol per serving. The food must also contain 10 percent of the recommended daily value of one of these nutrients: vitamin A, vitamin C, calcium, iron, protein, or fiber. "Healthy" individual foods must contain no more than 300 milligrams of sodium; prepackaged meals can't exceed 480 milligrams. There is no limit on the sugar content in "healthy" food.
- *"Natural flavors"* are defined by the Federal Food, Drug, and Cosmetic Act as "the essential oil, oleoresin, essence or extractive, protein hydrolysate, distillate, or any product of roasting, heating, or enzymolysis, which contains a flavoring constituent derived from a spice, fruit or fruit juice, vegetable or vegetable juice, edible yeast, herb, bark, bud, root, leaf or similar plant material, meat, seafood, poultry, eggs, dairy products, or fermentation products thereof whose significant function in food is flavoring rather than nutritional." This broad definition simply means that natural flavors are extracts from these nonsynthetic foods.
- *"Good source"* means a serving must contain 10 to 19 percent of the recommended daily value of a particular nutrient (e.g., vitamin A).

LABEL TERMS YOU SHOULD KNOW (CONTINUED)

- *"High"* (e.g., "high iron") means the serving contains 20 percent or more of the recommended daily value of this nutrient.
- *"Less"* (e.g., "less salt") means the food contains at least one-quarter less of this nutrient than the regular food to which it is being compared (e.g., contains at least one-quarter less sodium than the usual vegetable soup).

- *"More"* (e.g., "more vitamin C") means that a serving contains at least 10 percent more of the recommended daily value of a particular nutrient than the regular food to which it is being compared (e.g., more vitamin C than regular tomato juice).
- *"Energy"* (e.g., "energy drinks") refers to any product that contains calories. Just about any drink, except water, can meet that definition.

100 percent corn oil but along the way may have diluted it or hydrogenated it, changing it into a fat that will clog your arteries, not one that flows free and golden. Another common label lie is "made from natural . . ." This simply means the manufacturer started with a natural source, but by the time the natural food was processed, it may be anything but "natural."

- "Made with" can be very misleading. "Made with real fruit" is a good example. The law does not require the label to specify how much fruit. This boast is particularly prevalent in snacks for children, which may contain a grape or two in a snack that is otherwise mostly sugar. "Made with whole grains" is another little "white" label lie. The consumer is led to believe that this is a whole-grain product, but the package label is not legally required to say how much "whole grain" is in the product. Its main ingredient could still be refined flour — with just a small amount of whole wheat added. In that case, the food won't contain all the fiber and other nutrients associated with whole grains. "Made with vegetables" is another misleader; it sounds healthy but says nothing about how much nutrition is really in the box.

- Understand the real meaning of "fat free" on a label. For example, suppose a food is labeled

"95 percent fat free." This means that 5 percent of the total weight of the food is fat. This may not seem like much, but a single gram of fat contains 9 calories, compared to 4 calories in a gram of protein or carbohydrates. Five grams of fat in 100 grams (approximately 3½ ounces) of ground or dark-meat turkey without the skin represents one-quarter of the calories in that serving.

- "Enriched" is often a tip-off that something good was taken out of the food, requiring another process to put some of the good stuff back in. Enriched flour and enriched white bread are not as nourishing as their whole wheat counterparts.

- "Smoked" legally describes the flavor of the food, not how it was made. The consumer imagines the food is smoked in a backyard barbecue or an old-fashioned smokehouse. In fact, the food could have been artificially or chemically smoked and/or just contain smoked flavoring and still legally be labeled "smoked."

- Beware of fruit "drinks," which may contain little or no real fruit juice. Look at the ingredients to find out what's really in there. "Drink" in the name of the product tells you that this is not 100 percent juice. It may, in fact, be mostly sugar and water, with added vitamin C. This enables the manufacturer to say an orange drink is "high in vitamin C," even if it's a long way from being real orange juice.

- The terms "organically grown," "organic," "pesticide free," "all natural," and "no artificial ingredients" say very little about the nutritional value or safety of the product. Trust only labels that say "certified organically grown." These are the only words that mean the food was grown without chemical fertilizers and pesticides, in soil free of these substances. (For the meaning of "organic," see page 223.)

There are plenty of other terms to be skeptical about, too. Experienced label readers look right past the banners and big type on the front of the food packages and look instead for the facts in small print on the back. And even here they practice healthy skepticism.

HOW TO READ A PACKAGE LABEL

Now that you can wisely evaluate the claims on the front of the package, here is the information you need to be able to interpret the large and small print on the sides and back of the package. "Nutrition Facts" is the most useful part of the food label. This is where you can find out, for example, exactly how much fat the food contains, how much protein, and how much fiber. This breakdown of the nutritional content of the food is prepared by the food maker's nutrition department, and the information listed there is what it says: factual. The facts that must be included in this box and the way they are presented are regulated by law. The box follows the same format wherever it appears, making it easy to compare foods. While it's not perfect, the "Nutrition Facts" box is a big improvement on the piecemeal nutrition information that used to be included on food

packaging. Once you learn how to read the information in this box and, more important, interpret it, you can make informed choices about what you're eating. Each line of the "Nutrition Facts" box gives you information you can use. If you take the information on each line and then read between the lines, you can decide how a particular food fits into your eating plan. Let's dissect a sample "Nutrition Facts" label not only to learn what each listing means but also to read between the lines for hidden nutrition facts (see page 121).

SERVING SIZE

This line reflects the amount that the average person eats in one helping. Serving size is expressed in kitchen terms — cups, tablespoons, slices, and so on — and also in grams. Serving size is set by the FDA, not by the manufacturer, for all similar products (e.g., all yogurts), so you can make comparisons without having to do a lot of math. But be aware that your average serving may be more or less than this amount.

SERVINGS PER PACKAGE

The next line tells you how many servings the package contains, enabling you to compare similar products on the basis of cost per serving. Multiply this number by the serving size, and it should equal, or come close to, the total volume of the package.

CALORIES

This line tells you the number of calories per serving. Remember to adjust this (and other nutrient amounts, too) if your idea of a serving size is different from that stated on the package. If a ½-cup serving has 50 calories, but you usually eat a 1-cup serving, you'll be getting 100 calories. When shopping, compare the nutrient values to the *total calories* of the same size serving of each food. For example, a cereal that contains 4 grams of protein in a 100-calorie serving is more nutritious than a

LABEL ENDORSEMENTS

Americans have grown to trust organizations such as the American Heart Association (AHA) and the American Cancer Society (ACS) as benevolent benefactors of our general health and well-being. Not necessarily true. The ACS has gradually lost its credibility for two reasons: devoting precious little of their resources to cancer prevention and selling their endorsement to product manufacturers for a pricey sum. The AHA is also not so pure. When you see a label displaying a big red heart with the words "This product meets AHA guidelines . . . ," don't assume that this is a low-fat healthy food. You might be surprised at how loose these guidelines really are and how the junkiest of foods can display this label and meet the AHA's guidelines. The following are AHA guidelines for "heart-healthy eating":

- Total fat intake should be no more than 30 percent of total calories.
- Saturated fatty acid intake should be 8–10 percent of total calories.
- Polyunsaturated fatty acid intake should be up to 10 percent of total calories.
- Monounsaturated fatty acids should be up to 15 percent of total calories.
- Cholesterol intake should be less than 300 milligrams per day.
- Sodium intake should be less than 2,400 milligrams per day.
- Carbohydrate intake should make up 55–60 percent or more of calories, with emphasis on increasing sources of complex carbohydrates.
- Total calories should be adjusted to achieve and maintain a healthy body weight.

There are problems with these guidelines:

- Many nutritionists believe 30 percent fat of total calories is too high for many people.
- The AHA guidelines are so clogged with cholesterol recommendations that they've omitted some more important nutritional issues. For example, the AHA omits advising people to shun hydrogenated or fake fats, which are actually more damaging to the body than "cholesterol" in the foods. If this were the case, many of the common household foods would have to remove the red heart so proudly and misleadingly displayed on their label.

NUTRITIP
Cholesterol Free Does Not Mean Fat Free.

When fast-food establishments boast that their french fries are "cooked in cholesterol-free, 100 percent vegetable oil," they are often referring to hydrogenated vegetable oil. This stuff stands up better both to life on a shelf and the heat of the fryer, but the effect on your blood-cholesterol levels is similar to that of lard.

cereal with 2 grams per 100 calories. A food with 4 grams of protein in 100 calories is less nutrient dense than one with 3 grams of protein in a 50-calorie serving of the same volume.

CALORIES FROM FAT

This line tells you how many calories in each serving are from fat. Use this and the "Total Fat" line below to decide if the food fits your goals for fat consumption. If this food gets a lot of its calories from fat, you'll want to eat it sparingly or not at all.

NUTRITION FACTS

Serving Size ½ cup (31g/1.1oz.)
Servings Per Package About 17

Amount Per Serving

Calories	80
Calories from Fat	10

	% Daily Value**
Total Fat 1.0g	2%
Saturated Fat 0g	0%
Cholesterol 0 mg	0%
Sodium 65 mg	3%
Potassium 390 mg	11%
Total Carbohydrate 24g	8%
Dietary Fiber 10g	40%
Sugars 6g	
Other Carbohydrate 7g	
Protein 4g	
Vitamin A	15%
Vitamin C	25%
Calcium	15%
Iron	25%
Vitamin D	10%
Thiamin	25%
Riboflavin	25%
Niacin	25%
Vitamin B-6	25%
Folate	25%
Vitamin B-12	25%
Phosphorus	35%
Magnesium	30%
Zinc	25%
Copper	15%

** Percent Daily Values are based on a 2,000-calorie diet. Your daily values may be higher or lower depending on your calorie needs:

	Calories	2,000	2,500
Total Fat	Less than	65g	80g
Sat. Fat	Less than	20g	25g
Cholesterol	Less than	300mg	300mg
Sodium	Less than	2,400mg	2,400mg
Potassium		3,500mg	3,500mg
Total Carb.		300g	375g
Fiber		25g	30g

Calories per gram:
Fat 9   Carbohydrate 4   Protein 4

Ingredients: Wheat bran, sugar, malt flavoring, calcium phosphate, salt, sodium ascorbate and ascorbic acid (vitamin C), niacinamide, zinc oxide, reduced iron, pyridoxine hydrochloride (vitamin B-6), riboflavin (vitamin B-2), vitamin A palmitate, thiamin hydrochloride (vitamin B-1), folic acid (folate), vitamin B-12, and vitamin D.

NUTRITIP
"Not from Concentrate"

When this label appears on a fruit juice package, many consumers believe it means a nutritionally superior juice. Not necessarily so. "Concentrated" simply means that the water has been removed, and the consumer adds it back in before drinking. Concentrating juice is more an economic change than a nutritional one: Smaller packages are cheaper to transport and store. The juice you buy that is not from concentrate may contain more vitamin C than "made from concentrate" juice. Of course the juice you squeeze at home is always more nutritious, since it has not been subjected to pasteurization, processing, or storage.

% DAILY VALUE (DV)

This section tells you what percentage of the total recommended daily amount of each nutrient (fats, carbs, proteins, major vitamins and minerals) is in each serving, based on a 2,000-calories-per-day diet. If you eat more or less than 2,000 calories, adjust this value proportionally.* These daily values are for adults and children four years of age or over. *These values cannot be applied to infants or children under four.*

TOTAL FAT

This line tells you how many grams of fat are in one serving, and what percentage that is of the recommended daily value (DV). For example, "Total Fat 1 gram, 2%" means that one serving contains 1 gram of fat, which is 2 percent of the

---

* *The average active woman (nonpregnant and nonlactating) needs about 2,000 calories per day. The average active man needs 2,500 to 2,800. An athlete may burn between 3,000 and 4,000 per day.*

LABELS THAT SHOULD BE AGAINST THE LAW

If you don't ask, the food manufacturer won't tell. The consumer has a right to know what type of ingredients make up the food, and the manufacturer has an obligation to tell the truth. Don't buy foods containing these misleading terms:

- *"No-name" labels* (e.g., "vegetable oil" or "vegetable shortening"). You have a right to know which type of vegetables are used in the oil, as some are more nutritious than others. "Vegetable shortening" sounds more appealing and more healthy than "lard," but most of these shortenings are made with hydrogenated oils, which act in the body as a fat worse than lard. You will find this term deceivingly used in packaged foods and fast-food outlets. Hydrogenated fats can be buried in the fine print. Look for a more explicit label, such as "saturated-fat free."

- *"And/or"* (e.g., "contains soy and/or palm kernel oil" or "contains partially hydrogenated and/or . . ." or "contains corn and/or cottonseed oil"). And/or labeling gives the manufacturer leeway to substitute cheaper, often less nutritious, and even unhealthy oils without changing the printing on the label. Since the price of different oils fluctuates, this allows the manufacturer to put the cheapest oils in the food.

- *"Cold-pressed."* This is a term that is used on oils to give the consumer the impression that the oils have been pressed more naturally, since some consumers know that heat hurts oils. "Cold-pressed" has no legal, biochemical, or technological meaning. The actual press that was used to squeeze the seeds into oil may not be heated (because it doesn't have to be), yet the heat generated by friction when the seeds are compressed may be enough to harm the oils. Except for some virgin oils, most commercially pressed oils are heated during their pressing process, even though the press itself was "cold." A more useful and truthful label would be "protected from heat, light, and oxygen during processing."

- *"Cholesterol free."* "Cholesterol free" tops the list of labels that lie. It should be changed to "contains no cholesterol-raising ingredients," since many of the hydrogenated fats buried in the ingredients list can raise cholesterol even though the food still qualifies as cholesterol free because these fats do not biochemically fit the definition of cholesterol.

- *"High in polyunsaturated fatty acids."* "Polyunsaturated" is one of the more recent nutritionally incorrect buzz words, since the public is being led to equate the word with "healthy." In fact, it depends on the polyunsaturate. Some polyunsaturates are healthy, such as essential fatty acids; others, such as that found in margarine, are not, because they are chemically altered by hydrogenation.

- *"Made from* or *made with natural ingredients."* This is no great claim. Most processed foods are made from natural ingredients, which simply means that the food starts out on a vine somewhere. Even the drug heroin is made from the natural ingredients in the poppy plant.

ANATOMY OF A LABEL FOR A NUTRITIOUS CEREAL

Sugars. The 2 grams of sugars indicate a rather small amount of sweetener relative to the 25 grams of total carbohydrates.

Vitamins and Minerals. Many of the most nutritious cereals do not have a lot of added vitamins and minerals, yet some of the top junk cereals do. Perhaps it is cheaper to add synthetic vitamins and minerals than it is to use whole grains.

Ingredients. Notice the magic word "whole" in the grain list. Since makers of more nutritious cereals know that their consumers are sugar savvy, they usually do not put the term "sugar" in the ingredients list, but rather disguise it as "evaporated cane juice." This is simply sugar with a nicer name. But in this case we're happy that there are only 2 grams per serving.

NUTRITION FACTS		
Serving Size ⅔ cup (30g)		
Servings Per Container About 12		
Amount Per Serving		
Calories	120	
Fat Calories	5	
	% Daily Value	
Total Fat 0.5g	**1%**	
Saturated Fat 0g	**0%**	
Cholesterol 0 mg	**0%**	
Sodium 60 mg	**3%**	
Total Carb. 25g	**8%**	
Dietary Fiber 4g	**16%**	
Sugars 2g		
Protein 3g		
Vitamin A 0%	Vitamin C	0%
Calcium 0%	Iron	6%

Ingredients: Organic **whole** oat flour, organic **whole** wheat flour, organic wheat bran, organic **evaporated cane juice,** organic oat bran, organic corn meal, organic brown rice flour, organic barley malt extract, organic whole wheat sprouts, and a trace of sea salt.

total recommended daily intake of fat. Even the factory fats ("hydrogenated" and "partially hydrogenated") must legally be included in the total fat amount.

SATURATED FAT

This subheading under "Total Fat" tells you how much of the fat in each serving is saturated fat and what percentage that is of your recommended daily value (DV). Current nutritional recommendations are that less than one-third of the fat in your diet (that is, less than 8 percent of your total daily calories) should come from saturated fat.

CHOLESTEROL

This line tells you how many milligrams of cholesterol are in one serving, and what percentage of the recommended daily value for cholesterol that is.

Reading between the lines. Even though the label may say "no cholesterol," what it doesn't tell you is the amount of cholesterol-raising fats ("partially hydrogenated") in each serving. Hydrogenated fats (also known as "trans fatty acids") can be as hazardous to your health — or more so — than saturated fat or cholesterol. So, as a novice

---

ANATOMY OF A TRICKY LABEL

The following is an analysis of some of the tricky label listings from a leading cereal:

Fat. A consumer looking at the 0.5 grams of saturated fat and 0 cholesterol might be favorably impressed. Yet, looking at the fine print of the ingredients list, you'll notice the term "partially hydrogenated." Since partially hydrogenated oils are really more harmful than saturated fats and have been shown to raise blood-cholesterol levels, they really should be included on the "Saturated Fat" line. Instead, they are buried in the "Total Fat" listing. The consumer has no way of knowing how much of the 2.5 grams of Total Fat is actually the hydrogenated stuff.

Cottonseed and/or soybean oil. The "and/or" listing should be illegal. Consumers have a right to know which of the oils, cottonseed or soybean, they are eating, since these two oils have vastly different nutritional properties. Cottonseed oil has much less nutritional value,

NUTRITION FACTS	
Serving Size	1 box (43g)

Amount Per Serving		
Calories	160	
Fat Calories	20	
		% Daily Value
Total Fat 2.5g		4%
Saturated Fat 0.5g		3%
Cholesterol 0 mg		0%
Sodium 110 mg		5%
Total Carb. 34g		11%
Fiber 2g		10%
Sugars 12g		
Protein 3g		

Ingredients: whole oats, whole grain wheat, brown sugar, raisins, rice, corn syrup, almonds, glycerin, **partially hydrogenated cottonseed and/or soybean oil**

and in addition, cotton crops may be sprayed with lots of pesticides.

---

food-label detective, if you look at the fine print in the ingredients list and see, for example, "partially hydrogenated soybean oil," then assume that "trans fatty acids" is missing from the fat facts. A consumer has a right to know not only the amount of fat, but also the breakdown of nutritious and unnutritious fats. A more factual and truthful label would break the total fat into monounsaturated, polyunsaturated, saturated, and trans fatty acids.

SODIUM

This line refers to salt. The recommended daily value for sodium is less than 2,400 milligrams.

POTASSIUM

The recommended daily value for potassium is 3,500 milligrams.

TOTAL CARBOHYDRATE

Dietary Fiber
Sugars
Other Carbohydrate

Total Carbohydrate: This line tells you how many grams of carbohydrates are in each serving and the percentage of the recommended daily value that represents. This number includes

ANATOMY OF A JUNK LABEL

Here's a dissection of part of the label from a popular children's cereal:

AHA seal of approval. The unwary consumer might conclude that since this particular food is endorsed by the American Heart Association, it must be healthy. Wrong!

Dietary Fiber. One gram of fiber is relatively low for a "multigrain" cereal.

Sugars. Fifteen grams of sugar per serving is a lot of sweetener.

Protein. The cereal is low in protein. That should give you a hint about the nutritional quality of the grains used.

Corn, wheat, and oat flour. Even though the front of the box boasts "multigrain," since these flours are not described as "whole wheat" or "whole-grain," you can assume that they are refined flours with much of the nutrients processed out.

sugar. In the ingredients list, sugar is listed as the second ingredient after grains, confirming a high content of added sugar.

partially hydrogenated vegetable oil. Hydrogenating oil provides little nutrition and possibly does physiological harm.

one or more of: coconut, cottonseed, and soybean. Consumers have the right to know which oil they are eating, since these oils greatly differ in nutritional quality.

natural orange, lemon, cherry, blueberry, raspberry, lime, and other natural flavors. "Natural" has limited legal meaning. The consumer may imagine that these flavors come from ground-up fruits, but that is not necessarily true. (For the official meaning of "natural," see page 117.)

yellow #6, red #40, blue #2, and blue #1. Artificial food colorings are in the GRAS (generally recognized as safe) category. This means that no one really knows for sure. In fact, they may be harmful to children who are food-coloring sensitive.

Meets **American Heart Association** food criteria for saturated fat and cholesterol for healthy people over age 2.

Diets low in saturated fat and cholesterol may reduce the risk of heart disease.

NUTRITION FACTS

Serving Size	1 cup (32g/1.1 oz)
Servings Per Container	About 13

Amount Per Serving	**Cereal**
Calories	120
Calories from Fat	10
	% Daily Value
Total Fat 1.0g	2%
Saturated Fat 0.50g	3%
Cholesterol 0 mg	0%
Sodium 150 mg	6%
Potassium 35 mg	1%
Total Carbohydrate 28g	9%
Dietary Fiber 1g	4%
Sugars 15g	
Other Carb. 12g	
Protein 2g	

Ingredients: Corn, wheat, and oat flour; sugar; partially hydrogenated vegetable oil (one or more of: coconut, cottonseed, and soybean); salt; sodium ascorbate and ascorbic acid (vit. C); **yellow #6;** niacinamide; zinc oxide; reduced iron; **natural orange, lemon, cherry, blueberry, raspberry, lime, and other natural flavors; red #40,** turmeric color; annatto color; **blue #2;** pyridoxine hydrochloride (vit. B6); **blue #1;** riboflavin (vit. B2); vit. A palmitate; thiamin hydrochloride (vit. B1); BHT (preservative); folic acid (folate); vit. B12 and vit. D.

starches, complex carbohydrates, dietary fiber, added sugar sweeteners, and nondigestible additives. The following three carbohydrates all add up to the total carbohydrate value.

Dietary Fiber: This figure represents the number of grams of fiber in each serving.

Sugars: This figure represents the number of grams of added sweeteners, which may appear in the ingredients list as sugar, corn syrup, honey, brown sugar, and so on.

Other Carbohydrate: This line reveals the number of grams of complex carbohydrates, not including fiber, but including nondigestible additives, such as stabilizers and thickening agents. Theoretically, this number should reflect the amount of the more nutritious sugars, that is, the ones naturally present in the food.

Reading between the lines. As a general guide, the greater the discrepancy between "Total Carbohydrate" and "Sugars" on the label, the more nutritious are the carbohydrates the food contains. This means that the package contains more of the food's natural sugars than added sugars. The closer the number of grams of "Sugars" is to the "Total Carbohydrate" in each serving, the closer the food gets to the junk quality (sort of like junk bonds — they are a risky investment). The "Total Carbs" minus the "Sugars" value is particularly helpful in comparing the nutritional value of cereals. For example, a serving of regular All-Bran contains 24 grams of total carbohydrates and 6 grams of sugars, resulting in 18 grams of complex healthy carbohydrates. A serving of a popular "fruit" cereal, on the other hand, contains 28 grams of total carbohydrates, 15 grams of which are sugars — over 50 percent of the total carbohydrates in the junk cereal are added sweeteners, versus 25 percent in more nutritious ones.

When comparing juice labels, you will notice that even in "100 percent juice," the "Total Carbs" and the "Sugars" values are the same, since juice is nearly all natural sugar.

When you're buying cereal, bread, or crackers, look for complex carbohydrates without a lot of added sugar. There is no line in the "Nutrition Facts" box for complex carbohydrates, but you can get a rough idea of the amount of healthy carbs in a food by comparing the "Total Carbohydrates" line with "Sugars." The greater the difference between the two, the more grams of complex carbohydrates in the food.

PROTEIN

This line tells you how many grams of protein are in each serving. You will notice that the percentage of recommended daily values is missing from the protein label because protein insufficiency is not generally thought to be a problem. The average daily protein requirement for most adults is between 50 and 75 grams a day. So, a serving that contains 3 grams of protein would give you around 4 to 6 percent of the DV for protein.

VITAMINS AND MINERALS

This list includes the percentage of the recommended daily values for vitamins A and C, calcium, and iron in each serving. The food may provide significant amounts of other vitamins and minerals, which may also be listed, but they are not required by law.

INGREDIENTS

The ingredients list tells you, usually in fine print, what ingredients the food contains. These are listed in order, starting with the ingredient found

---

NUTRITIP
Show Me the Freshness.

Become accustomed to looking for and reading the "use by" date on packages, especially on perishables, such as prewashed salad makings, meat and poultry, and dairy products. Check "on sale" items carefully.

NUTRITIP
Be Wary of Desserts Labeled "Low-fat."

The manufacturer often compensates for the fat by adding more sugar. "Low-fat" is not the same as "low-calorie."

in the largest amount by weight, and progressing to the ingredient present in the smallest amount. The ingredients list may be the most important information on the box to someone with food allergies or to a parent wary of the effect of food colorings or preservatives on a child's behavior. Here you can find out if a food contains eggs, soy, milk, corn, or whatever you must avoid eating. It's important, even critical, to know the lingo. Casein, caseinate, lactalbumin, whey, and whey solids are all derived from cow's milk, though their names don't reveal this. Albumin comes from eggs. Dextrose and glucose may originate in corn. Hydrolyzed vegetable protein starts with

soybeans, and some of the products used to thicken or stabilize food texture, such as acacia gum, are legume products.

Pay attention to where and how various kinds of sugar are included on the ingredients list. Use your good sense. Ketchup, for example, should contain mainly tomatoes, and tomatoes, not sugar, should be first on the ingredients list. A cereal in which sugar is the first, second, or third ingredient would certainly be less nutritious than one in which two or three types of grains are listed before the sugar.

From time to time it's good to check the ingredients list of foods you buy regularly. Manufacturers' recipes change, depending on all kinds of factors. Some changes may make the food less acceptable to you than it once was. The flavor advertised as "better than ever" may come from more sugar. Or, the oil in a salad dressing that once was corn oil may now be less nutritious cottonseed (which is why they use "and/or" — so they don't have to change the label).

13

Good Grains

DID YOU EVER WONDER why grains received top billing (or should it be bottom billing?) in the USDA's Food Guide Pyramid? Purely and simply, grains are great foods. Grains are also the world's most plentiful food and enjoy first place in the diet of nearly every culture, except perhaps fish-loving Eskimos.

What makes grains so good? Around two-thirds of the calories in grains come from carbohydrates, the complex kind. This is right in line with current dietary recommendations that 60 to 65 percent of daily calories should come from carbohydrates. Grains are also a rich source of protein. In most cultures, except beef-eating Western, most of the protein in people's diet comes directly from grains. (In our culture, it's the cattle that get their protein from grains.) Yet, the body cannot live on grains alone. Most are not complete proteins, since they are missing one or more of the essential amino acids, usually lysine. No problem — who eats dry cereal anyway? Mixing grains with dairy, legumes, or just about any other protein source completes the minimal amino acid deficiency of grains. Also, grains are great sources of fiber, zinc, iron, folic acid, minerals, and B vitamins. And there's more great news about grains: They're naturally low in fat.

Even before the grain-heavy new Food Guide Pyramid was put out by the USDA, grains were becoming the "in" food, and names of "new" grains are cropping up all the time. While all grains are nutritious, some are more nutritious than others. Here is what you should know about the most common grains, the greatest grains, and some interesting ones you may not have heard of.

GETTING TO KNOW YOUR GRAINS

Wonderful Wheat

In American diets, wheat is the top grain. Not only is it the most plentiful — the wheat belt stretches over the middle of the United States, and we export as much as we consume — it is one of the most versatile grains. What gives wheat its unique baking value is the protein called "gluten," the elastic substance that allows bread to stretch and pasta to hold its shape during cooking.

Wheats are rated according to the "hardness" of the grain, which is determined by the amount of gluten it contains. Harder wheats have more gluten, and therefore a higher protein-to-carbohydrate ratio. They are used in foods that need to retain their shape and have a firmer texture, such as bread and pasta. Softer wheats, such as in pastry flour, are used in pastries, cakes, and pies. "All purpose" flour is a blend of hard and soft wheats.

READING BREAD LABELS

In comparing bread ingredient labels, the shorter the ingredients list, the better the bread. The most nutritious bread may be made from only whole wheat flour, water, yeast, and salt, with possibly a touch of molasses or honey, or the addition of other "whole" grains. The key word on the bread label is "whole." Be particularly careful of the most recent little white label lie called "wheat flour," which does not mean the same as whole wheat. Wheat flour, which gives bread a light brown color and therefore more health appeal, is 75 percent white flour and only 25 percent whole wheat. So it's only 25 percent healthy bread instead of 100 percent. Breads can be grouped into three categories:

- **Best breads** are 100 percent whole grain. Whole wheat flour is the first ingredient on the label. Enriched flour does not appear in the ingredients list. If it doesn't say "whole wheat," it's not. Wheat flour, as listed on labels, officially should mean 75 percent white and 25 percent whole wheat, but it may not. All white bread is "wheat flour," so this term is misleading, at best. A truthful label would state what percentage is whole wheat. If a label says "wheat flour," assume it's not *whole* wheat.
- **Better breads** list "whole-grain flour" as the main ingredient but may include white flour, too.
- **Downright junk breads** list "bleached, enriched flour" first in the ingredients list. Leave these on the shelf, where they belong. If it doesn't say "whole" on the label, it's wrong for your body.

Here are some wheat terms you may not be familiar with:

- The *wheat bran* is the outer layer of the wheat kernel that covers the grain inside. It is removed when wheat is refined into white flour. Bran is the part of the wheat kernel that is highest in fiber, primarily the insoluble type, which has been shown to lower the risk of colon cancer. Bran is also the part of the wheat plant that contains most of the minerals and vitamins.

- The *wheat germ* is the nutrient-dense embryo of the wheat plant, which is power-packed with protein, minerals, and iron, and contains most of what little fat there is in the wheat plant. (Processors like to remove it from flour since the fat shortens the shelf life.) Wheat germ is often used as a dietary supplement because it is rich in iron, B vitamins, vitamin E, and the antioxidant selenium.

- The *endosperm* is the largest part of the wheat kernel and the least nutrient dense. Yet, because by weight the endosperm is about 80 percent of the whole wheat kernel, it contains the greatest amount of proteins and carbohydrates.

- *Cracked wheat* starts as the whole kernels of hard varieties of wheat. The kernels are then cracked into small pieces, which add a crunchy texture when added to bread or cereal. Or, you can cook cracked wheat in water like rice.

- *Wheat berries* are the whole kernels of wheat. They take longer to cook than the cracked variety. When cooked they can be eaten like rice or added to bread dough.

- *Bulgur wheat* is a form of cracked wheat. The whole wheat kernels are cooked, dried, and cracked into a coarse grain that is usually used in cooked cereal, pilaf, or a popular Middle Eastern grain dish, tabbouleh.

NUTRITIP
Weigh Your Bread.

As a general guide, the heavier the bread, the more nutrition it contains. When shopping, compare breads by holding a loaf in each hand. The loaf that weighs more is more loaded with nutrients. Bread made with whole wheat flour is naturally heavier, firmer, and more nutrient dense than airy white bread.

- *Spelt* is a high-quality European whole wheat.

- *Wheatgrass* (sprouts) results when the wheat kernel has been allowed to grow, or germinate. Whether or not sprouted wheat is more nutritious than an unsprouted wheat is uncertain. During the sprouting process, much of the fat and carbohydrates in the seed is used for growth. The sprout still contains a lot of protein and, possibly, an increased amount of vitamins and minerals. The nutritional benefits depend upon eating a large volume of the sprouts, since they are now mostly water rather than protein by weight.

- *Stone-ground whole wheat* is ground the old-fashioned way — between rotating stones, so that the bran, germ, and endosperm remain together. Wheat purists believe that stone grinding produces a more nutritious flour than the conventional high-speed roller milling, which, they claim, may overheat the grain and cause deterioration of some nutrients. Stone-ground flour usually needs to be refrigerated once opened, since the oil released during grinding makes it spoil more quickly. It's best to store any kind of whole-grain flour in the refrigerator if you won't be using it up within a month or two. Depending on the heat produced during milling, nutritionally, stone-ground and roller-milled flour should be about the same.

Humans do not live by wheat alone. Do not deprive yourself of the unique tastes of other grains, or of the variety of nutrients they contain that complement one another. Below are some less familiar, but nutritious, grains that you should know.

Oats

Next to wheat, oats are the most popular grain found in breads and cereals such as granola and muesli. While oats are nutritionally similar to whole wheat, the oat kernel has not been taken apart like the unfortunate wheat, so some oats are nutritionally superior to some forms of wheat.* The most nutritious and practical way to use oats is to purchase oat bran and sprinkle it on cereal or add it when baking goods. One-third of a cup of oat bran provides the following:

- 130 calories
- 7 grams of protein
- 6 grams of fiber
- iron, zinc, vitamin E, and B vitamins

The fiber in oat bran is a perfect complement to that in wheat bran. The fiber in wheat bran is primarily insoluble (the kind that reduces the risk of colon cancer), while the primary fiber in oat bran is the soluble, cholesterol-lowering kind.

Rolled oats, the kind you use in oatmeal, are made by rolling and heating whole-grain oats so they cook more quickly. In bread, rolled oats appear as pale flecks and give bread a chewy, moist texture. Uncooked rolled oats appear in cereals like muesli and granola.

Barley

Barley is a popular grain in cereals and, because of its easy digestibility, is used as an alternative to

---

* *If you see the word "groats" applied to grains, don't think it's a misprint. "Groats" is the term given to the whole kernels of any grain in the raw state — before any processing.*

ANATOMY OF A GRAIN

The edible seed of the grain, called the "kernel," is composed of three parts, each with a different nutritional value.

- The *bran* is the outer layer of the kernel and the part that contains most of the minerals, especially calcium, riboflavin, niacin, iron, and a lot of protein. It contains most of the grain's fiber.
- The *germ,* even though it is the smallest part of the grain kernel, is the most nutrient dense, meaning it contains more nutrients per weight than any other part of the kernel. The germ is the seed part of the kernel, which sprouts other kernels if planted. So, when a grain is called "sprouted" (or "germinated") it means the germ part of the kernel has reproduced itself, adding more nutrients to the kernel. The germ also contains what little fats are in the kernel, which is one reason that food factories like to remove this pesty, but nutritious, part of the grain: to keep it from turning rancid and shortening the shelf life of the loaf of bread.
- The *endosperm* is the largest part of the kernel, and it is the least nutrient dense of the three parts, meaning it contains the least nutrients per volume of weight. Yet, because it makes up around 80 percent of the kernel, it contains the most proteins and carbohydrates.

This anatomy lesson is important to learn before buying a loaf of bread. When you see the term "whole" on a grain, it means that all three parts of the kernel have been left in: the bran, the germ, and the endosperm. Otherwise, it's usually only the endosperm that is left in the resulting white flour. You'll know that has happened by the terms "enriched," "refined," "bleached," or when the label doesn't include the term "whole."

---

rice in baby cereals. Yet, because barley does contain some gluten, it is a less intestines-friendly cereal for gluten-sensitive children and adults. Unfortunately, most Americans get most of their barley in beer, since barley malt is a popular grain in beer making. Most of the barley commonly used in cereal or bread making is *pearled,* which means it has been refined to remove the germ and the bran, much like the degrading of whole wheat to white. You'll find barley in many soups. It can also be cooked and used in main dishes as a substitute for rice.

Buckwheat

Despite its name, buckwheat is actually neither a wheat nor a grain. Botanically a fruit, this favorite pancake ingredient got its name from the Dutch word *boekweit.* Buckwheat enjoys a few nutritional perks over wheat: It is much higher in the amino acid lysine, somewhat higher in vitamin E, and is much lower in gluten, an important difference to gluten-sensitive individuals. Buckwheat does have some fiber, primarily of the soluble

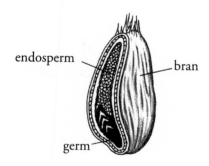

Wheat Kernel

type, but it is less good as a source of fiber than wheat and many of the other grains. Buckwheat is the main ingredient in a ricelike Eastern European dish called "kasha," which is often served as a pilaf. In pancake batter, the combination of eggs and buckwheat makes buckwheat pancakes a complete protein.

Amaranth

Botanically amaranth is a seed, but it has the nutritional profile of a grain. It surpasses whole wheat in calories, protein, iron, zinc, copper, and nearly all nutrients and is the grain highest in folic

acid, calcium, and vitamin E. Also, like buckwheat, amaranth is rich in the amino acid lysine. It even contains a bit of vitamin C. Even though this overlooked and underappreciated food is expensive and found only in nutrition stores, it is a grain with a future. Amaranth can be added to other grains, used as a thickener, garnish, popped like popcorn, or added to homemade bread. Because it is one of the most nutrient-dense foods, we have placed it at the top of our greatest grains list (see "Ranking Grains," page 136).

Quinoa

Like amaranth, quinoa (pronounced *keen-wa*) is botanically a veggie, but it has the nutritional profile of a grain and similar uses. It ranks along with amaranth as a supergrain. It is higher than other grains in protein and iron, folic acid, and some B vitamins. Though it is deficient in the amino acids tyrosine and cystine and lower than some grains in fiber, it is a nutritious addition to other grains. It can be mixed and served in a pilaf or sauce or cooked as a cereal similar to oatmeal but with a firmer, slightly gooey texture and a much more distinctive flavor.

Millet

A popular grain used in Asian and Middle Eastern flatbreads, millet is lower than wheat in fiber but a rich source of B vitamins and trace metals. Because it's gluten free, it isn't used as the main grain in leavened breads. It can be used in its raw state as a healthy addition to some wheat breads, where it appears as crunchy, white beads, or cooked like rice.

Rice

Rice enjoys a popularity similar to that of wheat. In Asia, it's the main grain. It is much less nutrient dense than wheat, being lower in protein, fiber, iron, folic acid, calcium, zinc, vitamin E, and B vitamins. Rice's claim to fame is that it contains the most carbohydrates, which makes it a popular energy food in many cultures. Rice, a good accompaniment, is much more palatable than some of the more nutritious grains that overpower the senses with their taste and aroma. Also, rice is one of the more intestines-friendly grains. Since it is low in fiber and gluten free, it is often the grain of choice for persons, especially infants, recovering from diarrheal illnesses or who are gluten sensitive.

White rice. The processing that refines natural brown rice into the white stuff removes many of the nutrients, similar to the way that milling factories disassemble wheat. As with so many food trade-offs, white rice is more popular than brown because it is blander and quicker to cook. White rice belongs in the same nutritional category as white bread.

Brown rice. Brown rice is much higher than white (even the enriched variety) in the following nutrients: protein, fiber, zinc, folic acid, vitamin E, B vitamins, and calcium. Brown rice has over fifteen times the amount of vitamin E as white rice.

Wild rice. Botanically not really a grain but rather a grass, wild rice is more nutritious than even brown rice, being much higher in protein, zinc, folic acid, and vitamin E. It has a texture and flavor that far surpass those of any other form of rice, which accounts for its popularity in finer restaurants. Once considered a delicacy, it is now so widely available that for the nutrition-minded person it is really the healthiest form of rice. Wild rice has gotten an unfair rap by being dubbed "too expensive." Not true. After cooking it swells to three or four times its initial volume, so a little wild rice goes a long way. One cup of dried wild

rice becomes three or four cups of rice on the plate, enough for six to eight servings.

Rice Terms

Besides white, brown, and wild, there are other terms that you will see associated with rice that have more to do with taste, appearance, and mode of preparation than with nutritional differences.

- *Rice bran.* Rice bran is nutritionally similar to oat and wheat brans, but contains more calcium, iron, zinc, and folic acid. Like other brans, it is a rich source of fiber, some of which is in the cholesterol-lowering soluble form. Since rice bran is higher in fat and less palatable than some of the other brans, it spoils quickly and is not a popular addition to foods, though it is often added to rice cakes and cereals and sprinkled on other foods.

- *Long-grain, medium-grain,* and *short-grain* refer to the length of the rice particle. The longer the grain, the more fluffy the rice, and the less it clumps together. Long-grain rice is the most popular variety in the United States and accounts for most of the domestic-grown rice. Medium- and short-grain rice is more popular in Asian cooking. One reason is that the short kernel size and the higher percentage of starch make the kernels clump together, so it is easier to eat with chopsticks.

- *Enriched rice* means that the B vitamins niacin and thiamin have been added, as well as iron, to make up for the nutrients lost when brown rice is refined into white. This is a bad nutritional deal, since more good stuff was taken out than is put back in. Better to just eat brown rice.

- *Rice cakes* are made of puffed rice, which is mostly air and very low in nutrition. But rice cakes are an alternative to bread as a vehicle for nutritious spreads, such as peanut butter and fruit spreads. Rice cakes, made with either white or the more nutritious brown rice, are a

favorite melt-in-the-mouth starter food for infants and a good snacking food.

- *Converted* or *parboiled* means the rice has been
soaked and steamed before milling, which prevents some of the nutrients in the grain from
being lost in the refining. Converted rice retains
a bit more of the folic acid and B vitamins, but
otherwise it is essentially the same as white rice.
This rice may actually take longer to cook than
white rice, and it may yield a fluffier grain.

- *Instant rice* (available in white or brown) shortens
the cooking time from twenty or thirty minutes
to five minutes. Yet, as happens so often with
processed foods, you trade away some nutrition
for a gain in convenience. Compared with regularly cooked rice, the instant variety has a bit less
of the following nutrients (though the differences
may be insignificant): selenium, zinc, vitamin B-
6, folic acid, and many of the amino acids. Instant rice also loses a bit of its texture.

- *Basmati* rice is a slightly nutty-flavored rice. It is
used in Indian cuisine, available as brown or
white.

Rye

Rye flour contains twice as much fiber, iron, zinc,
vitamin E, B vitamins, and calcium as whole
wheat flour. The amino acid profile of rye flour is
also better than that of whole wheat. Does that
make rye bread better for you than whole wheat?
Not exactly, for two reasons. In its original form,
or dark variety, rye flour is much more nutritious
than wheat. But by the time the rye is refined, the
"light rye" contains around half the nutrients of
the original natural dark rye. In addition, most
American rye bread is not 100 percent rye, but a
mixture of rye flour and refined wheat flour. So,
by the time the factory turns rye into bread, the
product that reaches the supermarket is either
similar to, or less nutritious than, a slice of whole

NUTRITIP
Sweet Breads

Even the best breads contain a bit of
sweetener, such as sugar, honey, molasses, or
fructose. Sugar makes the bread more tender
and helps the crust brown. Don't be a
sweetener purist when it comes to bread or
else you'll wind up with a mouthful of dry,
gooey, tasteless grain. Ditto this for salt. Salt
helps control the rate at which the bread
rises and adds flavor. A pinch of salt and a
bit of sweetener are necessary to get the
bread chemistry working right.

wheat bread. A mixture of whole rye flour (also
called "dark rye flour") and whole wheat flour
would be a terrifically nutritious bread.

RATING BREADS AND CEREALS

Some grains, like rice, make it to the table on
their own, but most of the grains in the American
diet appear in bread or cereal. Supermarket
shelves are full of many varieties of both, a sign of
the growing role of grains in people's daily diet.

NUTRITIP
Storing Whole Grains

Because whole grains still have their germ
(which contains natural oils), they can turn
rancid and are more likely to get moldy if
left at warm or room temperature. Whole
grains keep longer and stay fresher if kept in
tightly closed containers, such as plastic bags,
and in cold places. They keep longest in the
refrigerator or freezer.

All breads and cereals are not created equal. Some pack plenty of nutrients; others are little more than empty calories. Knowing which are the most nutritious requires some careful label reading. Here is what you need to know about flours, bread, and cereals.

Bread Basics

Even in biblical days, bread was known as the "staff of life." Each culture has brought to the table its own breads, from pitas to pumpernickel. There is French bread, Italian bread, English muffins, and, well, American bread — the airy, nutrient-poor, white enriched stuff. Here are the facts you should know about various breads and how to select them.

Bread is basically flour and liquid. The liquid is usually water or milk, but there are many different types of flours that can be used to make bread. The nutrient quality, color, texture, and overall appeal of breads are all affected by the quality of the flour.

So, let's build a bread from scratch to learn about how bread gets its nutritional value and taste appeal.

Wheat Flour

Flour, the main ingredient of bread, is ground-up grain. The nutritional quality of the grain and how it's affected by processing determine the nutritional quality of the bread. Start with a good grain and don't mess with Mother Nature and you'll get a loaf of nutritious bread.

Wheat is the most popular flour used in bread making, due to its unique protein, gluten. Gluten allows the dough to stretch. Yet, for a few people, it's not the most intestines-friendly protein and may cause a diarrhea-producing condition called "gluten sensitivity." Some varieties of wheat contain more gluten than others, and the gluten content determines the firmness of the bread. A wheat high in gluten is known as "hard wheat"

and yields a firmer bread. Hard wheat is also used to make pasta; durum, farina, and semolina are all varieties of hard wheat used in pasta making. Soft-wheat flours contain less gluten and are used for cakes and pastries. On the supermarket shelf, you'll find an all-purpose flour, a blend of soft and hard wheat, that works well in most recipes. A natural foods store may even have whole wheat pastry flour, which produces baked goods with a softer texture than regular whole wheat flour.

The wheat seeds, called "kernels," contain three parts. The *bran* is the tiny covering of the seed. The *germ* is the tiny embryo of the wheat plant and the source of the essential fatty acids in wheat. The *endosperm* is the largest part of the kernel and is mostly starch — food for the growing wheat plant.

Flour is made by grinding wheat kernels, resulting in a powdery substance that comes from the endosperm, coarser pieces of the bran, and the germ. Centuries ago, grains were ground between stone wheels powered by wind, water, or oxen. The result was a coarse flour that made a heavy, brown, and very nutritious bread. Sometimes, however, flour was "bolted" after milling; that is, it was sifted through a silk-cloth strainer, removing the coarse particles. This produced a more-refined flour that made a lighter, whiter, but less nutritious bread. Because this bread was more expensive to make, it became a status symbol. The rich people ate white bread, the poor got the coarser bread. Nutritionally, the poor people were better off than the rich ones. In the mid-nineteenth century, high-speed roller mills were invented. These were able to crack the grains, grind the flour, and blow off the excess particles of bran and germ. This brought down the price of white flour, so that rich and poor alike could now eat white bread every day. Before, those who had more got less for their money. Now those who had less also got less. White flour actually became cheaper to use than whole-grain flour. Without the germ of the wheat, it even had a longer shelf life.

RANKING GRAINS

It's misleading, if not impossible, to rank grains. Their relative value depends on what nutrients you are looking for. Is one nutrient more important than another? Is fiber more important than protein? Maybe if you're a senior citizen, but not if you're a child. Do you judge nutritional value by nutrients per ounce or by nutrients per calorie? When you see any rating system for food, take it with a grain of salt and remember that variety is also an important key to healthy eating.

In spite of the difficulty, we've rated the twelve most common grains according to the following nutrients: protein, fiber, iron, zinc, folic acid, vitamin E, riboflavin, niacin, thiamin, and calcium. If you assign one point for each of these nutrients, the ratings come out as follows:

Total Nutrient Points (highest to lowest)	Fiber Content (grams per serving)	Protein (grams per serving)
1. amaranth	1. barley	1. amaranth
2. rye	2. amaranth	2. oats
3. oats	3. whole wheat	3. rye
4. wild rice	4. rye	4. wild rice
5. millet	5. buckwheat	5. millet
6. barley	6. millet	6. quinoa
7. quinoa	7. oats	7. barley
8. buckwheat	8. wild rice	8. whole wheat
9. whole wheat	9. quinoa	9. buckwheat
10. brown rice	10. corn	10. corn
11. white rice	11. brown rice	11. brown rice
12. corn	12. white rice	12. white rice

The grains highest in calcium, ranked in order, are amaranth, quinoa, oats, barley, rye, and whole wheat. Gluten-free grains (or flours) are corn, rice, and soy. (Buckwheat may contain a small amount of gluten.) The top six grains for iron are quinoa, amaranth, oats, enriched rice, millet, and barley. The top grains for zinc (an important immune-system booster) are wild rice, rye, amaranth, oats, and quinoa. The top grains for folic acid are millet, wild rice, rye, amaranth, and oats.

Even though according to our ranking system amaranth ranks as the greatest grain nutritionally, overall, the top grain in our book is whole wheat. Other grains may have slightly more nutrients, but wheat is a whole lot more useful in a whole lot more foods. Whole wheat comes out as top grain.

When the bran and the germ are removed from the flour, the amounts of twenty-two vitamins and minerals are highly diminished. Fiber and protein content suffer as well. Because so many nutrients are removed from white flour and white bread, by law, manufacturers must "enrich" the white flour with added B vitamins and iron, and sometimes calcium, vitamin D, and folic acid. The result makes good label copy: "enriched flour"; but really, white bread is a bad nutritional deal. The milling process has taken out far more nutrients than are put back in.

Flour that comes directly from the endosperm of the wheat kernel is a slightly yellow color, not pure white. Flour is not naturally white. Decades ago bread makers discovered that consumers equated white with purity and health, so they started adding chemicals to the flour to bleach it. The result: a whiter, more popular flour. You can find unbleached white flour on the shelf at the supermarket, but you'll have to look hard for it and pay a slightly higher price — even though it's had less done to it. Most of today's whole wheat flour is ground with the same kind of roller mill used to make white flour, but the germ and the bran are put back in at the end of the process.

Non-wheat Flours

The term "flour" doesn't necessarily refer to wheat. Flour, and therefore bread, can be made from any grain. But since other flours don't contain as much, or any, gluten, most of these appear in bread in combination with wheat flour. They may appear on their own in other types of baked goods. Popular non-wheat flours are:

NUTRITIP
Take a Whole Look at "Wheat."

Bread marketers, hip to nutritional fads, know that consumers believe "wheat" to be healthier than white. White anything has gotten a well-deserved bad-nutrition rap. So they use terms like "wheat bread" and "multigrain" to attract buyers to breads that are made with mostly refined flour. Choose breads, cereals, and other grains that say "whole wheat" or "whole grain." This means the husk and germ have been left in, along with all their nutrients.

- *Buckwheat flour.* Despite its name, buckwheat contains minimal wheat (or gluten) protein and is digestible by most gluten-sensitive persons. It's a popular pancake flour, combined with wheat.

- *Oat flour.* Oat flour is more commonly used in cereals than in bread. When used with whole wheat flour, it makes a moister whole-grain bread.

- *Rye flour.* Rye is a high-protein, high-fiber grain of at least equal nutrition to wheat flour and is often used for breads. (See "Comparing Breads," page 138.) Look on the label for "unbolted" rye if you want a whole-grain rye flour.

- *Cornmeal.* This is made from white or yellow corn. You'll find it in breads, pancakes, and muffins. If there is an American bread, cornbread would be it. It was a staple of early pioneer diets. Like other flours, cornmeal comes either bolted ("degermed") or unbolted. *Corn flour* is finely ground cornmeal.

- *Soy flour.* Defatted, ground soybeans make a flour high in protein. You can substitute soy flour for a small amount of the wheat flour in recipes to boost the protein content of the finished product.

- *Arrowroot flour.* Unlike the protein-rich wheat, arrowroot is primarily starch. It comes from the root of a tropical plant called "maranta." Because it is easy to digest, it's a popular ingredient in starter cookies for infants and children.

Liquids

Most breads use either water or milk as their liquid component. Most commercial breads are made with water, since it is inexpensive. (This is good news for people with milk allergies, though bread made with milk may not be a problem anyway since the baking process itself is likely to make milk proteins less allergenic.) Instead of water, milk is a popular ingredient in homemade or bakery bread, since it adds protein and produces a richer flavor, a browner crust, and a softer, smoother crumb. Milk also acts as a preservative to help keep the bread fresh, and it makes bread a complete protein by providing lysine, the amino acid that is lacking in wheat flour. Nonfat milk, or nonfat dried milk, is often used in bread making since fat tends to coat the flour particles and interfere with the elasticity of gluten.

Yeast

Yeast is a live fungus that gets a rise out of bread. When put in a warm, moist environment with carbohydrates to feed on, yeast begins to bud and produce enzymes that ferment the sugars in the flour into carbon dioxide and alcohol. The CO_2 is trapped in the elastic network of the gluten, which has been well developed by kneading the dough. These organisms continue to multiply, release more CO_2, and the dough rises. Some of the alcohol from the sugar fermentation evaporates during baking, and the rest of it contributes to the flavor of the bread. (Too much yeast causes overrising of the dough and results in excessive production of alcohol, which makes the bread taste disagreeably "yeasty.") Besides making dough rise, yeast reacts with the gluten to make the dough hold together better and gives bread its characteristic flavor and aroma. Sourdough breads use a longer yeast-fermentation process to give the bread a special flavor.

Yeast increases the nutritional value of the loaf of bread, adding a trace of vitamins, minerals, and some high-quality protein. (In fact, one typical package of yeast, the amount used in baking one loaf of bread, contains 3 grams of protein and as many essential amino acids as a quarter cup of kidney beans.)

RANKING BREADS

As with grains, ranking breads is very difficult. We have attempted to rate them according to the following nutrients: protein, fiber, calcium, iron, zinc, folic acid, niacin, riboflavin, and vitamins B-6 and E (assigning one point each), and factoring in nutrients per calorie. Using this point system, the breads rank:

1. multi whole-grain
2. whole wheat
3. pita, whole wheat
4. pumpernickel
5. rye, American
6. white

Comparing Breads

No matter how you slice it, whole wheat bread is more nutritious than white because whole wheat bread contains the following:

- nearly one-third more protein
- three to four times the amount of fiber
- four times more zinc
- more folic acid
- more iron
- more chromium (an important mineral that regulates sugar and fat metabolism — especially important in hyperactive children)

Although whole wheat bread is reported to have the same glycemic index (see page 35) as white bread, because of the extra nutrients the carbohydrates in whole wheat bread may have less of a roller-coaster effect on blood sugar.

The nutritional content of bread is not affected by the bread's shape or presentation. Whether it's rolls, bagels, sliced bread, or pita, what matters

LOOK FOR "MULTI WHOLE-GRAIN"

Packing many grains together into one food will give you the benefit of many different nutrients. Is whole wheat bread deficient in lysine? No problem — add some amaranth. Need more niacin in the bread? Boost it with barley. What's great about grains is that one plant's nutritional deficiency is another one's strength. Multigrain breads and cereals teach your tongue to enjoy more than just plain old wheat or rice and help you appreciate more nutritional variety. Take some whole wheat, sprinkle in some amaranth (for more protein and fiber), add a touch of quinoa (for iron) and a bit of barley (for fiber), add a few flecks of millet (for folic acid), add a dash of rye (for vitamin E), and you have the makings of a six-grain cereal that has the best that each grain has to offer. But don't forget to read the label carefully. "Multigrain" is not the same as "whole grain."

most is the kind of flour in the bread: The main nutritional difference is whether breads are made with whole wheat or white flour.

Choosing Cereals

Now that you know your grains, you are ready to navigate the maze of cereals in the supermarket and make an intelligent decision about the best box for your buck. Take a stroll down cereal lane in any supermarket and you'll be overwhelmed by the overdose of colorful boxes. The variety, the catchy names, and the fabulous graphic designs are a tribute to the creativity of American advertising firms. But to choose the most nutritious cereal for your family, you'll need to look past the

NUTRITIP
Impoverished Flour

"Enriched" on the flour label means the thiamin, riboflavin, niacin, and iron lost during processing have been put back in. Manufacturers are not required to replace any other vitamins or minerals, so you get less nutritional benefit from enriched products than from the unrefined originals. Refining is a factory process, and not a nutritionally advantageous one.

glitz. Here are some guidelines to help you select a nutritious cereal.

Rule #1: Don't let the kids decide. Children are influenced by box designs and TV ads, and they care nothing about the nutritional content of cereal. Let them make decisions, but give them healthy choices: pick three cereals that you would select anyway and let them choose one. At least this way they have a choice. Children are more likely to eat cereal they select themselves, but parents must prescreen.

NUTRITIP
Add Your Own Oats.

If you're eating oat bran for your heart, rather than looking for the small amounts that may be added to cereals such as granola (which may also contain hydrogenated oils that can raise your cholesterol), buy a package of oat bran and sprinkle it on your choice of cereal. Or add oat bran to home-baked goodies.

NUTRIMYTH

The darker the bread, the more healthy it is. Not necessarily. Certainly, whole wheat bread is healthier than white, but bread sellers, catering to consumer perception that darker bread is healthier, now bake bread in various shades of tan. Actually, some wheaty-looking bread is nothing more than white bread with a chemical tan. It's made by adding caramel colorings to white bread. So, look beneath the tan and read the label. If "flour" or "enriched flour" is the first ingredient, it's white bread in disguise. If the bread is whole wheat, the term "100 percent whole wheat" will appear first on the ingredients list.

Rule #2: Read the "Nutrition Facts" box and the ingredients list on the back or side of the package. This information is clearer and more accurate than claims on the front of the box. Because these parts of the label follow a standard format, you can use them to make meaningful comparisons between products. Ignore the hype on the front of the box (e.g., the cereal that boasts that it is "low-fat" — nearly all cereals are low-fat).

Rule #3: Think about why you are buying cereal in the first place. Yes, cereal is a favorite family breakfast food, but consider which nutrients cereals are the best source of. The list includes fiber, protein, folic acid, zinc, iron, and B vitamins. Most other nutrients can be found just as readily, if not more easily, in other foods. You don't need to get your daily vitamin C or calcium from your cereal bowl. Choose cereals that are highest in the nutrients that cereals do best.

Guidelines for Reading Cereal Labels

To help you decide whether a particular product merits a place in your pantry or is better left on the shelf, consider these six criteria for a healthy cereal:

- The grains should be *whole* (e.g., "whole wheat," or "wheat bran," not just "wheat").
- Protein content should be at least 3 grams per serving.
- The total carbohydrate-to-sugars ratio should be no less than four to one.* This means if the "Total Carbohydrate" line says 24 grams, the sugars should have a value of 6 grams or less. That tells you that most of the carbs come from the grain and fibers, not from the added sugars. On the other hand, a cereal with 28 grams of total carbohydrate and 15 grams of sugars would fall into the "junk cereal" category. Supernutritious cereals have a carb-to-sugars ratio of six or seven to one (e.g., 23 grams to 3 grams). Also look for the "five and five" rule: Less than 5 grams of sugar and at least 5 grams of fiber.
- Zinc content should be 25 to 40 percent of the recommended dietary amount.
- Iron content should be 25 to 40 percent of the RDA.
- Other vitamin and mineral content should be 25 to 40 percent of the RDA.

There are also ingredients that a nutritious cereal should *not* contain. Check the ingredients list for these:

- hydrogenated oils
- dyes or artificial colors
- chemical preservatives

---

* *Another way to evaluate the amount of sugar in a cereal is to look at the number of grams of sugar per 1-ounce serving. As a general guide, more than 7 grams of sugar (1.5 teaspoons) per 1-ounce serving is too much. Some cereals, especially those in our junk category, have 3 or 4 teaspoons of sugar added per 1-ounce serving. Even your kids might say "Too sweet!"*

A TALE OF TWO CEREALS

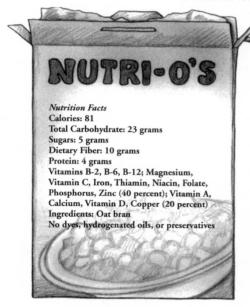

NUTRI-O'S

Nutrition Facts
Calories: 81
Total Carbohydrate: 23 grams
Sugars: 5 grams
Dietary Fiber: 10 grams
Protein: 4 grams
Vitamins B-2, B-6, B-12; Magnesium,
Vitamin C, Iron, Thiamin, Niacin, Folate,
Phosphorus, Zinc (40 percent); Vitamin A,
Calcium, Vitamin D, Copper (20 percent)
Ingredients: Oat bran
No dyes, hydrogenated oils, or preservatives

JUNK-O'S

Nutrition Facts
Calories: 120
Total Carbohydrate: 28 grams
Sugars: 15 grams
Dietary Fiber: 0.6 grams
Protein: 1 gram
Vitamins A and D (10 percent); Calcium (1
percent); Riboflavin, Vitamin B-6, Vitamin
B-12, Vitamin C, Iron, Thiamin, Niacin,
Folate, Zinc (20 percent)
Ingredients: Corn, wheat, and oat flours,
sugar, partially hydrogenated vegetable oil
(one or more of coconut, cottonseed, and
soybean) . . . yellow #6, red #40 . . . blue
#2 . . . blue #1 . . . BHT (preservative)

The labels make it obvious how far ahead you'll be nutritionally if you choose the Nutri-O's, but you wouldn't know this from the front of the package. The front of the Junk-O's box says "All natural fruit flavors" and "sweetened multigrain cereal." Junk-O's even displays the seal of the American Heart Association and proudly notes: "This product meets American Heart Association dietary guidelines for healthy people over age two when used as part of a balanced diet." No such American Heart Association seal appears on the Nutri-O's. Don't be taken in by the hype.

Other Label Facts Cereal Consumers Should Know

- Don't be deceived by a fruity name and little red berries floating all over the front of the box. In most cereals there's very little fruit. Dried fruit may be heavier than grain, so it may be listed near the top of the ingredients list, leading consumers to believe they are getting a lot of fruit in the cereal. It's more nutritious to buy only grains and add your own fruit.
- When comparing the nutrient density of cereals it's best to make comparisons based on the calories per serving rather than the volume or weight of a serving. For example, an ounce of a nutrient-dense cereal such as All-Bran with extra fiber would contain fewer calories and take up less volume than a more light and airy puffed rice. You'll get more calories if you

eat the bigger bowl of puffed rice, but you'll get more nutrients per calorie in the bran cereal.

- As a general guide to the nutrient density of a cereal, look at the weight of a serving (grams) in relation to the volume (e.g., ½ cup). If it takes a greater volume of one cereal than another to come up with the same weight in grams of fiber, protein, or other nutrients, choose the cereal with the lower volume per serving. The heavier cereal is usually the more nutritious. The extra space taken up by the lighter cereal is just a lot of expensive air.
- The quality of the grain is more important than the percentage of the vitamins listed on the box. Synthetic vitamins may be cheaper to add than nutritious grains. For example, a cereal listing "corn" or "wheat" but containing lots of vitamins may not be as nutritious as a cereal listing "whole wheat" or "whole bran" yet containing a lower percentage of vitamins.
- Outrageous names on cereal boxes usually mean that a lot of good nutrition has been left out. This is particularly true of cereals targeted at children, who are most influenced by the catchy name and hype on the front of the box and in the TV commercials. Children are too young to read the "Nutritional Facts" box and the ingredients list on the side of the box. They rely on their parents to look out for their nutritional best interest.

CHOOSING INFANT CEREALS

In selecting cereal for your baby, use criteria similar to those you use in choosing your own. What are the main nutrients you want your baby to get from this cereal? Try these shopping tips:

- Protein: at least 1 gram per serving
- Iron: at least 3 milligrams per serving. Remember, after infants and toddlers are weaned from breast milk or formula, cereals may supply about half of their daily requirement for iron, which averages around 6 to 10 milligrams a day. Infant cereals generally contain more iron per serving than adult cereals since they are enriched with iron.

PASTA

Pasta is one of the greatest things that ever happened to grains. Pasta may have its origins in Asia and the Mediterranean, but its growing popularity has made it truly an American food. Here are the most common questions asked about this favorite family food.

What is pasta?

Pasta is the Italian word for "paste." All pasta is made from a dough of grain flour mixed with water. There are many different shapes and sizes of pasta. While most are made from wheat, other grains can also be used on their own (for people who are gluten intolerant) or combined with wheat.

What do the different names for pasta mean?

Take a dough made from grain, force it through a variety of different-shaped molds, and out come nifty noodles of varying shapes — flat, smooth,

SLOW GOING?

One of the most important components of cereals is fiber, which acts like an intestinal broom and sponge, soaking up water and sweeping out waste in the form of softer stools. A high-fiber cereal will prevent constipation.

Look for cereals that contain high-fiber grains, such as barley, buckwheat, millet, oats, rye, and whole wheat. Avoid white rice cereals, since rice is low in fiber. Many cereals advertising high fiber have extra bran (and/or wheat) and include a grain called "psyllium," which is very high in fiber. A word of caution: Psyllium is powerful. It will cure constipation, but eating too much too fast will cause gas and bloating. If you are using psyllium as a supplement (it's available in health stores), begin with the equivalent of ½ tablespoon a day, and gradually build up to 1 tablespoon, which provides a whopping intestines-cleansing dose of 8 grams of fiber, about a third of the RDA.

For fiber to work, you must take extra fluids to help soften the stools. Otherwise, the extra fiber turns to sludge in the bowels and actually contributes to constipation. (For more on fiber, see Chapter 9.)

solid, hollow, and twisted. Give to these wiggly forms melodious Italian names, and you have the many kinds of pasta that sit on the supermarket shelf. In many cases, the shape of the noodles determines the name of the pasta:

- *Spaghetti,* from *spago,* "cord"
- *Linguine,* "little tongues"
- *Vermicelli,* "little worms"
- *Conchiglie,* "shells"
- *Rigatoni,* "furrows," short, wide fluted tubes

WHY CEREALS ARE GREAT FOR KIDS

Most children love cereal and willingly eat a lot of it. Add to this the nutrition found in cereals and you'll agree that grains are great kid foods. One cup of a nutritious cereal can supply as much as half the daily nutritional requirements for fifteen of the top vitamins and minerals. Add milk or yogurt to the cereal, and it boosts the nutritional content even higher. Plain and simple, cereal is a great way to get a lot of nutrition into a child at one sitting. In fact, a nutritious cereal is like a multivitamin/multimineral supplement in a tasty, attractive package.

- *Lasagne,* broad, sometimes ruffled, ribbons of pasta (from Latin for "pot")
- *Fettuccine,* "small ribbons"
- *Ravioli,* "little turnips"
- *Rotini,* "spirals" or "twists"
- *Capellini* (angel hair), "fine hairs"
- *Fusilli,* "little spindles" (spirals)
- *Penne,* "quills"
- *Tortellini,* "little cakes"
- *Cannelloni,* tube- or cane-shaped pasta

Is one pasta more nutritious than another?

The nutritional quality of a pasta, and often its taste and texture, depend upon the flour. Those made with whole-grain flours, usually found in nutrition stores, are naturally the most nutrient rich, because the bran and germ of the grain have been left in. Most pasta is made with *durum* wheat, a hard wheat high in protein and gluten, which makes a dough that sticks together well and holds its shape, a feature so important to pasta makers. Most of the familiar dried pastas are made with *semolina* or *farina,* or a combination of

NUTRITIP
Juicy Cereal

Usually we think of milk and cereal as being married to one another. In one sense, this is an ideal marriage, since the proteins in the milk make up for the few amino acid deficiencies in the grain. Milk and cereal together mean that a person gets a complete protein meal. However, milk can somewhat decrease the absorption of iron from the cereal. Juices high in vitamin C, such as orange, grapefruit, or tangerine, can increase the absorption of iron. If you're consuming cereal primarily for calories and protein, milk is a better choice than juice. If you're serving cereal primarily for iron absorption (e.g., to a baby who drinks enough milk or formula as a beverage), then juice in the cereal may be a better nutritional choice.

the two. In these flours, the germ and bran have been removed, and the fiber and nutritional values are lower. Semolina is made from durum wheat and may have more protein than farina flour, which is made from a softer wheat. So, as with all foods, look at the label. Here are some words to look for:

NUTRITIP
Flecks in the Flakes

Here's another observation from a cereal lover: While many less nutritious cereals have thin flakes (we call them "see-through flakes"), more nutritious cereals have a rich, brown, thick appearance, with white or brown flecks of grains embedded within each flake.

NUTRITIP
Cereal for Two

Moms-to-be should enjoy only cereals that meet the "best list" criteria, since these cereals are most likely to contain the nutrients growing moms and babies need, such as protein, folic acid, iron, and zinc. "Best-list" cereals also contain a lot of fiber, which helps the slow-going bowels of late pregnancy.

NUTRITIP
Salty Cereals

Cereal manufacturers know that children like salt. One cup of some of the leading children's cereals contains the total daily requirement (around 300 milligrams) for sodium in the preschool child. Once children get used to salty cereals, you may have trouble enticing them to try healthier and less salty alternatives. Read the label carefully.

- *Whole wheat* means what it says: the whole grain.
- *Macaroni* means the pasta is made with semolina, farina, and/or flour made from refined durum wheat. Macaroni comes in many shapes: spaghetti, elbow macaroni, shells, etc.
- *Egg noodles* are made from flour, water, and egg (either egg white or whole eggs). At least 5.5 percent of the weight of the noodle must be from egg.
- *Corn pasta* has less protein than wheat pasta, but it is more easily digested by gluten-sensitive persons.
- *Multigrain pasta* adds dense grains, such as amaranth, quinoa, or flour from Jerusalem artichokes or soy, to wheat flours to make the pasta richer in protein. Rye pasta is also known as

"spelt" and is particularly high in protein, fiber, zinc, and iron.
- *Flavored pasta* includes vegetables, such as spinach and tomato, to add taste, variety, and nutrition to plain old pasta.
- *Couscous* is a cross between a grain and pasta. It is made from cooked and dried semolina. The tiny grains are cooked like rice, absorbing all the cooking liquid. The refined flour it's made from is not enriched with vitamins, so couscous is low in nutrients.

When evaluating pastas, use the same criteria that you would use in comparing cereals:

NUTRITIP
Good Grazing

Munching on healthy cereal is a good way to snack, especially for toddlers who don't like to sit still and eat big meals but prefer nibbling throughout the day.

NUTRITIP
Fat Cereals

Grains are naturally low in fat, unless, of course, you do something unnatural to them, such as add hydrogenated oils in processing. Be wary especially of granola cereals, which may contain 4 to 9 grams of fat per serving, especially if it's hydrogenated.

NUTRITIP
Eat Your Cereal Fast.

Ever watch kids eat cereal? They tend to down it quickly, yet they may dawdle with other foods. Let them scarf it down. Cereals quickly dissolve into mush. They need to be eaten fast. Better some inelegant eating habits than a sticky, blobby mess left in the bowl.

NUTRITIP
Be Picky About Your Pasta.

When was the last time you went into your favorite Italian restaurant and asked what kind of wheat they use to make their pasta? The amount of protein and other nutrients in the pasta depends on the wheat used. Restaurants usually use pasta made from semolina. Depending on how friendly you are with the chef, ask and you might receive whole wheat pasta.

- Is the starter grain whole or refined?
- What is the protein content?

Judge the ingredients list for pasta in the same way you judge the ingredients list on bread labels. It's hard to find whole wheat pasta without a bit of semolina added (remember, semolina is little more than a nice Italian-sounding word for "enriched white flour"), since the addition of semolina gives the pasta a more acceptable taste and texture.

Because they are made from refined flour, most pastas, ounce for ounce or calorie for calorie, are less nutritious than the same amount of whole wheat or multigrain bread or cereal, especially in

the following nutrients: fiber, vitamin E, B vitamins, zinc, and folic acid. They may also be lower in protein if eggs are not included. Still, pasta is a good low-fat source of protein since semolina is high in protein.

Isn't pasta fattening?

Not necessarily. Pasta itself is low-fat because grains are low-fat. It's what you put on the pasta that makes it fattening. The calories and much of the nutritional quality of pasta dishes depend, for better or worse, on the sauce you put on top of the pasta. Sauces that contain cream, lots of high-fat cheese, and lots of oil contribute far more calories to a pasta dish than the pasta itself. Choose your sauce wisely, and pasta can be a nutritious medium-calorie meal. Pasta tossed with a bit of olive oil, steamed vegetables, and perhaps a small amount of white-meat chicken or seafood can be a nutritious entree. Noodles coated with cream and cheese are a high-fat disaster.

NUTRITIP
Sprinkle On the Hard Stuff.

Parmesan cheese contains less fat than many cheeses. That's what makes it a hard cheese. Hard cheeses are higher in calcium. One ounce of freshly grated hard parmesan cheese contains a bone-building 336 milligrams of calcium. Parmesan also packs a lot of flavor. That's what makes it a favorite pasta topper.

14

Fabulous Fruits

LET'S FACE IT, our food preferences are based on taste, not nutrition, which is why fruit is such a great food. Fruits taste sweet and interesting. They have agreeable textures — crunchy apples, smooth peaches, juicy oranges, and so on. And most fruits are surprisingly nutritious. Though not as nutrient dense as vegetables, fruits are an important source of vitamins, minerals, and enzymes. Some fruits are more nutritious than others, but with fruits, as with vegetables and grains, variety is the spice of life. Nutrients that one fruit lacks, another fruit provides. Fructose is the principal sugar in most fruits; in the case of certain others, such as oranges, melons, and peaches, sucrose is the principal sugar. Fructose is absorbed slowly into the bloodstream, so fruit gives you energy without triggering the ups and downs of the insulin cycle.

A GLOSSARY OF FRUITS

Apple. An apple a day may not keep the doctor away entirely, but apples have a lot to recommend them. They are nutritious, convenient, and always available. Apples get an A+ in fiber content, since they contain a lot of the soluble fiber pectin, which helps to lower cholesterol. They also con-

tain some cancer-fighting flavonoids. Eating a whole apple is more nutritious than drinking apple juice, since the fiber, vitamins, and minerals may be processed out of the juice. When the flesh of an apple turns brown, it means some of the nutrients have oxidized and are lost. As with any fruit, to get the best that an apple has to offer, eat it fresh.

Apricot. Five apricots contain around the same number of calories as one apple, but they have much more protein, calcium, iron, vitamin K, zinc, vitamin A, and folic acid. Apricots are high in beta carotene, too, as well as potassium and fiber. You'll find them on our list of the top ten nutritious fruits (see page 151).

Apricot, dried. Dried apricots are a particularly good source of beta carotene, potassium, and fiber (3 grams per 10 dried apricot halves). When purchasing dried apricots, read the label. Preservatives, such as sulfites or sulfur dioxide, are often used to maintain apricots' orange color. These will be listed on the label. Sulfites can be an allergen for some people. You can purchase sulfite-free apricots in health food stores. Even though they are a less appealing brownish color, they are equally nutritious. It is not worth consuming sulfites just so the apricots look more orange.

FRUITS THAT ARE KIND TO THE INTESTINES

Allergies or illness can make the intestines more sensitive. Some fruits contain sugars that are easily absorbed into the bloodstream, while the sugar in other fruits may ferment and cause gas to build up in the intestines. This is hard on an intestinal lining already irritated by allergens or viruses. The ratio of fructose to glucose in the fruit as well as the fiber content determine how much of the sugar is absorbed. The higher the glucose-to-fructose ratio, the more intestines-friendly the fruit. Here's how these fruits rank:

Most Kind to the Intestines	Least Kind to the Intestines*
• white grapes†	• prunes
• strawberries	• pears
• raspberries	• sweet cherries
• blackberries	• peaches
• pineapples	• apples
• oranges	

* *The reason these fruits are less intestines-friendly is they contain a higher fructose-to-glucose ratio and some sorbitol (an intestines irritant), in addition to some being higher in fiber. If you are suffering from sluggish bowels or constipation, then use this nutritional quirk to your advantage, since juices, such as prune and pear nectar, tend to be laxative in effect.*

† *The most intestines-friendly fruit, especially if you are suffering from a diarrheal illness, is white grapes, since they contain equal amounts of fructose and glucose. The high glucose content helps all the fructose be absorbed so little is left over to ferment into intestinal gas. And, white grape juice contains no sorbitol.*

Avocado. Avocados are usually thought of as a vegetable, but they are really a fruit, with more nutrition than any other fruit. Avocados are high in protein, fiber, vitamin E, niacin, thiamin, riboflavin, folic acid, and zinc. Avocados get the lion's share of their calories from fat, and while these are the heart-healthy monounsaturated fats with no cholesterol, you pay a caloric price. While weight-conscious adults might want to stick to an apple a day rather than an avocado a day, the high calorie content of avocados makes them a good food for growing children. The fat content of avocados depends upon the variety. Avocados contain a trace of omega-3 fatty acids. Because avocados are so nutrient dense, we include them in our "Top Twelve Foods" list (see page 108) as well as in our "Top Ten Fruits" list (page 151).

Buying and serving tips: Avocados ripen after picking. Buy the avocado when it is underripe, meaning, it is firm, but not hard — squeezing it gently does not leave a dent. Store avocados at room temperature until they are soft enough to dent by squeezing. To speed ripening, place the avocados in a paper bag and store at room temperature until they are ready to eat (three to five

NUTRITIP
Storing Guacamole or Half an Avocado

Avocado turns brown after it's been exposed to air. To prevent this, sprinkle lemon or lime juice on the cut side of half an avocado and cover it tightly with plastic wrap. Include lemon or lime juice in your guacamole recipe to keep it from turning brown.

days). Including an apple in the bag speeds up the process even more.

For easy eating, halve the avocado by running a knife lengthwise around the middle of the avocado. Hold the avocado in both hands and twist at the cut. The halves will separate easily, leaving the pit in one half. Spoon out the flesh and enjoy. Mash avocados into dip for children. For adults, add tomatoes, onion, and garlic to make guacamole.

Banana. Bananas mash easily for baby food and blend nicely into a sweet smoothie. They contain a lot of potassium, so eating a daily banana is helpful to people on certain medications, such as diuretics, which may deplete the body of potassium. Pesticides are not a problem because the easy-to-peel feature of a banana makes it easy to peel the pesticides off.

Blueberries. On the surface, blueberries don't seem to pack any particular standout nutrient. Yet recent studies have shown that blueberries have healthy stuff in their skin — an antioxidant, cancer-fighting phyto called "anthocyanin." Blueberries are an excellent fruit for making smoothies. Their sweet taste and rich purple color give any smoothie a more appealing taste, texture, and color.

NUTRITIP
Avocado Sandwich

A favorite sandwich for growing children (and genetically lean adults) is whole wheat bread, a thin layer of organic peanut butter, thinly sliced tomatoes, a thick layer of guacamole, and a mound of alfalfa sprouts. For added richness, add a thin layer of low-fat mayonnaise. Enjoy!

Boysenberries. Boysenberries are a great source of fiber.

Cantaloupe. Cantaloupes are high in vitamin C, beta carotene, and potassium.

Cherries. Cherries contain some beta carotene, and sour cherries contain more beta carotene than sweet cherries.

Dates. Dates are a good source of fiber, iron, and niacin.

Figs, dried. Dried figs are high in calories and high in carbs, but they also contain abundant amounts of other nutrients, such as calcium, fiber, protein, and potassium. They make an excellent snack and add fiber when they're chopped up and included in cookies. Because of the high fiber and high calcium content, they get an honorable mention on our "Top Ten Fruits" list. Their high carbohydrate and sugar content could be a drawback for sugar-sensitive individuals, but for athletes, figs would be a great addition to a pre-game meal.

Grapefruit. Grapefruit is a great fruit, low in calories, high in fiber, with lots of vitamin C. If you get the pink or red variety, grapefruit is also rich in beta carotene. Half the fiber is the insoluble type (good for the intestines), and half is soluble pectin fiber (good for the heart). Remember, though, that a lot of fiber is in the stringy walls that separate the segments. If you're digging out grapefruit segments with a spoon, you'll miss out on much of the fiber.

Grapes. The skin of red and purple grapes contains cancer-fighting anthocyanin pigments similar to the ones in blueberries. Green, seedless grapes are not exactly nutritional standouts, but kids love to snack on them, especially on hot days. They're a popular alternative to soda or candy.

Guava. Guavas are hard to find, but gobble them up when you can. They rate high among fruits for fiber and vitamin E. Guava juice is readily available in the juice section of most supermarkets, but it contains added corn syrup, which dilutes the nutritional value compared to the raw fruit.

Honeydew melon. Honeydew melon is not nearly so nutritious as cantaloupe. Cantaloupe contains half the number of calories, nearly twice the protein, slightly more fiber, more calcium, and a lot more beta carotene, compared with only a trace in honeydew.

Kiwi. Kiwi is a great source of vitamin C. Try cutting it in half and eating it out of the peel with a spoon.

Lemon and lime. Lemons and limes are a moderately good source of vitamin C, with lemons containing about one-third more vitamin C than limes. Lemon and lime juice add flavor to dishes, which can be helpful if you're cutting back on salt.

Mango. Mangoes are high in fiber, high in beta carotene (similar to apricots and cantaloupe), and high in vitamin C — but much higher in calories than equal servings of similar fruits, such as cantaloupe and papaya.

Orange. Oranges are known for their vitamin C content, but they're also a good source of folate and fiber. They even contain some calcium. As with grapefruit, the white pith under the skin of the orange contains more vitamin C than the flesh and provides a lot of the pectin fiber. When peeling the orange, try to leave the white inner peeling on and eat it with the flesh (if you don't mind the slightly bitter taste).

Papaya. High in calcium, folic acid, vitamin C, fiber, and carotenoids, this near-perfect fruit is becoming more widely available and affordable.

Peach. The best peaches are tree-ripened and therefore locally grown. They contain some carotenoids and a tiny bit of vitamin C.

Pear. A high sorbitol content plus extra fiber makes pears ideal for persons suffering from constipation. Most of the vitamin C in pears is concentrated in the skin, as is some of the fiber, so peeled, canned pears are less nutritious than fresh.

Persimmons. Persimmons are high in fiber, carotenoids, and vitamin A. Some varieties are extremely high in vitamin C.

Pineapple. Its claims to fame are that it is the fruit highest in the essential nutrient manganese and that it has digestive enzymes, as does papaya.

Plum. Plums contain a bit of carotenoids and some vitamin C. There are many varieties from which to choose.

Prunes. Prunes get an honorable mention on our "Top Ten Fruits" list because they contain at least some of many different important vitamins and minerals. Compared with other fruits, prunes are especially high in fiber (half of it the soluble type), protein, potassium, vitamin A, vitamin E, calcium, and iron. They contain a touch of zinc and

---

NUTRITIP
Skin Deep

Much of the fiber in fruit is in the skin, especially when it comes to apples, pears, peaches, and nectarines. To get the full benefit of fiber, wash the fruit well and then eat the fruit whole — with the skin.

niacin, and some prunes even contain a bit of beta carotene. Prunes are known for their ability to move the intestines, thanks to their high fiber content and large amounts of the stool-loosening sugar sorbitol.

Raisins. This favorite snack food is high in fiber and iron but also high in calories and sugar. You can get the iron and fiber at a lower caloric cost in other fruits.

Raspberries. Of all the fruits, raspberries pack the most fiber into the fewest calories. They're also higher in folic acid and zinc than most fruits. It is difficult to wash raspberries thoroughly, making pesticides a concern.

Strawberries. Strawberries have two nutritional claims to fame: They are higher in vitamin C per calorie than any other fruit and they are high in fiber. Like raspberries, strawberries lose points be-cause of the pesticide issue. You don't peel them, and because of their rough texture, they are hard to clean. Only organic strawberries make it onto our "Top Ten Fruits" list.

Tangerine. This member of the orange family contains much less vitamin C, folate, and fiber than an orange, but more vitamin A and carotenoids.

Watermelon. Watermelon is the top fruit source of the carotenoid antioxidant lycopene.

RANKING FRUITS

How you rank fruit depends upon the reason you're eating the fruit and your individual tastes. The four most valuable nutrients in fruits are fiber, vitamin C, carotenoids (e.g., beta carotene), and phytonutrients (health-building substances).

BERRY GOOD

Colorful berries (blueberries and blackberries) are full of phytonutrients, which contain powerful antioxidants called "anthocyanins" (from the Greek for "dark blue flower") and other cancer fighters. Blueberries are a prime example of our color rule: The deeper the color, the better the berry. Similar antioxidants are found in other reddish-purple fruits and vegetables, such as cherries, red cabbage, and plums. These are the type of antioxidants that are responsible for the much-touted heart-healthy effect of red wine. (You could probably get the same health benefits from munching on red grapes.) Blueberries have the highest antioxidant capacity of all fruits, mainly because of the high level of anthocyanins in their skin. But all blueberries are not created equal. The smaller, wild blueberries have more skin and less water than the plump, cultivated blueberries. Because most of the health-promoting pigment is in the skin, the smaller the berry, the more anthocyanins, so when it comes to these blue benefits, bigger is not better. Bilberries, which resemble blueberries, have anthocyanins in their flesh as well as in their skin. Blueberries are great in pancakes, muffins, on cereal, and blended into smoothies (see "School-Ade," page 309). The health properties of these often underrated berries are well worth the stain you may get on your fingers.

Here are our rankings — an overall "Top Ten Fruits" list and, on page 152, our top choices for fiber and vitamin C.

Top Ten Fruits

Our top ten ranking of fruits is based upon their content of these nutrients: vitamin C, fiber, carotenoids, calcium, and folic acid. Availability, safety, and versatility also influenced these choices.

1. avocado
2. papaya
3. guava
4. cantaloupe
5. orange
6. apricots (dried, unsulfured)
7. mango
8. strawberries (organic)
9. kiwi
10. grapefruit (pink or red)

TOP TEN FIBER-RICH FRUITS

Fruit	Calories	Grams of Fiber per 100 calories*
1. Raspberries, 1 cup	60	8.0
2. Blackberries, 1 cup	74	7.6
3. Strawberries, 1 cup	45	3.4
4. Prunes, ½ cup, cooked	113	7.0
5. Papaya, 1 medium	118	5.5
6. Orange, 1 medium	50	3.0
7. Apple, 1 medium	81	3.7
8. Pear, 1 medium	98	4.0
9. Figs, dried, 5	237	8.5
10. Avocado, half	150	4.0

Rankings are based on grams of fiber per 100 calories, not on fiber per ounce of fruit.

TOP SEVEN VITAMIN C–CONTAINING FRUITS

Fruit	Calories	Milligrams of Vitamin C
1. Guava, 1 medium*	46	165
2. Papaya, 1 cup, cubed	55	87
3. Strawberries, 1 cup	45	84
4. Kiwi, 1 medium	46	74
5. Cantaloupe, 1 cup	56	68
6. Orange, 1 medium	60	75
7. Grapefruit, half	39	42

Guava is actually a top source of fiber and other nutrients, but the raw fruit is not readily available in U.S. supermarkets.

15

Juice and Juicing

KIDS LOVE JUICE, and it is a healthy source of nutrients. But too much juice can be unhealthy for children. Here's what families should know about the wise use of juice and its abuse.

FACTS ABOUT JUICE

When choosing juice for your children, what you serve, how much you offer, how you prepare it, and how you store it all have implications for their nutrition and growth. Keep these nutrition facts in mind:

- Be label savvy. Buy juice that is labeled "100 percent fruit juice." Avoid the stuff we call "junk juice." Juice "drinks," "cocktails," and "punches" contain relatively little juice, and usually are nothing more than a small amount of juice and a great deal of added sugar and corn syrup and water. Yet they can cost as much as real fruit juice. Instead of buying diluted juice with sugar water, buy the real thing and dilute it with plain or carbonated water.

- The vitamin C content of juices depends upon preparation and packaging. Freshly squeezed juice contains more vitamin C than "made from concentrate" canned or frozen juices. The vitamin C content of canned juices deteriorates upon exposure to air. To preserve the vitamin C content of juice, refrigerate and tightly seal opened containers.

- Orange juice is one of the most nutritious juices for many reasons: It contains more vitamin C than other juices, and it contains cancer-fighting phytochemicals called "flavonoids." Compared with apple juice, orange juice is

---

NUTRITIP
Natural Juice

To be labeled "natural," the FDA requires only that the food contain no artificial sweeteners, preservatives, or colorings. A juice drink can be touted as "natural" even if it contains added white sugar or corn syrup, or if it was extracted using chemical methods. Ignore the big type on the front of the package and look at the small print in the list of ingredients. It should say "100 percent juice" in order to be truly natural. Most fruit "drinks," "cocktails," and "punches" are not natural juices.

RANKING JUICES

We've ranked the following juices on the basis of nutrients per volume, also taking into consideration the calorie content of the juice:*

Juice	Comment
1. Carrot	Highest in vitamin A
2. Tomato	Most nutrient-dense juice per calorie; downgraded to number 2 because of high sodium content
3. Apricot nectar	High in vitamin A, and also contains a bit of iron and zinc; avoid brands with added corn syrup
4. Prune	Highest in iron, zinc, fiber, and niacin
5. Orange	Highest in vitamin C
6. Grapefruit	Second highest in vitamin C
7. White grape juice	High in vitamin C. Most intestines-friendly, best juice for healing the intestines
8. Apple	No nutritional advantage over other juices; good for flavoring water because it dilutes well

Juice blends are not rated.

higher in protein, vitamin A, B vitamins, vitamin C (it contains over ten times as much), calcium, iron, and potassium. Because orange juice contains equal amounts of fructose and glucose and no sorbitol, it is also less likely to cause diarrhea than apple juice.

• During diarrheal illnesses, use intestines-friendly juices to keep a child's fluid intake high. White grape juice is the best juice to offer a child with a diarrheal illness because it is better absorbed and contains equal amounts of fructose and glucose and no sorbitol. Juices with a high ratio of fructose to glucose and that contain sorbitol (e.g., prune, pear, and apple, in that order) can aggravate diarrhea, especially in intestines made sensitive by irritation or infection. The higher the fructose-to-glucose ratio, the more likely the excess fructose will be fermented in the large intestine, contributing to diarrhea or abdominal pain. Sorbitol is a nonabsorbable sugar that naturally occurs in prune, pear, cherry, peach, and apple juice. For this reason, the American Academy of Pediatrics' Committee on Nutrition discourages the use of these juices during diarrhea-producing illnesses. Citrus juices and others (pineapple, strawberry, raspberry, blackberry, and white grape juice) do not contain sorbitol. These juices also tend to have equal parts of glucose and fructose, and are thus more intestines-friendly. Drinking too much (more than 12 ounces a day) apple or pear juice or their nectars can be a cause of chronic diarrhea. Infants and young children, because their immature intestines allow more unabsorbed sugar to reach the colon, where it ferments, are particularly prone to gas and diarrhea from excessive juice.

- High-fructose corn syrups added to drinks can aggravate intestinal malabsorption, especially in those juices that already have a high fructose-to-glucose ratio. Shun those juices to which high-fructose corn syrup has been added, especially during episodes of diarrhea.

- As a refreshing alternative to juice, drink nectar, which is more nutritious. Generally, the thicker the juice, the more nutritious it is. Apricot nectar is especially healthy, since it contains a lot of beta carotene and almost 1 gram of protein per 8 ounces and is higher than apple or orange juice in vitamin A, vitamin B-6, and iron.

- Prune juice retains more of the nutrients from the whole prune than the juice made from other fruits. It is the only juice that is a concentrated source of iron (3 milligrams per cup) and is higher than apple or orange juice in protein, fiber, vitamin A, beta carotene, niacin, calcium, iron, potassium, and zinc. It is also relatively

---

NUTRITIP
Show Me the Juice.

Generally, the cloudier the juice, the more nutritious it is. If you can see through it, you're buying mostly water. There should be some sediment at the bottom, a reminder of the juice's origins.

---

high in calories (double the calories of apple juice). While prune juice is one of the most nutritious juices, it can be hard on the intestines because it contains large amounts of sorbitol. This is what accounts for its laxative effect. Drink prune juice in small, frequent portions — adults, no more than 4 ounces at a time.

- Vegetable juices tend to be more nutrient dense than fruit juices, meaning they pack more nutrition into every calorie. Carrot juice, for example, contains around the same number of calories as common fruit juices but is much higher in pro-

---

BEGINNER JUICE

When, what, and how much juice to give your infant depends a lot on your feeding philosophy and your infant's individual taste. Here are some healthy starter tips:

When? Resist the juice temptation until your infant is at least six months of age, preferably nine months. Introduce juice when your infant is able to drink from a cup. Juice doesn't contain any nutrients that your baby won't get more of from breast milk or formula. Consider juice as a delivery system for extra water, which your baby needs once she is eating solid foods, since extra water helps baby's kidneys handle the extra salt from solids.

What? White grape juice is the most intestines-friendly juice, since it is better absorbed and the sugar profile is easier on growing intestines.

How much? Best not to exceed these amounts:

- 6 to 12 months: 4 ounces per day
- 1 to 4 years: 6 ounces per day
- 4 to 12 years: 8 ounces per day

To avoid filling your child up with juice and displacing more valuable calories, dilute the juice at least with an equal amount of water.

tein, fiber, vitamin A, beta carotene, many other vitamins, iron, and zinc. Tomato juice contains less than half the calories of apple or orange juice, but it is higher than apple or orange juice in protein, most vitamins, iron, potassium, and many of the important amino acids. The bad nutritional news about tomato juice is that it is overloaded with sodium (around 1,000 milligrams per 8 ounces). Try to buy a low-sodium variety. Because of the sweeter taste, children tend to prefer fruit juice to vegetable juice. This is one reason for getting children hooked on the taste of vegetables in early infancy — so they learn to accept a variety of flavors, not just sweet fruits and juices.

MAKING YOUR OWN JUICE

Fresh foods are more nutritious than packaged foods, and this is especially true of juices. A lot can happen to valuable nutrients as fruit travels from the tree to a package on the grocery store shelf. The fruit is juiced at a processing plant, and the water is removed to make a concentrate, which is shipped to another manufacturer, who may put water back into the juice (water that may be more or less safe than the water Mother Nature originally put in the fruit). The juice is pressure-pasteurized to kill any bacteria in it, and then it travels to the store, where it sits on the shelf in one of several kinds of container with varying degrees of air-tightness. Throughout all these steps, vital nutrients, such as vitamins and enzymes, deteriorate. Also, much of the nutritious part of the fruit is right under the skin, the skin itself, or in the pulp. These parts of the fruit, as well as much of the fiber, are lost in commercial juicing.

Juice manufacturers are more interested in making their product economical and safe than nutritious. To prolong shelf life, preservatives may be added, chemicals that the government has cate-

---

THE JUICE-OBESITY CONNECTION

Drink your juice — but not too much! Studies have shown that children two to five years of age who habitually drink 12 ounces or more of fruit juice a day have a greater chance of being short and obese than children who consume less juice. Excessive fruit juice consumption can malnourish a child enough to interfere with growth for two reasons. First, fruit juice is not a nutrient-dense food. Most fruit juices contain nearly as many calories per ounce as low-fat milk. But nearly all of the calories in juice come from carbohydrates, so juice is not, by itself, a source of balanced nutrition. Children who drink large amounts of juice consume a lot of calories that take the place of calories from more nutrient-dense foods, such as those containing protein, minerals, and healthy fats. Studies have shown that the more juice children drink, the less milk they consume. Juice drinkers simply substitute juice for more nutritious foods. The second reason that juice can interfere with growth is that the high fructose and sorbitol content of some juices (e.g., pear and apple) can lead to chronic diarrhea and diminished absorption of vital nutrients.

You can avoid malnutrition by limiting your child's juice consumption to less than 12 ounces a day and diluting the juice your child consumes with at least equal parts of water. Offer your children water instead of juice when they are thirsty. Children have a natural sweet tooth and will prefer juice to water unless they are discouraged from doing so. Get your children in the habit of drinking water as a thirst quencher or, as a second choice, diluted juice.

gorized as safe. This means that the substance in question has been tested by feeding a bunch of the stuff to rats. If an acceptable percentage of the rats don't die or get sick, and over many years humans aren't apparently harmed by it, the chemicals are "generally recognized as safe," or GRAS. The testing agencies hedge by saying "generally." The truth is, they do not know for certain, since subtle and long-term harmful effects in humans cannot be detected by these testing methods.

There are two easy methods for making your own juice: juicing and blending.

Juicing

Millions of people own a juicer, yet these expensive appliances sit tucked away in pantries because busy people don't have the time or energy to use them. Once you realize the health benefits of juicing, however, you may be more willing to make the effort.

Proponents of juicing tout the nutritional efficiency of consuming juice versus eating raw fruits and vegetables. They claim that the process of juicing separates out the fiber, which concentrates the other nutrients in the juice, and that the absence of fiber in the juice increases the intestinal absorption of the nutrients from fruits and vegetables, so that more can get into the bloodstream. Specifically, the benefits of fresh juicing over commercial juices include the following:

- *The preservation of live enzymes in the food.* Live enzymes are often killed in commercial processing, especially during heat processing.

- *Safer water content.* The water in fruits and vegetables grown organically will be safer than those grown with chemical pesticides and fertilizers. Also at issue is the safety of the water used by manufacturers to reconstitute concentrated juice.

- *Convenience.* While drinking juice is not exactly the same as eating fruits and vegetables (the

fiber content is altered during juicing), it is certainly easier to drink an 8-ounce glass of juice than it is to eat the bunch of vegetables it took to make that juice.

When you make your juice at home, you know what goes into the final product. You can select the type of fruits or vegetables you want to juice. You can choose high-quality produce, organically grown if you wish. You can even pick vine-ripened fruits and vegetables yourself. You have no say, no knowledge, about the quality of juice in a can or carton.

Juicing Tips

- While the peels and skin of most fruits and vegetables are packed with nutrition, they may not always be safe. It's best to peel nonorganic imported produce.

- When peeling citrus fruits, such as oranges and grapefruit, leave on the white pithy part beneath the peel, since it contains nutritious bioflavonoids.

- Remove the peels of any waxed fruit or vegetable.

- In general, remove the pits before juicing. Because apple seeds can contain cyanide, they should absolutely be removed before juicing. Lemon, lime, melon, and grape seeds can be left in.

- As you're getting used to fresh juice, drink it slowly. Bolting down too much juice too fast may give you indigestion, since your intestines may not be used to such a concentrated package of fresh stuff. Drink juice slowly and in small, frequent portions to let your intestines get used to the new juice and allow time for the digestive juices to dilute and process it.

JUICE ABUSE

Not only is excessive juice not healthy for growing intestines, it's not good for growing teeth. Don't let toddlers walk around with a baby bottle filled with juice. Excessive juice consumption is a cause of malnutrition (see "The Juice-Obesity Connection," page 156). It can also cause tooth decay. Don't put your baby or toddler down to sleep sucking on a bottle of juice (or formula). When a baby falls asleep, saliva production and the natural rinsing action of the saliva slow down, allowing the sugary juice to bathe the teeth all night and contribute to bacterial growth, plaque, and eventual decay, a condition called "juice bottle syndrome." If your infant is hooked on the nighttime juice bottle, remove the bottle promptly as soon as baby falls asleep and brush his teeth as soon as he awakens in the morning. Dilute the juice with more and more water each night until baby gets used to all water and no juice — a technique we call "watering down."

NUTRITIP
Nicer Facts About Nectars

For a few extra calories, nectar is more nutritious than juice because more of the nutrients, especially fiber, have been preserved in the processing. Apricot nectar and the nectar of the three P fruits (peach, pear, and prune) are particularly nutritious.

NUTRITIP
Clean Juice

Commercial juices that are not pasteurized are required to say so on the label. This new law is a result of recent juice-borne bacterial illnesses that are especially harmful to immunocompromised persons. The new high-pressure pasteurization method increases the shelf life and significantly reduces the bacteria count, but it is reported not to affect the flavor or vitamin and mineral content of the juice.

Blending

Blending is nutritionally superior to juicing. With juice extractors (juicers), you do just that — extract the fluid from the pulp. Yet there is a lot of nutrition and fiber that goes down the drain with the wasted pulp. Blenders blend the fluid and pulp into a drinkable liquid. Despite what juicer makers claim, common sense tells us that the whole food must be more nutritious than a few of its parts. And studies on the discarded pulp from juice extractors confirm this suspicion: Much of the nutrients and juice remains in the discarded pulp.

Add to this nutritional benefit the energy-saving fact of kitchen life that a blender container can be cleaned in a few minutes, while disassembling, cleaning, and reassembling a juicer takes at least ten tedious minutes. The Sears family kitchen contains both a blender and a juicer. The blender gets used daily for healthy smoothies, soups, and frozen treats; the juicer gets used probably once a month. Nearly all fruits, especially high-water-content fruits such as strawberries and blueberries, blend easily in a blender. Because we have a lot of tummies to fill during morning rush hour, we make a half gallon of smoothies with our blender on school-day mornings. Fibrous foods, such as carrots and green, leafy vegetables, do better in a juicer. We use our blender for smoothies and our juicer to make carrot juice and beet green juice (a juice that tastes so earthy, you know it's got to be good for you).

16

Value Your Vegetables

YOUR MOTHER ALWAYS SAID, "Eat your vegetables," and, after devouring this chapter, you'll agree she was right — maybe in more ways than she knew. While you don't have to go whole veggie and become a strict vegetarian, one of the healthiest eating habits you can foster in your family is to make vegetables the centerpiece of your meals and let the other food groups accompany them. For many families this may be a switch of mind-set from MEAT and potatoes to POTATOES and meat. The animal food is more of a garnish, adding flavor and nutrition to the medley of vegetables and grains. A stir-fry is a good example. (Even better would be a combination of fish and vegetables.) If you aren't ready to relegate steak and meatloaf to second place, at least make vegetables equal stars in the meal. With interesting and tasty vegetable dishes on the table (and also a variety of starches), your family will gradually begin eating less meat.

SEVEN REASONS WHY VEGGIES ARE SO GOOD FOR YOU

Yes, you've been told all your life that vegetables are good for you. Perhaps you heard this so often that it's actually lessened the appeal. Eating vegetarian used to be considered healthy because of the bad stuff (e.g., saturated fats) vegetables didn't contain. New research is showing vegetables are healthy also because of the good stuff they contain. It really is true, but don't let all these nutritional advantages stand in the way of your eating pleasure.

1. Vegetables are nutrient dense. Vegetables pack a lot of nutrition into a minimum of calories. For a measly 35 calories (the amount in 1 little tea-

---

LOVE THOSE SWEET POTATOES

A good source of protein, fiber, beta carotene, vitamin C, folate, and calcium, sweet potatoes are a nutritious and tasty family food and merit a place in the "Top Twelve Foods" list (see page 107). Contrary to their name, sweet potatoes are not botanically a potato, but rather a root. Though white potatoes contain much more niacin, sweet potatoes are overall more nutritious: They are lower in carbs and higher in fiber, beta carotene, folic acid, and calcium. Like potatoes, sweet potatoes are best stored in a cool, dry pantry. If refrigerated, they lose their taste.

MONKEY SEE, MONKEY EAT

A nutritional perk that is a boon for busy parents and picky little eaters is the fact that if your child dislikes one food, chances are she has other favorites that contain the same nutrients. This perk is called "crossover." Fruits, grains, and dairy products will provide your child with everything a vegetable does except for the cancer-fighting phytos found mostly in vegetables. (Phytonutrients fight mostly against adult diseases anyway.)

Surveys have shown that children who eat a lot of fruits and vegetables when they are young tend to continue this eating habit when they're adults. But how do you get your children to eat vegetables? Eat them yourself. The more vegetables the adults in the family eat, the more the children are likely to eat. As they say, monkey see, monkey eat. And remember, tastes change with age — children who turned down vegetables as babies may eat them when they're toddlers. Keep offering, but don't force the vegetables. If baby refuses squash at six months, offer it again at nine months. Use modeling, not bribery or threats, to get your child to eat vegetables. Good eating habits, like good sleeping habits, can't be forced on a child. The best you can do is create a healthy eating attitude in your home and let your child catch the spirit. Your job is to serve and eat lots of vegetables, be excited about them, prepare them in a variety of appealing ways, and dress them up to have kid appeal. The rest is up to your child.

---

spoon of butter), you can get a half cup of vegetables that contains a wide variety of vitamins, minerals, and health-building substances called "phytonutrients" (see Chapter 36) — not to mention a lot of flavor. Load up on legumes (the family of beans, peas, and lentils). Second only to soy, legumes are the best plant source of proteins, fiber, and iron, in addition to being high in folic acid.

2. Veggies are a dieter's best partner. Vegetables get top billing on any fat-control diet because most are "free foods," meaning, you can eat an unlimited amount without having to count the calories. Why this indulgence? Because of the neat little biochemical quirk that only veggies enjoy: The body uses almost as many calories to digest vegetables as there are in vegetables in the first place. You'll use up most of the 26 calories in a tomato just by chewing, swallowing, and digesting it. The leftover calories don't even have a fighting chance of being stored in a fat cell. You'd have to eat entire platefuls of most vegetables before the calories begin to add up.

3. You can fill up for less. Because of the fiber in vegetables, you get fuller faster, which is another reason that it's nearly impossible to overeat veggies.

4. Vegetables are fat free and cholesterol free. All vegetables by definition are cholesterol free and, for all practical purposes, fat free. Over 95 percent of vegetables contain less than 1 gram of fat per serving, and even that insignificant gram is mostly unsaturated fats.

5. Variety, variety, variety. Let's face it, diversity makes life interesting. Adults, at least, like different foods prepared in different ways. There are dozens of kinds of vegetables available and many more ways to prepare them.

TERRIFIC TOMATOES

Tomatoes make the "Top Twelve Foods" list, not only for their nutritional qualities, which are many, but because they are so versatile and they're a kid favorite in ketchup and spaghetti and pizza sauce. While some green veggies rate higher on paper than red tomatoes, try getting any kale into kids. Here's why tomatoes are tops:

Like that lycopene. The very nutrient that makes tomatoes red — lycopene — is also a top antioxidant. Even though beta carotene gets all the press as a health food, the most powerful cancer-fighting carotenoid is really lycopene. Lycopene delivers twice the antioxidant power of another top antioxidant, vitamin E. Yet you'd have to eat a hundred times as many calories in vitamin E–containing foods to get the antioxidant power that's in one tomato. Even though lycopene can help lower the risk of all cancers, research to date shows that tomato-based foods are most effective in lowering the risk of prostate cancer.

Tomatoes are usually picked when green, and as they ripen off the vine in transit to your home, they make more lycopene as they get riper and redder. While lycopene is found most abundantly in tomato products, it is also found in guava, watermelon, and pink grapefruit. Tomato processing concentrates the amount of lycopene in the final product. The body absorbs more lycopene from tomatoes when they are cooked into sauce, paste, and salsa, and the lycopene in canned tomatoes is even better absorbed than in raw ones. (This is one of the few foods we can do something to to improve upon nature.) For salad lovers, an additional nutriperk is that a little oil eaten with the tomato pulls more of the lycopene out of the tomato and into the bloodstream. Cancer researchers believe that this combination is one of the reasons why people on a typical Mediterranean diet, which combines tomato products with olive oil, have one of the lowest rates of intestinal cancer and one of the longest lifespans.

Tomatoes are one of nature's most nutrient-dense foods. Tomatoes are reported to contain around four thousand phytonutrients, plant chemicals that pack powerful health properties. In addition to packing a powerful antioxidant profile, a tomato stores a lot of other good stuff in those pithy 26 calories, such as half a gram of fiber, 25 percent of the DV for vitamin A, 1 gram of protein, a bit of vitamin B-6, riboflavin, and niacin, almost half the DV for vitamin C (high among veggies), and even a pinch of the minerals zinc, iron, magnesium, manganese, and copper. It is even low in sodium and high in potassium, which is just what your body needs.

Tomato terms you should know (or may be curious about): Tomato puree is concentrated tomato juice and tomato pulp. If the tomato puree is seasoned, it's called *tomato sauce*. If the puree is superconcentrated, it is known as *tomato paste*, which is even a richer source of such nutrients as beta carotene and iron. *Sun-dried tomatoes* are dehydrated tomatoes. They are sometimes packed in olive oil, both to preserve them and to enrich their flavor.

6. Vegetables provide complex carbohydrates. The energy in vegetables is in the form of complex carbohydrates. These take some time to digest and don't cause the blood-sugar highs and lows that sugars do. (An exception is the sugar in beets or corn, which does have a high glycemic index and triggers the insulin cycle.)

7. Vegetables contain cancer-fighting phytos. On paper, a nutrient analysis of vegetables may not look all that special. Sure, there are lots of nutrients in vegetables, but most of these can also be found in other foods, such as fruits and grains. What you don't see in the nutrition charts or on the package labels are the hundreds of valuable nutrients called "phytochemicals" found in plants, which have as yet untold health-promoting properties. New research, especially in the field of cancer, is showing that vegetables are nature's best health foods (see Chapter 36).

TOP TEN VEGGIES

Taking into consideration the following factors — protein, fiber, beta carotene, vitamin C, B vitamins, folate, calcium, zinc, iron, and phytonutrients — here are our top ten veggies in alphabetical order:

Artichokes
Beans (kidney and black)
Beet greens
Broccoli
Chickpeas
Lentils
Spinach
Sweet potatoes
Tofu
Tomatoes

Honorable mentions: kale, sweet peppers, chili peppers, pumpkin.

TOP FIBER VEGGIES

Artichoke (1 medium)	16	grams
Beans, black, kidney, lima (½ cup)	5–8	grams
Lentils (½ cup)	8	grams
Chickpeas (½ cup)	5.3	grams
Pumpkin (½ cup)	3.5	grams
Peas (½ cup)	3.5	grams
Sweet potatoes (½ cup)	3.4	grams

DV

Children: 10 grams   Adults: 25 grams

There are as many ways to rank vegetables as there are reasons to eat them. See the boxes throughout this chapter for vegetables to eat when you're looking for particular nutrients (e.g., iron, protein, folic acid, etc.).

GROWING YOUR OWN GARDEN

Want to have some family fun — and teach your children about food, nature, hard work, and responsibility at the same time? Plant a family garden. While parents are, naturally, the overseers, children can feel that this is primarily their proj-ect. They take responsibility for the planting and the care, with a little parental guidance. Of course, they get first pickings in eating the fruits of their labors. Garden growing gives children a sense of responsibility and the pride of ownership, and they learn valuable lessons about how sun, water, seeds, and soil come together to make food. The big payoff is that kids are more likely to eat the veggies they grow. Our little 6 x 20-foot garden has rewarded us with not only hours of family fun but also produce we can trust. Here are some home-gardening tips to help you get started:

- Ask neighbors who have a garden what grows best in your part of the country and when to plant it. Or go to a garden store in your community for advice. The store personnel can tell you what you need to get your garden going, including tips on soil preparation, gardening tools, seeds, plants, gardening books, and main-tenance.

- Select an area in your yard that gets a lot of sun.

- Choose fruits and vegetables that will grow well under the conditions you have and that you most like to eat. Because children are impatient, choose at least some vegetables that grow big and fast. For our family, it's zucchini, which can

NUTRITIP
Red Hot Chili Peppers

Take the heat; it's worth it. Recent research shows that the same chemical that flames your throat, capsaicin, is also a potent anti-cancer phyto. Also, chili peppers are near the top of the list of vitamin C–containing vegetables. Prefer sweet peppers? Sweet peppers are an even better source of vitamin C.

TOP BETA CAROTENE (VITAMIN A) VEGGIES

Sweet potatoes (1)	11.0 mg.
Pumpkin (½ cup)	1.8 mg.
Carrots (1)	4.4 mg.
Asparagus (½ cup)	2.5 mg.
Squash, winter (½ cup)	2.4 mg.
Beet greens (½ cup)	2.0 mg.
Kale (½ cup)	1.5 mg.

DV: 6 mg.

TOP VITAMIN C VEGGIES

Sweet peppers (½ large)	170 mg.
Chili peppers (1)	109 mg.
Brussels sprouts (½ cup)	48 mg.
Broccoli (½ cup)	41 mg.
Artichoke (1 medium)	30 mg.
Sweet potato (1)	28 mg.

Honorable mentions: Tomato, cauliflower, kale, and a potato all have between 20 and 25 mg. of vitamin C.

DV
Children: 50 mg.
Adults: 60 mg.

TOP FOLIC ACID VEGGIES

Artichoke (1 medium)	153 mg.
Asparagus (½ cup, 6 spears)	131 mg.
Lentils (½ cup)	118 mg.
Spinach (½ cup, canned)	105 mg.
Chickpeas (½ cup, canned)	80 mg.

DV
Children under 4: 200 mg.
Adults and children over 4: 400 mg.
Pregnant/lactating women: 800 mg.

399.) Put as much color in your garden as you can, such as red tomatoes and peppers, yellow squash and corn, and purple peppers. Pole beans are fun, too. They'll climb a trellis or fence, or you can lean some poles against each other for a leafy teepee.

• Make a maintenance chart and help your children keep track of when they planted each vegetable, when they have watered the garden, and when they have taken care of other garden

grow bigger than a child's arm almost overnight, it seems. The vines have big impressive leaves and get into everything. You can make great zucchini pancakes or even muffins — a real family treat! (See recipe, page

NUTRITERM
"Vine-Ripened"

This is more of a marketing term than a technical term. It's meant to refer to vegetables, such as tomatoes, that have been left to ripen longer on the vine and, therefore, contain more phytonutrients and more flavor. In fact, many fruits and vegetables produce a natural ripening gas, ethylene, that helps them ripen off the vine. Fruits and vegetables in produce markets are usually slightly underripe. You can speed up the ripening process at home by putting fruits in a paper bag. Add an apple if you really want to speed things up.

TOP CALCIUM VEGGIES

Tofu (½ cup, firm)	258 mg.
Spinach (½ cup, canned)	136 mg.
Artichoke (1 medium)	135 mg.
Rhubarb (½ cup, unsweetened)	133 mg.
Beet greens (½ cup)	82 mg.

Honorable mentions: Kale, beans, chickpeas, pumpkin, and sweet potatoes have 30 to 50 mg. per serving.

DV
Children: 800 mg.
Adults: 1,200 mg.

TOP ZINC VEGGIES

Tofu (½ cup, firm)	2.00 mg.
Artichoke (1 medium)	1.47 mg.
Chickpeas (½ cup, canned)	1.25 mg.
Beans, kidney, lima (½ cup)	0.75 mg.

DV
Children: 10 mg.
Adults: 15 mg.

TOP IRON VEGGIES

Tofu (½ cup, firm)	5–10 mg.
Artichoke (1 medium)	3.9 mg.
Lentils (½ cup, boiled)	3.2 mg.
Beans (½ cup, canned)	1.5–2.3 mg.

Honorable mentions: Beet greens, chickpeas, pumpkin, and spinach* (½ cup, canned) all have 1 to 2 mg. per serving.

DV†
Children: 10 mg.
Adults: 12–18 mg.

* *Greens, such as spinach, beet greens, and chard, and some legumes and vegetables contain substances called "inhibitors," such as polyphenols and phytates, that bind iron, thereby lowering its absorption. The figures above represent the amount of iron in the food, but because of these inhibitors, the amount that actually gets into the body may be much less than the amount on paper. The percentage of vegetable iron absorbed can be increased by eating iron enhancers along with a meal, such as meat and vitamin C–containing foods. For practical dietary purposes, this iron-binding problem is significant only if you eat that food alone. Eating foods such as spinach along with a variety of other foods, especially those containing vitamin C, compensates for the theoretical problem of iron binding. Yes, grandmother was scientifically correct when she said "Eat a variety of foods together at a meal."*

† *This represents the daily amount of dietary iron, not the amount of iron that needs to get into the body. These DV's are based upon foods of medium bioavailability, meaning that around 5 to 10 percent of the dietary iron will actually be absorbed into the body (more or less, depending on the self-regulating system of the body's total iron needs). The average child needs to get 1 milligram of iron into the bloodstream every day. So, for the child who eats 10 milligrams of dietary iron, a sufficient amount of 1 milligram of the iron should get into his body.*

tasks, such as weeding. This record keeping adds to their sense of responsibility. As they see the fruits of their labor, watch their pride sprout.

• Keep a garden book (like Thomas Jefferson did at Monticello). Keep track of what you plant and when from year to year, how much you harvest, what grows well, and what fails. Take photos of your children at work in the garden and with their harvest.

• Make first pickings a special occasion. When that first zucchini comes off the vine, make zucchini pancakes the main course. Make a special salad with the first tender lettuce in the spring.

• If your yard is not suitable for vegetable gardening, you can still plant a mini garden in pots, small and large. This works well for apartment dwellers, too. You can keep your garden on a patio, a balcony, or even the roof. Tomatoes and peppers grow well this way, as do herbs. Set a window box in a sunny kitchen or bedroom window. Your local garden shop can help you create a mini garden.

• Sprout some sprouts. Sprouts are kids' favorites, since you can plant a seed on Monday, and by the following Sunday the kids can already see their sprouts growing. Radish sprouts should be ready in a week.

• Beets are fun. The leaves (tasty steamed or raw) are more nutritious than the beetroot, with gobs of beta carotene and other phytonutrients. They're a healthy alternative to lettuce on sandwiches, but don't forget to remove the chewy purple stem. Of course, it's fun to discover the deep red beets under the ground, too.

TOP VITAMIN E VEGGIES

Tomato paste (½ cup)	5.6 mg.
Tomato puree (½ cup)	3.0 mg.
Tomato juice (1 cup)	2.0 mg.
Hummus (½ cup)	2.2 mg.
Swiss chard (½ cup)	1.6 mg.
Greens, mustard (½ cup)	1.4 mg.
Kohlrabi (½ cup)	1.4 mg.
Spinach (½ cup)	1.4 mg.
Pumpkin (½ cup)	1.3 mg.
Broccoli spears (½ cup)	1.0 mg.
Beans, kidney (½ cup)	0.5 mg.

DV
Children: 7 mg.
Adults: 10 mg.

- If you have several little gardeners, divide the garden into plots and let them name their plants (e.g., "Susie's squash," "Tommy's tomatoes").

- To have fun with your garden, let the children draw faces with a marker on the produce still

NUTRITIP
Crucifers Against Cancer

Taking their name from the Latin word for "cross" *(crux)* because their leaves are cross shaped, cruciferous vegetables include broccoli, cabbage, cauliflower, brussels sprouts, kale, and collards. Sometimes they're also known by their botanical name, *Brassica.* Because of the cancer-fighting chemicals they contain, especially when eaten raw, these vegetables are at the top of the list of anti-cancer vegetables in the anti-cancer diet (see Chapter 38).

NUTRITIP
Better Ketchup

If your child is a ketchup addict, as many children are, replace the highly sugared red stuff with a healthier brand that is lightly sweetened with fruit concentrates. At least you'll be getting more tomatoes than sugar. Even ketchups that are touting "no refined sugars" contain about an equal number of carbohydrates from added sweeteners, such as pear or apple juice concentrate, as from the tomatoes. Ketchup is a great vehicle for delivering other nutritious foods, though, such as a sauce for whole wheat pasta, and as a dip for veggies. So, a few added carbs are okay to sweeten the red stuff.

Also try *ketch-oil* for your ketchup addict. Mix a tablespoon of flax oil with 3 tablespoons of ketchup. Be sure to stir vigorously to mix the oil and ketchup. You can spread it on a sandwich or pour it into a bowl for dipping.

on the vine. As the pumpkins or zucchini grow, the eyes get bigger and the smiles get wider.

Will you save money by growing your own produce? It depends on what you grow and how much money you spend getting started. Even if your produce winds up costing more than what's available at the grocery store, the extra money is worth it. Gardens are great for kids. As they help the garden grow, the garden helps them grow, too.

COOKING AND SERVING VEGETABLES

Serve your family a wide variety of vegetables and from all different parts of the plant — roots, stems, leaves, and seeds. The leaves, or greens, of some vegetables, such as beets and turnips, are equally nutritious if not more so than the veggie itself. These greens are high in beta carotene, fiber, vitamin E, calcium, and iron, but they contain only around 25 calories per serving (without added butter or oil).

How a food is processed affects its nutritional quality. Generally, the less processing the better. In nutrient value, fresh is better than frozen, and frozen is better than canned. But there are many exceptions. Much depends upon the time between harvesting and freezing and canning. A vegetable that is frozen hours after harvesting may contain more vitamins than a fresh veggie that has had to travel across the country to market. There are various nutritional trade-offs when you choose packaged and processed vegetables. For example, canned and frozen vegetables contain more sodium. A serving of frozen broccoli may contain more beta carotene, since the stalks have been removed, leaving only the florets in the package, but it will have less calcium and more sodium. As often as possible, serve fresh vegetables to your family, so they get used to the more varied and intense flavors.

Steaming vegetables preserves a lot more of the nutrients and the fresh vegetable taste than boiling, which releases some valuable nutrients into the water. Microwaving also preserves the nutrients in veggies. Consult a reliable cookbook to avoid overcooking. Cover them tightly so they don't lose moisture. Perk up the flavor with seasonings other than salt and butter. Try lemon juice, onion juice, honey, dill, cinnamon, nutmeg, basil, curry powder, oregano, and garlic. A bit of olive oil, a sprinkling of sesame seeds, or grated cheese adds interest.

Savvy salad.

When you're creating a salad, remember that the darker the leaves, the more nutritious the salad. The paler the greens, the fewer nutrients there are. Spinach leaves are a much more nutritious alternative to iceberg lettuce. Romaine lettuce contains about three times the amount of folic acid as iceberg. Although most lettuces and salad greens are similar in their traces of B vitamins and minerals, there are some differences. Here's how salad greens rank from most nutritious to least: spinach, arugula, watercress, endive, romaine, bib, Boston, and iceberg.

17

Eating Vegetarian: Why and How?

ONCE UPON A TIME, a vegetarian might as well have been someone from another planet, so different was this eating pattern from that of the typical meat-devouring American. Now, with studies showing that vegetarians can expect to outlive their beef-eating critics, the veggie is in and the meatball is out. Perhaps tofu burgers and grilled eggplant will one day replace hamburgers on cook-out menus across the country. Here are some questions you might have if you are considering a vegetarian diet for yourself or your family.

What does a "vegetarian diet" mean?

The term "vegetarian" is really a misnomer, since vegetarians eat more than just vegetables. Vegetarian simply means a plant-based diet. There are several kinds of vegetarian diets, defined by what types of foods are consumed. A strict vegetarian, or *vegan,* avoids all foods of animal origin, including meat, poultry, fish, dairy products, and eggs. *Lacto-vegetarians* include dairy products in their diet. *Lacto-ovo-vegetarians* eat dairy products and eggs. *Pesco-vegetarians* eat fish, dairy products, and eggs along with plant foods. Finally, there are *semi-vegetarians,* who cheat a little and eat a little poultry along with fish, as well as dairy products and eggs. Most veggie lovers are not strict vegans.

After more than fifty years as an overconsumer of meat and an underconsumer of vegetables, I am now a pesco-vegetarian, which, I believe, is the healthiest diet for most people.

MEATLESS SUBS

If you are trying to wean your family off meat as a main course, do so gradually by preparing dishes that emphasize vegetables and grains but still include small amounts of beef or poultry. The meat becomes an accent, not the centerpiece of the meal. Or, make meatless dishes that look like they might have meat in them but really don't, such as these:

- stir-fried vegetables with tofu cubes
- tofu in spaghetti sauce over pasta
- meatless chili with textured vegetable protein (a "meaty" processed soy product)
- lasagne with eggplant and chunks of soy "sausage"
- garden burgers instead of beef burgers
- black bean burritos (black beans have an almost meaty texture)
- vegetable pizza with minced mushrooms, basil, tomato paste, garlic, and cheese

Is the vegetarian diet automatically the healthiest way to eat?

Yes and no. Yes, a vegetarian diet is excellent for good health when you follow the general rules of a nutritionally balanced diet and be sure you get the nutrients from vegetables that you miss by giving up animal foods. On the other hand, avoiding meat won't keep you healthy if instead you consume a lot of high-fat, nutrient-empty junk foods. Vegetarians must also have an otherwise healthy lifestyle to harvest the full benefits of their plant eating. It does little good to eat a tomato and sprout sandwich on whole wheat bread if you also plant yourself on the couch in front of the TV set and smoke cigarettes several hours a day. The vegetarian who piles on the chips soaked in hydrogenated oil and consumes high-fat cheese and artificially sweetened or highly sugared beverages would be better off nutritionally if he had less of a sweet tooth, cut down on fat, and allowed a little lean animal flesh.

What's so good about a vegetarian diet?

Vegetarian cuisine is naturally low in saturated fats, and foods of plant origin contain no cholesterol. Plant foods are also much higher in fiber than animal foods. Many plant foods contain significant amounts of the vital B vitamin folic acid, and fruits and vegetables are powerful sources of phytochemicals — nutrients that help every organ of the body work better. Also vegetarians tend to eat fewer calories, since grains, legumes, fruits, and vegetables, volume for volume, tend to be lower in calories than meat and poultry. Studies have shown that, as long as their diet is balanced and nutritious, people who consume fewer total daily calories live longer and healthier lives. Veggie lovers believe that foods from plant sources, which are lower on the food chain, are safer than animal foods, since pollutants tend to concentrate in fatty tissues. While raw fruits and vegetables can carry harmful bacteria and pesticide residues just like meat, you can remove many of these pollutants by washing the plant foods. Trimming the fat from meat or chicken is less effective. Meat, poultry, and seafood are also more frequent carriers of food-borne illnesses, such as salmonella, than plant sources. Finally, environmental conservationists believe that having more plant-based diets is healthier for the planet. It takes less energy and less farmland to feed a vegetarian than it does to feed livestock.

Are vegetarians really healthier in the long run?

Absolutely, positively yes! Even though nutritionists disagree on many topics, all agree that plant eaters and fish eaters tend to live longer and healthier lives than do animal eaters. In every way, the broccoli munchers tend to be healthier than the beef eaters. Vegetarians have a lower incidence of cancer, especially of the colon, stomach, mouth, esophagus, lung, prostate, bladder, and breast. The protection against intestinal cancers is probably due to the fiber in a plant-based diet. In fact, vegetarians have a lower incidence of nearly all intestinal diseases and discomforts, especially constipation and diverticulosis. The phytonutrients in plant foods, especially antioxidants,

---

NUTRITIP
Best Breast Milk Fats

Because studies show that breastfed infants of vegetarian mothers have lower blood levels of DHA than the breastfed infants of meat-eating mothers, vegetarian breastfeeding mothers should supplement their diet with either DHA supplements or flax oil. Eating cold-water fish (e.g., salmon and tuna) is another way to add DHA to your diet.

---

flavonoids, and carotenoids, may also contribute to protection against cancer.

Plant food is better for your heart, since it is low in cholesterol and saturated fat and high in fiber. Vegetarians have a lower incidence of cardiovascular disease, namely, heart attacks and stroke. A study of twenty-five thousand Seventh-Day Adventists showed that these vegetarians had one-third the risk of dying from cardiovascular disease than a comparable meat-eating population. Another study showed that incidence of death from cardiovascular disease was 50 percent less among vegetarians. These statistics may be the result of more than just diet; vegetarians tend to have healthier overall lifestyles. Plant eaters are much less likely to get diabetes than animal eaters. And vegetarians tend to see better. An eye disease called "macular degeneration," which is deterioration of the retina leading to blindness, occurs less frequently in vegetarians.

NUTRITIP
Veggie Tooth Care

The calorie-dense foods in vegetarian children's diets, such as nut butters and dried fruit, tend to stick to the teeth, requiring extra brushing and attention to dental hygiene.

Vegetarians tend to be leaner than meat eaters, even those meat eaters who skin their chicken and trim the fat off their steak. And, in general, leaner persons tend to be healthier. Being lean does not mean being skinny. It means having a low percentage of body fat. Muscular weight lifters tend to be lean, though no one would call them skinny. You don't have to "beef up" at the dinner table to make muscle. Even the U.S. Department of Agriculture's dietary guidelines (see the Food Guide Pyramid, page 112) recommend eating more vegetables and grains and less meat, despite pressure from the politically connected meat industry to promote meat.

Does it cost more or less to eat vegetarian?

Except for a few delicacies, pound for pound, plant foods tend to be a bargain. Of course, iceberg lettuce, sugary ketchup, and french fries — the typical fast-food fare — do not qualify as healthy, vegetarian foods, even though they are cheap.

I worry about getting enough iron. Aren't vegetarian diets low in iron?

Not necessarily. Some vegans we know seem to be so thin and pale that sometimes we just want to treat them to a 16-ounce sirloin. Yet studies have shown that vegetarians who eat a balanced diet don't seem to have any more iron-deficiency anemia than meat eaters. Even though the iron in plant foods is not as well absorbed as the iron in animal foods, vegetarians usually eat a higher volume of iron-containing foods. Also, many plant foods naturally contain vitamin C, which aids the absorption of the iron. You don't have to eat red meat to make red blood cells. (See Chapter 6, "Pumping Up Your Iron.")

Do vegetarian diets contain enough calcium?

Yes. Dairy products are still the easiest available source of calcium, and there are plenty of foods

BEST PLANT FOOD SOURCES OF IRON*

	Milligrams of Iron
Tofu (½ cup)	7
Iron-fortified cereals (1 ounce)	4–8
Cream of Wheat (½ cup cooked)	5
Blackstrap molasses (1 tbsp.)	3.5
Pumpkin seeds (2 tbsp.)	3
Lentils (½ cup cooked)	3
Prune juice (8 ounces)	3
Chickpeas (½ cup canned)	2
Swiss chard (½ cup)	2
Dried fruits: apricots, peaches (3 ounces)	2
Beans: black, kidney (½ cup)	2
Tomato paste (2 ounces)	2
Figs (5)	2
Jerusalem artichoke (½ cup raw)	2

The average adult woman needs around 15 milligrams of iron per day. Men and postmenopausal women need around 10 milligrams. Children and pregnant or lactating women need more.

NUTRITIP
Iron Binders

Coffee and tea lovers beware. Chemicals known as "polyphenols" in coffee and tea can lessen the absorption of iron in plant foods by up to 70 percent. If you're eating a vegetarian diet with marginal amounts of iron, avoid drinking coffee or tea within an hour and a half of eating iron-rich foods.

that are calcium rich that don't come from a cow. Since so many foods are now fortified with calcium, even vegans are likely to get their daily requirement of this important mineral. For best plant (nondairy) sources of calcium, see page 56.

Can vegetarian diets lead to some nutritional deficiencies?

Only vegans are at greater risk of deficiencies of some nutrients than meat eaters are. Lacto-ovo vegetarians and pesco-vegetarians (who also eat eggs and dairy products) are unlikely to suffer from nutrient deficiencies, as long as they have a balanced diet, since there are no essential nutrients in meat that are not also found in eggs, dairy, and fish. A vitamin B-12 deficiency (which can lead to loss of peripheral nerve function) is of concern for vegans, since animal foods are still the best source of vitamin B-12, and plant foods do not naturally contain B-12. Soy foods, such as some forms of tempeh, may contain vitamin B-12, but soy B-12 is not as biologically active as the vitamin B-12 in animal foods. Check the B-12 content of soy products on the package label. Vegans need to consume foods fortified with vitamin B-12, such as tempeh, cereals, or brewer's yeast, or take B-12 supplements.

Don't worry about suddenly developing a vitamin B-12 deficiency after becoming a vegan. The liver stores so much B-12 that it would take years to become deficient in this vitamin. However, vegan infants and children do not have such rich stores and are prone to vitamin B-12 deficiency unless they get supplements. Zinc deficiency is another possibility for vegans, but a deficiency of this mineral can be made up by eating grains, wheat germ, seeds, soy foods, and multimineral supplements.

VEGGIE RESOURCES

As more and more families pass by the meat counter and head for the produce section of the supermarket, there is a garden of vegetarian information out there just for the picking. Here's a brief sampling:

- "The Vegetarian Pages," at http://www.veg.org/veg/, an Internet guide for vegetarians. The site contains many resources (books, articles, organizations, etc.).
- *Vegetarian Times* magazine, 800-829-3340 or www.vegetariantimes.com
- *The Vegetarian Child: A Complete Guide for Parents,* by Lucy Moll (Perigree, 1997)
- *Vegetarian Voice,* the main publication of the North American Vegetarian Society, 518-568-7970 or http://www.cyberveg.org/navs/
- *Essential Vegetarian Cookbook,* by Diana Shaw (Clarkson Potter, 1997)
- For a referral to a dietitian specializing in vegetarian nutrition, contact the American Dietetic Association at 800-366-1655 or http://www.eatright.org/
- *Vegetarian Journal,* a bimonthly publication of the Vegetarian Resource Group, PO Box 1463, Baltimore MD 21203; 410-366-VEGE or http://www.vrg.org

Do vegetarians get enough protein?

It's a nutritional myth that you have to eat muscle to make muscle. Vegetarians who eat fish, dairy products, and/or eggs get plenty of protein, and even a strict vegan can get enough protein by eating enough grains and legumes, which provide a feeling of fullness along with the necessary quantity and quality of protein (see the discussion of complete and incomplete proteins, page 48). There's no need to worry about vegetarian chil-dren not getting enough protein. Each day, for example, preteens can get all the protein they need from an egg, a peanut butter sandwich, a couple of glasses of milk, a cup of yogurt, and a black bean burrito.

Do vegetarians get enough fat?

If you eat eggs, dairy products, and/or fish, you get enough fat. Plant-based food is thought to be deficient in fats, but actually the richest sources of the fats that are good for you — unsaturated fats and essential fatty acids — are plant foods, such

NUTRITIP
Good Grapes

Red wine has recently been touted as a health food because of studies showing a lower incidence of cardiovascular disease in cultures that drink a lot of red wine. Red wine may help to lower cholesterol. But the health properties are probably not in the alcohol but rather in the grapes. Grape skins contain resveratrol, a substance that can lower cholesterol and prevent fats in the bloodstream from sticking together and clogging arteries. Eating grapes, drinking dark grape juice that is made with skins, or eating raisins may be just as heart healthy as drinking wine, without the health hazards of alcohol.

NUTRITIP
Red Tomato Makes Red Blood Cells.

Ounce for ounce, tomato paste contains four times the amount of iron as tomato sauce.

as nuts, seeds, and oils. There is no essential fatty acid that can be found only in animal-based foods. Yet strict vegans must guard against deficiency of some essential fatty acids, especially DHA. Because vegetables provide no preformed DHA, some vegans take supplements of DHA, since some people are not able to convert the essential fatty acid ALA in food to DHA in their bodies. Some vegans may have low blood levels of DHA. Seafood is the only food source of preformed DHA, which is another reason we believe a seafood plus vegetarian diet is the most healthy for most people.

As a confirmed meat lover, how can I learn to like vegetable dishes? Don't vegetarians eat weird food?

You'll be amazed at the number and variety of foods — some familiar and some new — that can be a part of a vegetarian diet. Ethnic food is a wonderful source of flavorful, appealing vegetarian dishes. Try Middle Eastern, Greek, or Asian restaurants to learn about tasty vegetarian cooking. Spices accent the flavors of foods, and the

mixture of vegetables and grains adds fullness and crunchiness that can win over even the most confirmed meat eater. Italian restaurants have meatless pasta and other dishes on the menu. There are also many excellent vegetarian cookbooks available at the library or bookstore. You may find that you've been missing a lot as a meat lover.

Is it safe to feed children a vegetarian diet?

Yes, you can raise a healthy vegetarian. It's relatively easy if your child's diet includes eggs, fish, and dairy products. Raising a little vegan requires more planning and nutritional know-how to ensure that your child gets enough calcium, vitamin D, iron, vitamin B-12, and some of the other B vitamins. Children can grow normally on a diet of grains, legumes, and greens, but it's a bit risky. A

STEPS IN RAISING A LITTLE VEGETARIAN

Just as there are stages in a child's development of motor skills or cognitive abilities, there are developmental stages in eating habits. You can make the most impact on your child's eating habits if you respond to his development in age-appropriate ways.

Stage 1: Infancy. Program your baby to appreciate the tastes of fresh fruits and vegetables. Every baby starts out as a vegetarian, since meat is usually the last food group introduced to new eaters. Between five and nine months, babies can be introduced to a variety of grains, fruits, and vegetables, such as rice, bananas, pears, avocados, barley, sweet potatoes, carrots, squash, and mashed potatoes. Between nine and twelve months, introduce tofu. As a dairy alternative, get your one-year-old used to the taste of soy beverages.

Stage 2: Toddler years. Toddlers love to graze, so make a toddler nibble tray (see page 274) with bite-sized fruits and vegetables, together with a yogurt and avocado dip. Your toddler will learn to snack on fresh fruits and vegetables instead of packaged stuff. Meat is not necessary, as long as you use an iron-fortified cereal or formula or continue to breastfeed. (Alternative sources of iron are green, leafy vegetables, raisins, black-eyed peas, blackstrap molasses, and beans.) During the first three years you have a window of opportunity to shape young tastes. Your toddler learns what fresh fruits and veggies are supposed to taste like and accepts this as the normal family fare. (See the related discussion "Shaping Young Tastes," page 277.)

Stage 3: Preschool and school years. Plant a vegetable garden. Children are more likely to eat what they grow. Gardening gives you a chance to talk about good food. Talk about all the different colors in the garden and why it's so important to have a lot of color in the food on your plate at dinnertime. (For more on gardening, see page 163.)

Children can appreciate the concept of a rainbow lunch. Frequent restaurants that have large salad bars, planting in your child's fertile mind the idea that salad bars are a real treat: all you can eat of a great variety of multicolored and multitextured foods. Also, encourage your children to help in the kitchen. They can wash fruits and vegetables, tear up lettuce, stir, pour, knead bread dough, and serve and eat their creations proudly.

Sandwiches made with peanut butter or other nut butters on whole wheat bread, with healthy fruit preserves and sprouts are a new twist on a traditional favorite for school-age children. This is a time to emphasize fish (salmon and tuna) and flax oil for essential fatty acids. School-age children can also begin to read labels. Teach your child to avoid foods with "hydrogenated" in the ingredients list. Steer your child away from packaged snack foods, especially those with hydrogenated oils, and provide tasty and attractive alternatives in school lunches. If your family is semi-vegetarian, use meat as an accent in stir-fry or grain dishes, avoiding the usual picture of a steak in the middle of the plate with only a garnish of vegetables. Or serve fish, plus a substantial vegetable side dish. Older school-age children can also appreciate ethical and ecological issues associated with eating meat. To our older children we have cited the inhumane treatment of calves raised to produce veal as a good reason not to eat veal.

Stage 4: Teen years. Teens will dabble with junk food, but they won't overdose on it. Unlike children who have grown up with a junk-food diet as their nutritional norm, teens raised on a vegetarian diet are able to make the connection between eating well and feeling well. Salad bars, vegetarian pizzas, bean burritos, and fruit snacks are likely to be vegetarian favorites for teens. When they go into a fast-food restaurant, they are more likely to seek out the salad bar than the greasy stuff.

wise parent should seek periodic advice from a nutritionist experienced in vegan diets.

Protein is no problem, since children can get all the protein they need from plant foods only, especially whole grains, soy products, legumes, and nuts. Calcium may present a challenge, since traditional plant sources of calcium are not big favorites with children. (Good luck getting your child to eat kale and collards.) But many foods today are fortified with calcium, including calcium-fortified soy milk and orange juice, so a vegan child can get enough calcium without relying on supplements. Fortified foods, such as cereals and soy beverages, can also be a dietary source of vitamin B-12.

Getting enough calories may be another challenge in vegan diets. Veggies have a lot of nutrients per calorie, but not a lot of calories per cup. Tiny tummies fill up faster on lots of fiber but fewer calories. One way to overcome this problem is to encourage your child to graze on small, frequent feedings that include higher-calorie foods, such as peanut butter and other nut butter sandwiches, avocados, nuts and seeds (for children over four years of age, who can eat them safely), pasta, dried fruits, and smoothies (see pages 309 and 396 for recipes).

Vegetarian children should get the nutrients they need from foods rather than from pills, since pills don't provide calories, and the nutrients in foods, through the process of synergy, are better for the body. The growth of some vegan children may appear to be slower because vegetarian children, like vegetarian adults, tend to be leaner. A child's position on the growth chart is not an accurate measure of the state of his or her health; where a child fits on the chart is influenced more by genes than by diet.

Maintaining a vegetarian diet can be more challenging during periods in a person's life when there are extra nutritional needs, such as pregnancy, lactation, childhood, and adolescence. Once a person reaches adulthood, nutritional deficiencies are less of a concern. Even if your children do not remain vegetarians for life, by getting their little bodies accustomed to the taste and feel of a vegetarian diet, you have programmed them with a healthy eating pattern that will benefit them throughout life. Vegetarian children, because they get used to the comfortable after-dinner feeling of a vegetarian meal, tend to shun, or at least don't overdose on, junk meats, such as hot dogs and fast-food burgers. But don't expect your child to go meatless all his life. Give your children a vegetarian start and, as they grow away from your nest, let them decide what eating pattern they will follow. They may find reasons, such as concern for the environment, that keep them on the veggie track. Model your excitement about eating a wide variety of plant-based foods, serve them tastefully, and the rest is up to your child.

18

Favorite Fish

SUBSTITUTING FISH FOR MEAT is one of the best dietary changes you can make for your family. Downgrade meat as a daily main course and use it instead as an ingredient in other dishes, a way to enhance the flavor and nutrition of a stir-fry, pasta, or casserole. Upgrade fish as the centerpiece several meals a week, as salmon "steak" or tuna salad. Fish is a top-of-the-food-chain nutrient-dense food. It's low in fat and high in many good things. Here are just a few of the reasons to choose fish:

- Fish is a nutrient-dense source of protein — most varieties contain around 20 grams of protein per 3-ounce serving, the same as meat.

- Some fish are high in brain-building omega-3 fatty acids.

- Some fish are high in heart-friendly, cholesterol-lowering fish oils. Omega-3 fish oils have been linked to reducing total blood fats, reducing LDL (bad) cholesterol, and raising HDL (good) cholesterol.

- Fish is a good source of vitamin B-12.

- Most fish are rich sources of iron.

FISH FACTS

There are a lot of fish in the sea and a lot to choose from at the supermarket. Here are some facts to consider in selecting fish for your family meals.

The colder the water, the more nutritious and safer the fish. Cold-water fish, such as salmon and tuna, contain more of the omega-3 fatty acids DHA and EPA (see page 9) than fish from warmer waters do, such as catfish, red snapper, trout, and pike. As a general guide, the warmer the water, the lower the oil content of the fish. Ocean fish tend to be safer to eat than fresh-water fish, which are more likely to contain traces of environmental pollutants.

Fish is good heart food. Fish oils are good for the heart. They help prevent heart attacks and strokes by keeping the platelets, the saturated fatty acids, and cholesterol from sticking together and clogging the arteries. After all, fish fats are called "oils," meaning they *flow* rather than sit. One study showed that one serving of salmon per week cut the risk of heart attack in half. In another study, researchers who followed more than twenty thousand male physicians between forty and eighty-four years of age for eleven years found

FORGET FISH STICKS

It's so tempting to open the package of fish sticks, put them in the oven, and serve those convenient little pieces of fish that are grabbed by willing little fingers. After all, isn't fish good for children? Not necessarily. Fish sticks are obese with problems. They may be cheap, but they're the least nutritious way to eat fish. Oftentimes the type of fish used in fish sticks contains little of the brain-building and heart-healthy omega-3 fatty acids that children need. The breading and frying process adds hydrogenated fats and extra salt, undermining the nutritional value of the fish itself. Add to these the fact that children often dip fish sticks into sugary ketchup or tartar sauce, and you have a high-fat, nutrient-poor meal. Read fish stick labels carefully, and buy only those made from a nutritious type of fish with no added hydrogenated or saturated fats. Or make your own "fish fingers" by cutting salmon or tuna fillets into strips and breading them with a batter made of eggs and whole-grain flour.

NUTRITIP
Tasty Tuna Salad

When you're serving tuna steaks for the evening meal, prepare an extra one and use it for the next day's tuna salad. Add low-fat mayonnaise (or a soy-based substitute), sliced pickles, minced hard-boiled eggs, favorite seasonings, garlic, sunflower seeds (for children over four), a few tomato slices, and alfalfa sprouts on a whole wheat bun, and you've got a nutritious lunch to enjoy. (See page 397 for a recipe for tuna salad.)

that those who ate fish once a week were 52 percent less likely to die of cardiac arrhythmia (irregular heartbeats) than those who consumed fish less than once a month. The heart-friendly effects of fish oil seem to be related to their ability to lower total cholesterol, raise HDL (good) cholesterol, and lower LDL (bad) cholesterol.

Since fish fat actually seems to be good for people, might this cast some doubt on the conventional nutritional wisdom that a high-fat diet contributes to heart disease? It would probably be more accurate to say that the right fats contribute to heart health, the wrong fats to heart disease. As evidence look at the Eskimos, who have a diet very high in fat yet have lower levels of cardiovascular disease. Is this because they eat a lot of fish? (It may also be true that Eskimos have a genetically different way of metabolizing extra fats that protects their heart.) It is also true that most people who eat fish regularly have healthier lifestyles and diet in general.

Fish is good brain food. Not only is fish good for the heart, it's good for the head. Fish oils are healthy because they contain the two essential omega-3 fatty acids EPA and DHA, which are particularly valuable as nutrients for the cells of the brain and nervous system, the eyes, and the adrenal and sex glands. Come to think of it, those are the organs that help us think, see, and enjoy sex.

Fish food = good brain and heart food

FARM FISH VS. WILD FISH

Are wild fish from oceans and lakes more or less nutritious than farm-raised fish? Let's go fishing for some facts.

As health-conscious American consumers have turned from meat to fish, the demand for fish has outgrown the supply. Some waters have become

NUTRIMYTH

Shellfish are high in cholesterol. Actually, shellfish such as lobster and king crab contain no more cholesterol, and sometimes less, than the skinless white meat of chicken, and a bit less than lean beef (around 60 milligrams per 3-ounce serving). Shrimp, on the other hand, contains around 160 milligrams of cholesterol per 3-ounce serving — but this is probably more of a theoretical than an actual concern. Shellfish is actually one of the lowest-fat fish, especially lobster, which contains less than 1 gram of fat in 3 ounces, as does the much maligned shrimp. And, shellfish contain no saturated fats or hydrogenated fats, which are more likely to promote heart disease than the cholesterol in the diet.

THE FRESHER THE BETTER

If it smells fishy, it will probably taste fishy. The fishier a fish tastes or smells, the less fresh it is. The smell is due to a chemical called "trimethylamine," which is produced as the fish begins to spoil. Also, the mushier the fish feels, the older it is. Fresh fish should have a meaty texture and easily flake after a brief cooking. Unless you live near the source, you may find that the freshest fish you can buy is fish that has been shipped frozen. If you're buying fresh fish, plan on cooking it the same day you buy it.

less, shall we say, fishy. In some parts of the world, populations of certain kinds of fish have been depleted, and fish prices have jumped sky high. One solution to the supply problem is to grow fish in "farms," where conditions are controlled and ecological balances are not upset by overfishing. Fish on farms are raised in pens filled with water and are fed factory-made fish food. Fish farming has brought down prices for some kinds of fish and has made fish supplies steadier and more dependable.

However, a 1992 study comparing wild coho salmon, rainbow trout, and catfish with their farm-raised mates found that the farm-raised catfish had five times more fat and the salmon two and a half times more fat than the wild fish, with no significant difference in protein or vitamin content. Different conditions produce different fish, even within the same species.

Wild fish have these benefits on their side:

- a higher level of omega-3 fatty acids
- a lower level of total fat
- no chance of containing antibiotics
- perhaps fewer pesticides and environmental pollutants (in ocean, not necessarily in lake, fish)

Benefits of farm fish include these:

- lower cost
- more control over the purity of the water, so they may have a lower level of pollutants
- more control over flavor and quality (a farmer can cater to specific tastes — so-called designer fish)
- an ecological alternative to depleting fish populations in certain already overfished waters

The jury is still out on whether wild fish is healthier and safer than farm fish. So, it's back to using your common sense. Here's a tale of two fish — one from the oceans of Alaska, the other from the farms of Alabama. Both are salmon (our favorite fish).

The Alaskan salmon is spawned in a very fast-moving fresh stream, the source of which is usually the meltdown of tons of snow and ice. In order to survive, the baby salmon must fight the raging waters and make its way out to the sea, where she finds a healthy diet of seaweed. The seaweed is rich in brain-building fatty acids, which are known among fishermen as "nature's antifreeze," because they allow the seaweed to grow in such frigid waters. The little salmon becomes a big salmon and becomes even bigger by eating little fish that are also rich in omega-3

fatty acids. Over an average of four years, that salmon travels thousands of miles, spending winters in the warmer Pacific and summers in Alaska. The combination of a healthy diet and exercise builds a healthier fish, containing healthier oils. Once that little salmon becomes a big salmon, following one of nature's most fascinating, yet least understood, homing instincts, the fertile fish navigates back to her original birthplace and fights her way upstream past the raging waters to deposit her eggs and spawn more salmon. Soon after spawning, she dies. Any little fish that survives such a life cycle is one smart and healthy fish.

Contrast this natural fish cycle with the little salmon in the farm-fish tank. That fish doesn't have to battle predators and raging waters to survive. Nor does he have to swim much to search for food. The farm fish just has to swim and eat, the fish equivalent of a couch potato. So it stands to reason that the muscle and the oil in that fish will be chemically, and therefore nutritionally, different — sort of like the nutritional difference between free-range chickens (and their eggs) and caged birds. And the farm fish's food is chosen by the farmer instead of the fish, and it is unlikely that the fish farmer will buy expensive DHA-enriched fish food. The wild fish gets a healthier menu.

Fish just do not grow as fast in a pen as they do in the wild. (Keep a goldfish in a bowl, and it stays a tiny goldfish. Take that same fish and put him in a backyard fish pond, and that fish will grow.) This slow-to-grow fish will, however, be pushed to grow more quickly so he can go to market as soon as possible. Enter the fish-fattening chemists, who may give him fish-building steroids or other growth-boosting chemicals. Antibiotics may also be added to the feed to keep the fish healthy, and the water will be filtered to keep the fish cleaner. Clearly, this farm-raised fish will be different from the one that lived in the wild.

But deciding whether the wild fish is always the healthier fish is not so simple, especially because of pollutants and chemicals. For example, wild fish caught near the industrial areas of the Great Lakes may contain a lot more pollutants than closely monitored farm fish do. And fish caught in smaller lakes that collect agrochemical runoff may also have high levels of pollutants. On the other hand, high pesticide residues have been discovered in commercial fish foods, and farm fish may be raised in pens filled with the same polluted waters that are home to the wild fish. True, both farm fish and wild fish are "regulated and inspected," and the FDA routinely samples commercially caught and farmed fish for pesticide and hormone residues to see "if limits are exceeded," but not every fish that goes to market is inspected. And, who decides what is the "safe" or "tolerable" limit of pesticide, antibiotic, and hormone residues? There's much we don't know.

What's a health-conscious fish eater to do?

- *Consider the source.* Ask your fish market where the fish came from. Ocean fish tend to be cleaner and healthier than lake fish. Ditto that for cold-water fish versus warm-water fish. Cold-water fish, such as salmon and tuna, are more "oily."

- *Consider the package.* If the fish are from the farm, they must be labeled "farm fish." Yet, even the finest restaurants do not label farm fish. You have to ask. Restaurants may prefer to serve farm fish because customers prefer the higher fat levels and sometimes milder flavor. But most of the extra fat in farm fish is the heart-sparing unsaturated type.

- *Consider the price.* Wild fish are more expensive than farm fish, and it's likely to stay that way or get worse.

NUTRITIP
Fish for Omegas.

You can get omega-3 fatty acids from plant sources such as walnuts, flax oil, and canola oil. But seafood is the richest source of the most nutritious omega-3, DHA.

TUNA FISH FACTS

A good old-fashioned tuna fish sandwich is a favorite and nutritious food the world over. Canned tuna is the largest selling seafood in the United States. Because tuna fish is a favorite family food, here are some fish facts you should know about what's in the can.*

Canned tuna may contain one or several kinds of tuna, such as albacore, bluefin, yellowfin, and skipjack. These vary considerably in texture and flavor. Albacore, the most expensive, is the only one that can be labeled "white" under federal regulations. What you see on the label is not always what you get in the can. Government regulations allow canned tuna to contain up to 18 percent other stuff, such as casein and soy proteins, and sometimes sulfites. The labels on tuna fish cans don't list the amount of omega-3 fatty acids in the tuna, which is unfortunate, since this is one of the reasons to eat tuna in the first place. (Among popular cold-water fish, tuna ranks just below salmon in omega-3-fatty-acid content.) There are several reasons for this omission. The tuna fish inside the can may be a mixture of tunas of various quality,

---

* *If you're fishing for more seafood information, consult Dave's Gourmet Albacore, PO Box 1904, Soquel, CA 95073 (phone/fax 408-475-5847 or http://davesalbacore.com), an informative resource for recipes and information on how different fishing techniques and food-processing techniques affect taste and nutritional content.*

OMEGA-3-FATTY-ACID CONTENT OF POPULAR FISH*

Fish	Omega-3 Fats (grams)	Fish	Omega-3 Fats (grams)
(Serving size = 6 ounces cooked, unless otherwise specified)			
Salmon, sockeye	4.0	Flounder	0.9
Salmon, Atlantic	3.1–3.7	Sole	0.9
Tuna, albacore	3.5	Rockfish	0.8
Sardines in sardine oil (3 ounces)	2.8–3.3	Halibut, Pacific	0.8
		Pike, walleye	0.6
Salmon, chinook	2.0	Perch, ocean	0.6
Salmon, coho	2.0	Squid	0.6
Salmon, king	1.9	Snapper	0.6
Trout, rainbow, wild	1.7	Cod, Pacific	0.5
Tuna, bluefin	1.5	Haddock	0.4
Anchovy, European (3.3 ounces)	1.4	Yellowtail	0.4
Swordfish	1.4	Catfish	0.3–0.4
Herring, Atlantic and Pacific (3 ounces)	1.2–1.8	Crab, Dungeness (3 ounces, steamed)	0.3
Oysters	1.1	Shrimp (3 ounces, steamed)	0.3
Shark	1.0	Tuna (canned, 3 ounces)	0.2–0.7
Mackerel (3 ounces, canned)	1.0	Lobster	0.2
Pompano, Florida	1.0	Clams (3 ounces, steamed)	0.2
Whiting	0.9		

* The omega-3-fatty-acid content can vary according to the mode of cooking and whether the fish is a wild or farmed variety.

making it difficult to determine the omega-3 content. Also, some tuna is bathed, precooked, and bleached nice and white before canning to remove the oil that makes it spoil faster. The healthy fish oils are then thrown out with the bath water. The fish is then packed in vegetable oil or water. The result of this process is a loss of omega-3 fatty acids. Some specialty tunas are packed in their own oils and contain omega-3 fatty acids.

RATING SEAFOOD

When you're deciding what kind of fish to buy, ask yourself, "What's the main nutrient I'm trying to get from this food?" What nutrients can you get from this food that you can't get as well from others? For fish, the "most valuable nutrient" status goes to omega-3 fatty acids. For this reason, we have placed the fish containing the most omega-3 fatty acids at the top of the list on page 181. These are not necessarily the fish that are the lowest in fat. Note that when you choose one fish over another, you are making some trade-offs. Some of these are small and insignificant; if you eat dairy products regularly, you don't need to worry about how much calcium is in your fish. Other choices matter more: Mackerel, for example, is high in omega-3 fatty acids, but it also derives half its overall calories from fat, including saturated fats. You would do better choosing salmon or tuna instead, even canned, unless you're on a tight budget. Here's how fish rate according to different nutrients.

- Best sources of omega-3 fatty acids: salmon, albacore tuna, mackerel, lake trout, Atlantic halibut, sardines, herring (for other fish, see the box on page 181)
- Fish highest in protein per serving: tuna, salmon, snapper, swordfish (most fish are similar in protein content); best source of protein in grams per calorie of fish: lobster, shrimp, tuna, cod
- Highest vitamin B-12 content: clams, mackerel, herring, bluefin tuna, rainbow trout, salmon
- Highest in iron: clams, shrimp, mackerel, swordfish
- Lowest in iron: orange roughy, snapper, sea bass
- Highest in zinc: crab, lobster, swordfish, clams
- Highest in calcium: canned salmon with bones
- Highest in total fat, saturated fats, and calories: mackerel
- Lowest in total fat and saturated fat: lobster, orange roughy
- Highest in cholesterol: shrimp, mackerel, lobster
- Lowest in cholesterol: yellowfin tuna, albacore tuna, snapper, halibut, grouper
- Most risky fish for pollutants: wild catfish, shrimp, lake trout (warm-water fish and those in lakes from agrochemical runoff)
- Least risky fish for pollutants: deep-water ocean fish, salmon, tuna

19

The Merits of Milk

OT MILK?" asks the ad. "Does my child really need milk?" ask parents. Milk may be overrated (or at least overpromoted), but it is also misunderstood. We have grown up with the belief that a glass of milk is the perfect all-American accompaniment to mom's apple pie, yet new insights into nutrition have exposed not only harmful fats in the piecrust but concerns about the cow juice, too. There is a place for milk and dairy products in the American diet, as long as you choose the right kinds.

QUESTIONS YOU MAY HAVE ABOUT MILK

NUTRITIONAL BENEFITS

Why is milk so good for children?

While cow's milk is really designed for baby cows rather than for baby humans, it is a nutritional staple in the diet of many cultures. For children who are not lactose intolerant or allergic to milk protein, milk is one-stop shopping for nutrition. It contains nearly all the basic nutrients that a growing child needs: fats, carbohydrates, proteins, vitamins, and minerals (except iron). While it is true that most of the nutrients in milk can be got-

ten easily from other sources, such as vegetables, legumes, and seafood, milk puts them all together in a convenient package. Realistically, children eat or drink dairy products in greater amounts and more consistently than other foods. While cow milk is not the only way to get calcium into a child's diet, it's the most practical one. Good luck serving your children a breakfast of calcium-rich broccoli, kale, and sardines. Specifically, the following are the nutritional benefits of milk, *per 8-ounce glass:*

- *Protein:* 8 grams
- *Carbohydrates:* lactose, 11 grams
- *Fat:* anywhere from negligible amounts in nonfat milk to 8 grams per 8-ounce glass of whole milk
- *Calcium:* 300 milligrams, or 35 percent of the DV for schoolchildren. (Note that the percentage of calcium absorbed from dairy products is much higher than that absorbed from most vegetables. Milk is fortified with vitamin D, which boosts calcium absorption.)
- *Vitamin B-2 (riboflavin):* one-half of the DV for children under age three, one-third of the DV for schoolchildren, and one-fourth the DV for teens and adults
- *Vitamin B-12:* 30 percent of the DV for children

COW'S MILK — NOT FOR HUMAN BABIES

While cow's milk may be the preferred first food for baby cows, it's not for baby humans, especially infants under one year of age. Because of the excess of some nutrients and deficiency of others, as well as concerns about iron-deficiency anemia, the American Academy of Pediatrics advises against using cow's milk as the primary beverage in infants under one year old.

Cow's milk contains too little zinc, iron, and vitamins E and C to support an infant's rapid growth. Cow's milk contains twice as much sodium and three times as much phosphorus as human milk or infant formulas, as well as excess proteins. These pose a problem for baby's immature kidneys, which have the job of getting rid of unneeded minerals and protein. And the protein curd of cow's milk is difficult to digest. Pediatric allergists also caution against giving cow's milk to infants under twelve months of age. Because of the immaturity of the tiny infant's intestinal lining, milk proteins may seep through and set the infant up for later milk allergies.

Another reason for not using cow's milk under one year of age is the risk of iron-deficiency anemia. Besides being a poor source of dietary iron, excessive cow's milk can irritate the lining of an infant's intestines, especially during the first year, causing microscopic intestinal bleeding, which, over a long period of time, further contributes to iron-deficiency anemia.

It's best to avoid using cow's milk as baby's primary beverage and give baby breast milk or formula until at least one year of age. (Yogurt and cottage cheese, however, are safe to introduce around nine months.) When you do introduce cow's milk around one year of age, take two precautions: Limit your toddler's milk consumption to no more than 24 ounces a day. If your toddler is a milk lover, be sure that he eats enough iron-rich foods to make up for the lack of iron in milk. And if your infant or child refuses to drink his milk, don't force it. He's probably trying to tell you that milk doesn't sit well in his stomach and he needs an alternative beverage.

- *Zinc:* 10 percent of the DV for children
- *Vitamin D:* 25 percent of the DV for children and adults
- *Vitamin A:* 10 percent of the DV for children and adults

While milk isn't the perfect food, it still delivers a lot of nutrition in all its various forms, which include cheeses, cottage cheese, and yogurt. Besides, milk and dairy products are foods that kids will eat and drink willingly. Despite the concerns about milk, it has a lot of good nutritional things going for it.

MILK ALLERGIES

We have a lot of allergies in our family, and I'm concerned that my child may develop an allergy to milk. How common is this, and how do I recognize it?

Milk allergies are overdiagnosed by the general population and underdiagnosed by doctors. The real incidence of milk allergies lies somewhere between the folklore and the skeptical view of many physicians. Around 5 percent of children and adults seem to be either allergic to milk or intolerant of it. One carefully controlled study showed that 75 percent of infants under one year of age were allergic to cow's milk. A cows-milk allergy is more likely to develop in children who have a family history of milk allergy. The good news is that most children will partially or completely outgrow this allergy by the time they are two or three years old.

The protein in cow's milk is what provokes an allergic reaction. Because milk is a species-specific protein, cow's milk is suited to bovine intestines. Exposure of human intestines to bovine protein can cause irritation and damage to the intestinal lining, allowing these allergenic proteins to be absorbed into the circulatory system. The immune system recognizes these proteins as foreign and attacks them, causing the usual allergy symptoms of wheezing, runny nose, or a red, rough, sandpaper-like rash, especially on the cheeks. An allergy to milk is often the underlying cause of repeated colds and ear infections, due to fluid building up

---

NUTRITIP
Concentrated Calcium

The firmer the dairy product, the more calcium it's likely to contain. Hard cheeses contain more calcium than milk. One ounce of parmesan cheese contains a bone-building 336 milligrams of calcium. One tablespoon of grated parmesan contains 70 milligrams of calcium. Melted, sliced parmesan cheese makes a chewy addition to any sandwich, and grated parmesan is a calcium-rich topping on salads and spaghetti.

---

in the respiratory passages, sinuses, and eustachian tubes of the ears. Milk allergy has also been implicated in subtle behavioral changes, such as irritability, and night waking. Research has shown that the allergenic proteins in milk

---

MILK TIPS FOR FEEDING YOUR CHILDREN

While milk is not absolutely necessary in a child's diet, and even less necessary in the diet of adults, milk is still a nutrient-dense food for little consumers — provided parents use the right milk at the right time, and in the right amount. Try these milk tips:

- Avoid cow's milk as a beverage for infants under one year of age. Use human milk and/or iron-fortified formulas instead.
- Yogurt is a better first dairy food than cow's milk and can be given to infants around nine months of age.
- Nonfat milk is not recommended for infants under two years of age because of the load of excess minerals on immature kidneys and the lower caloric densities of these milks.

- Unless otherwise advised by your doctor, give your child whole milk until at least eighteen months of age or until your toddler is getting enough dietary fats from other sources.
- Begin using low-fat milk between eighteen months and two years of age, especially if your child drinks a lot of milk.
- Limit the volume of milk to 24 ounces a day for most toddlers and children.
- The symptoms of milk allergy and/or lactose intolerance can begin at any age and may be dose related; your child may be able to drink one glass without any problem but may react to more.
- Yogurt is a healthier, more nutritious dairy product for children than cow's milk.

(beta-lactoglobulin) can even pass through a breastfeeding mother's milk into her baby and cause some babies to react with colicky symptoms. The colic–cow's milk connection should be suspected as a possible cause of fussy behavior in an otherwise normal breastfed baby. The allergic reaction between the milk protein and the intestinal lining can cause minute gastrointestinal bleeding (sometimes so slight that it is missed) and be a subtle cause of anemia in infants and young children.

Chronic milk allergy can also weaken the intestinal lining, allowing foreign substances into the bloodstream that would ordinarily be screened out, a condition known as the "leaky gut syndrome" (see page 374).

True milk allergy involves the protein in the

NUTRITIP
Fake Creams

Nondairy creamers are not healthy substitutes for coffee cream (half and half), which contains a measly 1.7 grams of fat per tablespoon. Substitutes are made from all kinds of frightful stuff, such as hydrogenated oil, stabilizers, and flavoring. Stick to the cream that comes from the cow (or better, switch to whole milk). Above all, don't give these dairy substitutes to children. They provide none of the nutrition of milk and plenty of fake nutrients, which kids should avoid.

MILK-NUTRIENT SUBSTITUTES

Suppose you and your children just don't like milk or cannot tolerate it. The five most valuable nutrients found in milk are protein, calcium, vitamin A, riboflavin, and vitamin D. Here are some alternative sources of these five nutrients:

- *Protein:* whole-grain cereal, eggs, poultry, beef, legumes, soy products
- *Calcium:* chickpeas, spinach, broccoli, salmon (with bones), beans, blackstrap molasses, yogurt, cheese (see page 56 for the best nondairy sources of calcium)
- *Vitamin A:* carrots, squash, sweet potatoes
- *Riboflavin:* eggs, whole-grain cereal, green, leafy vegetables, meats
- *Vitamin D:* salmon, vitamin D–fortified milk and cereals, egg yolk, sunshine

---

milk. The fat content of the milk should not affect allergy symptoms. Some people who are allergic to milk may be able to tolerate cheese or yogurt or milk in baked goods, since when milk is heated or fermented, the proteins become less allergenic.

LACTOSE INTOLERANCE

I hear a lot about lactose intolerance. Is this a common problem?

Like milk allergy, lactose intolerance is usually an overdiagnosed or a self-diagnosed problem. Lactose, the sugar in both human and cow's milk, is normally digested by the intestinal enzyme lactase, which breaks the lactose down into glucose and galactose. Some infants, children, and adults are deficient in this intestinal enzyme and thus cannot absorb lactose. When the amount of lactose in the diet exceeds the supply of lactase in the cells of the intestinal lining, the undigested lactose travels down the intestines. There bacteria digest some of the lactose, but the rest ferments and is converted into the gas carbon dioxide, which causes bloating, diarrhea, and abdominal pain, and to lactic acid, which accounts for the red, irritated, burnlike ring around the anus, especially noticeable in lactose-intolerant children. Other more subtle symptoms are headaches, fatigue, and bad breath.

Lactose intolerance is rare in infants but more common as people get older, so there is some biochemical basis for the idea that you outgrow your need for milk. There are degrees of lactose intolerance, depending on the supply of lactase in the gut. Some children and adults can tolerate one glass of milk but not two or three; or they can drink milk with a meal but not on an empty stomach. Many can tolerate yogurt and cheese but not milk as a beverage. (The lactose in fermented yogurt is somewhat predigested.) Lactose intolerance is more common than allergy to the protein in milk. Allergic symptoms usually involve the skin and respiratory system, whereas lactose intolerance is limited to abdominal symptoms. Lactose intolerance is especially prevalent among Asians, Hispanics, and African Americans. In fact, it is estimated that around three-fourths of the world's population may have some degree of lactose intolerance. Most learn to live with it either by consuming small amounts of dairy products or by omitting them entirely.

Lactose intolerance may appear after the intestinal lining has been injured by allergy or infection. This is called "secondary lactose intolerance," and it lasts only until the intestinal lining is healed. It is especially common in children after a diarrhea-producing viral illness and is the reason for delaying the introduction of milk during the recovery stage.

If you are lactose intolerant, try these strategies for getting the nutritional benefits of milk into your diet:

- Avoid lactose-containing dairy products for a couple of weeks and then gradually increase the amount you consume, beginning with 1 tablespoon of milk and doubling the amount every few days until you reach your tolerance level. Within a few weeks, lactose indigestion can turn into digestion.
- Drink your milk in smaller, more frequent servings.
- Drink lactose-free milk, such as Lactaid, or take a lactase capsule along with your milk.
- Drink or eat dairy products with meals rather than solo to give your intestines a better chance to digest the lactose. Anything that slows the transit of food through the intestines gives the lactase-containing cells more time to do their job.
- Some dairy products contain more lactose than others. Here's how they rank, from most to least in lactose content:

nonfat milk	cheese
low-fat milk	cottage cheese
whole milk	cream cheese
yogurt	butter (none or
ice cream	negligible amount)

FAT CONTENT

Does milk contain a lot of fat?

Yes and no, depending on whether you use whole, low-fat, or nonfat milk. Since milk is an animal product, most of the fat in milk is saturated. So you can scratch whole milk from a heart-healthy diet. An 8-ounce glass of whole milk contains 5 grams of saturated fat, 2-percent milk contains 2.9 grams of saturated fat, and a glass of 1-percent milk contains 1.6 grams. An 8-ounce glass of whole milk also contains 23 to 31 milligrams of cholesterol, and three glasses of whole milk contain about the same amount of cholesterol as one lean ground-beef patty. In contrast, a glass of

1-percent (low-fat) milk contains only 10 grams of cholesterol. Three glasses contain only 30 milligrams of cholesterol, only one-tenth of the maximum 300 milligrams a day recommended for an adult and only one-fifth of the maximum 150 milligrams a day recommended for an average preschool child.

Cow's milk contains little of the essential fatty acids necessary for brain and body growth in young children. Certainly the fat in milk is not as healthy as that obtained from seafood or plant sources. The essential fatty acids from the cow feed may be hydrogenated or saturated as they pass through the four compartments of the cow's stomach, with the result that the fats in cow's milk contain some heart-harming *trans fatty acids*. As you can see, there are many good reasons for choosing low-fat or nonfat milk over 2-percent or whole milk, and for obtaining the necessary dietary fats from seafood and plant sources instead of from milk.

MEDICAL PROBLEMS*

I've heard there is a link between cow's milk and diabetes. Is this true?

Possibly. Studies comparing people with diabetes with the general population have shown a statistical correlation between milk drinking among young children and the later onset of insulin-dependent diabetes. Further studies are needed, but researchers speculate that the early introduction of cow's milk may cause an immune reaction in the body. By some biochemical quirk, the

---

* *The studies implicating cow's milk in a child's diet with a higher incidence of later illnesses are preliminary and of concern, but they should not be interpreted to mean that children should not drink cow's milk (with some exceptions; see bulleted items on page 189). It's entirely possible that cow's milk loses by default; that is, the link between the consumption of cow's milk at an early age and the development of later illnesses may not be directly due to the cow's milk but rather to the absence of breast milk in the child's diet in the first one or two years.*

ALMOND MILK RECIPE

If you or your toddler doesn't tolerate cow's milk or soy "milk," here's an alternative. Almond milk or a prepared mix for almond milk can be purchased in a nutrition store, or you can make your own.

½ cup blanched raw almonds
2 cups water (more as needed)
salt, honey, pure maple syrup, pure vanilla or almond extract (optional)

Place the blanched raw almonds in a blender. Add 1 cup of the water and blend until smooth — about five minutes on high. Add the remaining cup of water to thin the milk to the desired consistency, using more water as needed. Chill before using for best flavor. You may wish to flavor the milk by adding a few grains of salt, a bit of honey or maple syrup, or a touch of vanilla or almond extract. Almond milk can be used as a beverage, on cereal, or in baking and cooking.

If you plan to use almond milk as a nutritional substitute for milk or dairy products, consult a registered dietitian, since these two milks do not share all nutrients equally. While almond milk is rich in calories, protein, fats, and carbohydrates, it is lower than cow's milk in vitamins A, B-2, B-6, B-12, and D, and calcium and zinc. Adding a daily multivitamin multimineral to your child's diet should suffice.

protein in cow's milk (bovine serum albumin) is similar to the natural proteins in the human pancreas, the organ that manufactures insulin. Researchers theorize that some people produce antibodies in reaction to cow's-milk protein and that these antibodies attach themselves to the insulin-producing cells in the pancreas, eventually

NUTRITIP
Does Milk Make Mucus?

Is the warning not to drink milk when you have a cold an old doctor's tale? Yes and no. Some people do make more mucus when they drink milk, and any high-fat food may produce a sensation of thicker secretions in the back of the throat. But the mucus producers are probably those who are allergic to milk. Separating out the milk-allergic persons, research fails to show any correlation between milk drinking and mucus production during a cold. You need extra fluids during a cold anyway, so, if you're not allergic, it's okay to drink a few glasses of low-fat milk.

NUTRIMYTH

Drink milk for calcium. While a glass of milk contains 300 milligrams of calcium, it is also high in phosphorus. Calcium absorption depends upon the calcium-to-phosphorus ratio, which in cow's milk is almost one to one, meaning that there is almost as much phosphorus in cow's milk as calcium. (In human milk the calcium-to-phosphorus ratio is 2.5 to 1.) The higher calcium-to-phosphorus ratio, the better the calcium is absorbed. So, foods with a higher calcium-to-phosphorus ratio are better sources of calcium than milk (see nondairy sources of calcium, page 56). However, vitamin D–fortification of milk aids in calcium absorption, and the various hormones that regulate calcium in the body also control how much calcium is absorbed from the intestines.

destroying them and leading to diabetes. In one statistical study, insulin-dependent children had elevated levels of anti–bovine serum albumin antibodies, but the control children had only a small amount of these antibodies in their blood.

It's prudent to breastfeed infants and to delay the introduction of cow's milk to children if any of the following are present:

- a strong family history of milk allergy
- a strong family history of Type 1 (i.e., insulin-dependent or juvenile-onset) diabetes
- any indication that the child may have a milk allergy

The possible connection between diabetes and cow's milk can't be all that strong, since over 99 percent of the baby boomers who were raised on cow's-milk formulas have not gone on to develop insulin-dependent diabetes.

Is it true that the more milk children and adults drink, the more medical problems they have?

Possibly. Compared with breastfeeding infants, cow's milk–fed (and formula-fed) infants have more middle-ear infections, more upper respiratory tract infections, and more intestinal infections. And there is the remote diabetes–cow's milk connection described above. There are those who would make milk the scapegoat for just about every ailment imaginable — from bed-wetting to hyperactivity — but there is no scientific evidence for a cause-and-effect relationship between milk drinking and these other conditions. In fairness to much-maligned milk, in our opinion, any connection between cow's milk and disease is probably more a result of the absence of breast milk in

RICE DRINKS

While rice is an intestines-friendly food, rice "milk" is not a healthy substitute for milk. The "milk" extracted from rice is mostly carbohydrates, or starch, unlike dairy milk, which is naturally a balanced source of protein, fats, carbohydrates, many vitamins, and calcium. What are now termed rice beverages or rice drinks (legally they can no longer be called "milk"; that is a term reserved exclusively for dairy products) are a composition of rice "milk," often with added oils and fortified with vitamins A and D and calcium so that, at least on paper, they resemble milk. Because they are more intestines-friendly than dairy products, rice drinks are particularly useful for children who are allergic or intolerant to dairy products or who are recovering from a diarrhea-producing illness in which the intestinal lining has been temporarily injured. Because of its low protein content, it is certainly not recommended as a substitute for formula in infants under one year and should not, unless recommended by the infant's doctor, replace milk in infants between one and two years.

the infant's diet than it is a reaction to the presence of cow's milk.

NUTRITIP
Healthier Milk

Buy certified organic milk. It doesn't contain antibiotics or added bovine growth hormone (BGH).

NUTRIMYTH

Lower fat means fewer problems. Low-fat milk means just that — "lower in fat" — and nothing else. While avoiding the greater amounts of saturated fat in whole milk may help prevent cardiovascular illness, other potential problems associated with milk are not affected by fat content. Nonfat milk can be just as allergenic as whole milk and just as upsetting to people with lactose intolerance.

I've been feeding my baby iron-fortified formula. When is it okay to switch to whole cow's milk?

Research comparing cow's milk– and formula-fed infants during the first year of life has shown that cow's milk is irritating to the intestines of a tiny infant. It causes infants to lose a tiny bit of blood in their stools, which contributes to iron-deficiency anemia. There is very little iron in cow's milk anyway, and the iron that is there is poorly absorbed. Concern about iron-deficiency anemia has led the American Academy of Pediatrics, backed by solid research, to discourage the use of cow's milk in children under one year of age. One of America's top pediatric blood specialists, the late Dr. Frank Oski, Professor and Chairman of the Department of Pediatrics at Johns Hopkins University (and co-author of a book entitled *Don't Drink Your Milk!*) advised parents to be cautious and not to rush into the use of cow's milk, even during the child's second year of life. At present it would seem prudent to continue giving your baby iron-fortified formula during the second year of life and very gradually wean him to dairy products, beginning with yogurt. If your toddler generally has a balanced diet, and routine hemoglobin tests show that he is not even close to being anemic, then switch from formula to whole milk sometime during the second year, but don't be in a hurry.

ADDITIVES

I've heard that milk can contain a lot of pesticides, hormones, and antibiotics. Is it safe?

The safety of milk depends on who's interpreting the data. While milk bashing is popular among consumer groups, the government (with the support of the American Dairy Council) has tried to foster a pure image for the sacred cow. Cow feed may contain pesticides, and cows are given antibiotics to keep them from getting sick and hormones to increase their milk production. Whether or not these substances show up in standard milk (which is supposed to be tested for detectable residues) is uncertain. Be sure. Buy certified organic milk, which means there were never hormones or antibiotics in the cow feed and the milk was protected from pollutants during processing.

GOT GOAT'S MILK?

What does goat's milk give you that cow's milk doesn't? In many parts of the world, goat's milk is preferred to cow's milk. Even in the United States, the goat is gaining popularity. Goats eat less and occupy less grazing space than cows, and in some families the backyard goat supplies milk for family needs. Goat's milk is believed to be more easily digestible and less allergenic than cow's milk. Does it deserve this reputation? Let's disassemble goat's milk, nutrient by nutrient, to see how it compares with cow's milk.

> **NUTRIMINDER**
> **Dairy Dates**
>
> - no cow's milk before age one
> - whole milk until two
> - nonfat or low-fat after that

Different fat. Goat's milk contains around 10 grams of fat per 8 ounces compared to 8 to 9 grams in whole cow's milk, and it's much easier to find low-fat and nonfat varieties of cow's milk than it is to purchase low-fat goat's milk. Unlike cow's milk, goat's milk does not contain the clumping substance agglutinin. As a result, the fat globules in goat's milk do not cluster together, which makes them easier to digest. Like cow's milk, goat's milk is low in essential fatty acids, because goats also have EFA-destroying bacteria in their ruminant stomachs. Yet, goat's milk contains more of the essential fatty acids linoleic and arachidonic acids, in addition to a higher proportion of short-chain and medium-chain fatty acids. These are easier for intestinal enzymes to digest.

Different protein. Goat's-milk protein forms a softer curd (the term given to the protein clumps that are formed by the action of stomach acid on protein), which makes the protein more easily and rapidly digestible. Theoretically, this more rapid transit through the stomach could be an advantage to infants and children who regurgitate cow's milk easily. Goat's milk may also have advantages when it comes to allergies. Goat's milk contains only trace amounts of an allergenic casein protein, alpha-s1, found in cow's milk. Goat's-milk casein is more similar to human milk, while cow's milk and goat's milk do contain similar levels of the other allergenic protein, beta-lactoglobulin. Scientific studies have not found a decreased incidence of allergy with goat's milk, but, as sometimes happens, parents' observations and scientific studies are at odds. Some parents are certain that their child tolerates goat's milk better than cow's milk, and parents are more sensitive to their children's reactions than scientific studies are.

Less lactose. Goat's milk contains slightly lower levels of lactose than cow's milk does (4.1 percent versus 4.7, respectively). This may be a small advantage for lactose-intolerant persons.

Different minerals. Although the mineral content of goat's milk and cow's milk is generally similar, goat's milk contains 13 percent more calcium, 25 percent more vitamin B-6, 47 percent more vitamin A, and 134 percent more potassium. It is also three times higher in niacin and four times higher in copper. Goat's milk also contains 27 percent more of the antioxidant selenium than cow's milk. Cow's milk contains five times as much vitamin B-12 as goat's milk and ten times as much folic acid (there are 12 mcg. in cow's milk versus 1 mcg. in goat's milk per 8 ounces; the recommended dietary allowance for children is 75 to 100 mcg.). The fact that goat's milk contains less than 10 percent of the amount of folic acid contained in cow's milk means that it must be fortified with folic acid in order to be adequate as a formula or milk substitute for infants and toddlers. Some popular brands of goat's milk advertise "Fortified with Folic Acid" on the carton.

Goat's-Milk Formula vs. Commercial Formula for Allergic Infants

Parents of babies allergic to cow's-milk and other commercial formulas often ask if it is safe to use goat's-milk formula as an alternative. Though some people believe goat's milk is less allergenic and more easily digestible than cow's milk, it should not be used as a substitute for infant formula. Like cow's milk, it can cause intestinal irritation and anemia. Infants *under one year of age*

who are allergic to cow's milk–based formulas should try either a soy-based formula or one of the hypoallergenic formulas discussed on page 258. If your baby can't tolerate either soy or hypoallergenic formulas, *after consultation with your doctor and/or a pediatric nutritionist* try the following recipe for goat's-milk formula:

12 ounces evaporated goat's milk, fortified with folic acid and vitamin D (Evaporated milk has been heat processed, which increases the digestibility and lessens the allergenic properties of the protein.)
24 ounces sterile water
a carbohydrate source: either 3½ tbsp. corn syrup or 7 tbsp. dextrin maltose

This formula has stood the test of time. One batch contains 715 calories and 19 calories per ounce, which is essentially the same as cow's-milk formulas. This is sufficient for an infant of six to twelve months. A baby on goat's-milk formula should also receive a multivitamin with iron supplement prescribed by her doctor.

In infants *over one year of age,* goat's milk can be readily used instead of cow's milk. Be sure to buy goat's milk that is certified free of antibiotics and bovine growth hormone (BGH). For more information about goat's milk call 805-565-1538 or 800-343-1185.

NUTRITIP
The Fresher, the Better

The longer the time between the milk's coming out of the cow and going into the human, the more bacteria there will be in the milk. It's best to drink milk that is fresh and to keep it cold. Refrigeration slows down bacterial growth, but it doesn't stop it completely.

As more and more is learned about the nutritional uniqueness of goat's milk, its use in cow's milk–allergic infants, children, and adults is sure to grow.

NUTRIMYTH

Women must drink milk to prevent osteoporosis. It's true that the body needs calcium in order to prevent osteoporosis, but that calcium does not have to come from milk. For other sources of calcium than milk see page 56.

20

Yummy Yogurt

YOGURT IS ONE of the oldest health foods, dating back thousands of years. It is surrounded by legends as rich as its creamy texture. One tale is that an angel revealed to Abraham how to make this fermented-milk product. A more likely explanation of yogurt's origin is that it was accidentally discovered in the Middle East by desert travelers who found that the hot sun turned bags of milk into a substance with a firmer texture. Cultured-milk products gradually became treasured foods in ancient cultures and now enjoy as much supermarket shelf space as milk. Yogurt became popular again in the seventies.

WHAT IS YOGURT?

Yogurt is a good example of the nutritional principle of "synergy": Add two nutrients together, and you get a product better than both of them — sort of like 1 + 1 = 3. According to industry standards developed in 1985, in order for a product to be called "yogurt," it must meet these three criteria:

1. The main ingredient must be milk.
2. It must go through a fermentation process.
3. It must be fermented by live and active cultures, primarily bacteria from the *Lactobacillus* family.

How Yogurt Is Made

Milk gets a dose of culture. Two bacterial cultures, *Lactobacillus bulgaricus* and *Streptococcus thermophilus,* are added to pasteurized milk. While the milk is kept warm, the bacteria convert the milk's sugar to lactic acid, which gives yogurt its unique flavor. The acid curdles the proteins, forming a delicate gel. Another culture, *Lactobacillus acidophilus,* is added to some yogurts to increase the health benefits. The culturing process also changes the lactose, proteins, and minerals (and to a slight degree the fats) into more digestible forms. The bacterial cultures use up around 30 percent of the milk sugar, lactose, as a

---

NUTRITIP
Best Bugs for Your Bowels

Even though *L. bulgaricus* and other strains of the *Lactobacillus* organisms are typically present in yogurt, *L. acidophilus* is not. It must be added. Acidophilus is superior to *L. bulgaricus* in its value to colon health. Look for *Lactobacillus acidophilus* on the yogurt ingredients list.

---

source of energy for their own growth but leave the final product richer in lactase, which explains why the live and active cultures in yogurt may be enjoyed by persons who are lactose intolerant (i.e., lactase deficient) and can't tolerate milk. The byproduct of the fermentation process, called "lactic acid," acts as a preservative, giving yogurt a much longer shelf life than milk. Lactic acid also improves the digestibility of the protein and the absorption of the minerals.

All yogurts are not equally cultured. Some yogurts are pasteurized again, after the fermentation process. This kills the beneficial bacteria cultures and decreases many of the health benefits of yogurt, which depend on live and active cultures being present after pasteurization. The National Yogurt Association (NYA) has developed a "Live and Active Cultures" (LAC) seal for the yogurt label to identify yogurt that contains significant levels of live and active cultures. Be aware that a label stating "made with active cultures" does not mean the same as the LAC label. The LAC label means that the yogurt contains at least 100 million cultures per gram of yogurt at the time of manufacture and *after* pasteurization. Frozen yogurt with this seal contains at least 10 million cultures per gram at the time of manufacture. Some yogurt products may have live cultures but not carry the LAC seal, but without the LAC seal, there is no

---

NUTRITIP
Low-Lactose Yogurt

To get the most out of the low-lactose properties of yogurt, be sure the yogurt contains live and active bacterial cultures. Look for the LAC seal on the label of the yogurt container, certifying that a large amount of live and active bacterial cultures are present.

---

way to be sure that live and active cultures are present.

Look for the LAC seal on the label. Also avoid yogurt that says "heat treated after culturing" on the label. This means that the yogurt was pasteurized after the healthful organisms were added, which dilutes the health benefits of the yogurt. Pasteurization deactivates the lactase and kills the live cultures, thereby obliterating two health benefits of yogurt. Heat treating yogurt trades economic gain for nutritional loss. It prolongs yogurt's shelf life but spoils its nutrition and health-food value. Lactose-intolerant persons who can tolerate yogurt containing live and active cultures may not be able to digest the kind that has been heat treated. Yogurt-based salad dressings and yogurt-covered raisins, pretzels, and candy typically do not contain live and active cultures.

The U.S. National Yogurt Association has been urging the FDA not to allow products that do not contain live and active cultures to be called "yogurt." The LAC label ensures consumers that the healthful properties of the organisms are present at the time they eat the yogurt, not just at the time of manufacturing.

TEN REASONS YOGURT IS A TOP HEALTH FOOD

We have included yogurt in our list of top twelve foods not only because it is tasty but also because it is a versatile and nutritious food.

1. Yogurt is easier to digest than milk. Many people who cannot tolerate milk, either because of a protein allergy or lactose intolerance, can enjoy yogurt. The culturing process makes yogurt more digestible than milk. The live and active cultures create lactase, the enzyme that lactose-intolerant people lack. Another enzyme (beta-galactosidase) contained in some yogurts also helps improve lactose absorption in lactase-deficient persons. In

LOVE YOUR LACTOBACTERIA!

Healthy bacteria reside in everybody's colon, and in return for food and a warm place to live, these resident bacteria contribute to your health. Among the most intestines-friendly resident bacteria are those of the family *Lactobacillus,* so called because they thrive on lactose sugars. The resident germ you will read most about is *L. acidophilus,* which means "acid-loving," because these organisms grow best in an acidic intestinal environment. Here are some healthy things lactobacteria do for your body:

- *Improve digestion.* Lactobacteria, as the name implies, help digest the lactose in dairy products, preventing lactose overload and lessening problems with lactose intolerance. Lactobacteria also help with the absorption of valuable nutrients and stimulate peristalsis, the movement of food through the intestines that leads to regular bowel movements.
- *Manufacture vitamins.* Just as rich soil grows vitamin-rich foods, lactobacteria produce B-complex vitamins along with vitamin K.
- *Manufacture nutrients.* These friendly bacteria help manufacture essential fatty acids called "short-chain fatty acids" (SCFA's). These are valuable nutrients for intestinal cells and also produce cancer-fighting substances.
- *Boost immunity.* Lactobacteria inhibit the growth of harmful bacteria and fungi, such as candida (yeast). They help keep the intestinal environment acidic and compete with harmful bacteria and the toxins they produce. They even produce hydrogen peroxide, which has a natural antibiotic effect.
- *Protect against carcinogens.* Lactobacteria bind potential carcinogens, preventing them from damaging cells. *L. bulgaricus,* the main lactobacteria used in yogurt, has anti-tumor activity. Specifically, lactobacteria bind heavy metals and bile acids, which are potential carcinogens. These bacteria inhibit the growth of nitrate-producing bacteria (nitrates can be a carcinogen). They also metabolize flavonoids, producing natural anti-tumor substances.
- *Protect against cardiovascular disease.* Lactobacteria help regulate cholesterol and triglyceride levels in the blood.

Be kind to the bugs in your bowels. They do good things for you.

---

addition, bacterial enzymes created by the culturing process partially digest the milk protein casein, making it easier to absorb and less allergenic. In our pediatrics practice, we have observed that children who cannot tolerate milk can often eat yogurt without any intestinal upset. While the amount of lactose varies among brands of yogurt, in general, yogurt has less lactose than milk. The culturing process has already broken down the milk sugar, lactose, into glucose and galactose, two sugars that are easily absorbed by lactose-intolerant persons.

2. Yogurt contributes to colon health. There's a medical truism that states, "You're only as healthy as your colon." When eating yogurt, you care for your colon in two ways. First, yogurt contains lactobacteria, intestines-friendly bacterial cultures that foster a healthy colon and even lower the risk of colon cancer. Lactobacteria, especially acidophilus, promote the growth of healthy bacteria in the colon and reduce the conversion of bile into carcinogenic bile acids. The more of these intestines-friendly bacteria in your colon, the lower your chance of colon diseases. Basically, the friendly bacteria in yogurt seem to deactivate harmful substances (such as nitrates and nitrites before they are converted to nitrosamines) before they can become carcinogenic.

Second, yogurt is a rich source of calcium (see below) — a mineral that contributes to colon health and decreases the risk of colon cancer. Calcium discourages excessive growth of the cells lining the colon, a condition that can place a person at high risk for colon cancer. Calcium also binds cancer-producing bile acids and keeps them from irritating the colon wall. People who have diets high in calcium (e.g., Scandinavian countries) have lower rates of colorectal cancer. One study showed that an average intake of 1,200 milligrams of calcium a day is associated with a 75-percent reduction of colorectal cancer. As a survivor of colon cancer, I have a critical interest in the care of my colon. My life depends on it.

3. Yogurt improves the bioavailability of other nutrients. Culturing of yogurt increases the absorption of calcium and B vitamins. The lactic acid in the yogurt aids in the digestion of the milk calcium, making it easier to absorb.

4. Yogurt can boost immunity. Researchers who studied sixty-eight people who ate 2 cups of live culture yogurt daily for three months found that these persons produced higher levels of immunity-boosting interferon. The bacterial cultures in yogurt have also been shown to stimulate infection-fighting white cells in the bloodstream. Some studies have shown that yogurt cultures contain a factor that has anti-tumor effects in experimental animals.

5. Yogurt aids healing after intestinal infections. Some viral and allergic gastrointestinal disorders injure the lining of the intestines, especially the cells that produce lactase. This results in temporary lactose-malabsorption problems. This is why children often cannot tolerate milk for a

---

NUTRITIP
A Chaser for Antibiotics

Antibiotics kill not only harmful bacteria; they also kill the healthy ones in the intestines. The live bacterial cultures in yogurt can help replenish the intestines with helpful bacteria before the harmful ones not killed by the antibiotics take over. I usually "prescribe" a daily does of yogurt while a person is taking antibiotics and for two weeks thereafter.

---

month or two after an intestinal infection. Yogurt, however, because it contains less lactose and more lactase than milk, is usually well tolerated by healing intestines and is a popular "healing food" for diarrhea. Many pediatricians recommend yogurt for children suffering from various forms of indigestion. Research shows that children recover faster from diarrhea when eating yogurt. It's also good to eat yogurt while taking antibiotics. The yogurt will minimize the effects of the antibiotic on the friendly bacteria in the intestines.

6. Yogurt can decrease yeast infections. Research has shown that eating 8 ounces of yogurt that contains live and active cultures daily reduces the number of yeast colonies in the vagina and decreases the incidence of vaginal yeast infections.

7. Yogurt is a rich source of calcium. An 8-ounce serving of most yogurts provides 450 milligrams of calcium, one-half of a child's recommended dietary allowance and 30 to 40 percent of the adult DV. Because the live and active cultures in yogurt increase the absorption of calcium, an 8-ounce serving of yogurt gets more calcium into the body than the same volume of milk can.

8. Yogurt is an excellent source of protein. Plain yogurt contains 10 to 14 grams of protein per 8 ounces, which amounts to 20 percent of the daily protein requirement for most persons. In fact, 8 ounces of yogurt that contains live and active cultures has 20 percent more protein than the same volume of milk (10 grams versus 8 grams). Moreover, the culturing of the milk proteins during fermentation makes yogurt's proteins easier to digest. For this reason, the proteins in yogurt are often called "predigested."

9. Yogurt can lower cholesterol. There are a few studies that have shown that yogurt can reduce the blood cholesterol. This may be either because the live cultures in yogurt can assimilate the cholesterol or because yogurt binds bile acids, which has also been shown to lower cholesterol. Or both.

10. Yogurt is a "grow food." Two nutritional properties of yogurt may help children with intestinal-absorption problems grow: the easier digestibility of the proteins and the fact that the lactic acid in yogurt increases the absorption of minerals. And even most picky eaters will eat yogurt in dips and smoothies and as a topping.

Perhaps we can take a health tip about yogurt cultures from those cultures that consume a lot of yogurt, such as the Bulgarians, who are noted for their longer lifespan and who remain in good health well into old age.

WHAT KIND OF YOGURT SHOULD YOU BUY?

As when you purchase any food, read the label, both the "Nutritional Facts" panel and the list of ingredients. Look specifically at the following:

The length of the ingredients list. The best nutritional deal is plain yogurt, which has only two ingredients: live cultures and milk (whole milk, low-fat, or nonfat). The longer the list of ingredients (e.g., added fruit, sweeteners, corn syrup, sugar, fillers, emulsifiers, etc.), the more calories you get and the less yogurt nutrition. In some fruit- and sweetener-filled containers, you're getting more calories in the sweetener than you are in the yogurt. That's a bad nutritional deal. Look at the protein and sugar values in the "Nutrition Facts" box. The higher the protein and the lower the sugar content, the more actual yogurt you're getting in the container. Add your own flavoring.

The calcium content. The best yogurts provide 35 to 40 percent of the recommended dietary allowance for calcium in an 8-ounce container. Once the calcium gets below 30 percent of the DV, it's a good bet that the container is filled with a lot of less-nutritious filler.

Yogurt Terms to Watch For

There's a dizzying array of yogurts in the supermarket dairy aisle. Here's a key to the different types.

- *Whole-milk yogurt* contains approximately 7 grams of milk fat per 8-ounce serving.
- *Low-fat yogurt* contains between 1 and 4 grams of milk fat per 8-ounce serving.

BEST YOGURT	OKAY YOGURT	DON'T-EVEN-BOTHER YOGURT
It contains only live and active cultures (LAC seal) and milk.	It contains live and active cultures (LAC seal), milk, and some filler ingredients.	It might as well be pudding. It says "heat treated" on the label, and it may contain added sugar and stabilizers — and more!

NUTRITIP
Feeling Fuller Longer

Foods that take longer to make the journey from one end of the intestinal tract to the other help you feel full longer. The nutrients in them may also be better absorbed, since the food is in contact with the intestinal lining longer. Yogurt has an intestinal transit time twice as long as milk's.

NUTRIMYTH

All foods made with yogurt are created equal. Not so. In fact, the yogurt used to coat nibble foods such as raisins, nuts, and fruit bits is often so highly sugared that you're really eating more sugar than yogurt.

- *Nonfat yogurt* contains less than ½ gram of milk fat per 8-ounce serving.
- In *Swiss* or *custard-style yogurt,* fruit and yogurt are mixed together. To ensure firmness, a stabilizer, such as gelatin, may be added. This is also called "blended yogurt." Swiss yogurt is fermented in vats and then transferred to cups. This process breaks the gel, so that artificial binders and stabilizers must be added.
- *Fruit-added* or *plain yogurt* has a runnier consistency. The whey, the clear liquid at the top, should be stirred into the solids. (For a comparison of the nutritional content of fruit-added and plain yogurt, see the following page.)
- Yogurt also comes in *liquid form,* called "kefir," which may contain added sweeteners such as corn syrup.
- *Heat treated.* Some yogurt manufacturers market "heat-treated yogurt" to prolong the yogurt's shelf life or decrease its tartness and produce a more pudding-like texture. While perhaps more appealing to some consumers' tastes, the heat treatment of the yogurt after the cultures have been added kills many of the health benefits of the yogurt.

NUTRITIP
Yogurt — Good for Young and Old

Yogurt is a valuable health food for both infants and elderly persons. For children, it is a balanced source of protein, fats, carbohydrates, and minerals in a texture that kids love. For senior citizens, who usually have more sensitive colons or whose intestines have run out of lactase, yogurt is also a valuable food. Also, the declining levels of *bifidus* bacteria in elderly intestines allow the growth of toxin-producing and, perhaps, cancer-causing bacteria.

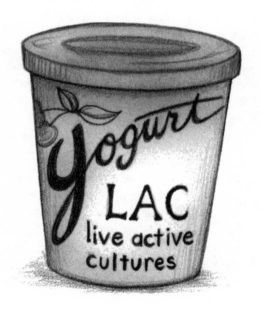

The Benefits of Plain Yogurt

Ounce for ounce, plain yogurt is more nutritious than fruit-added preparations. Notice the differences on the labels:

- Plain yogurt contains around one-half of the calories of the same amount of fruit-added yogurt.
- Plain yogurt contains almost twice the amount of proteins.
- Plain yogurt contains fewer fillers.
- Plain yogurt contains more calcium.
- Plain yogurt contains no added sugar.

If plain yogurt doesn't appeal to you, it's best to buy plain yogurt and flavor it with your favorite fruit. This way you control the sweeteners.

USING YOGURT AS A NUTRITIOUS SUBSTITUTE

Yogurt is one of the most versatile foods, especially for children who love dips and toppings. It can substitute for many high-fat foods. Here are some suggestions.

Use yogurt in place of mayonnaise. Nonfat plain yogurt contains less than 10 percent of the calories, less than 1 percent of the fat, and around 3 percent of the cholesterol of an equal amount of regular mayonnaise. Combining equal amounts of low-calorie mayonnaise and low-fat yogurt works

---

NUTRITIP
A Favorite with Toddlers

Yogurt makes a tasty and nutritious dip for toddlers, who love to dip their exploring fingers into new foods. It is also a favorite topping for toddler foods and a time-honored bait to entice toddlers to try new foods.

---

well for many dishes, including potato salad, coleslaw, pasta salad, tuna salad, dips, and appetizers.

Try whole plain yogurt as a healthy alternative to sour cream. It is much lower in calories, fat, and cholesterol. If you're adding it to a sauce in place of sour cream, heat it over very low heat so it doesn't curdle. After a while, switch to low-fat.

Try yogurt in baking recipes. Plain yogurt can often be substituted for milk, buttermilk, or sour cream in recipes for waffles, pancakes, and muffins.

Substitute yogurt for ice cream. Yogurt shakes and smoothies are a low-fat alternative to ice cream (see "School-Ade," page 309).

NUTRIMYTH

Frozen yogurt is a healthy substitute for regular yogurt. Actually, frozen yogurts, even those that contain live and active cultures, may not be as healthful for you as nonfrozen yogurt, since refreezing the yogurt can destroy the digestive enzymes and the beneficial bacteria.

21

The Joy of Soy

OTHER CULTURES HAVE KNOWN the secrets of soy for centuries. Now, many food-savvy Americans are switching to soy as a healthier alternative to meat and dairy. Of the many foods for health we discuss throughout this book, the soy story is the most exciting to tell.

SEVEN REASONS THAT SOY IS SO GOOD FOR YOU

The seven secrets of soy are just a few of the reasons more Americans are trading their sirloin for soy foods.

1. Soy is a nutrient-dense food. Few foods contain as much nutritional bang for the buck as this bountiful bean. Ounce for ounce, calorie for calorie, the soybean gets top billing as a rich source of protein, unsaturated fats, fiber, B vitamins, folic acid, potassium, calcium, zinc, and iron — and it's cholesterol free. There is no other single food that supplies so much nutrition in such a tiny package. While TV and print ads tout milk as the perfect food, the soybean actually deserves this title. Soy *really* does a body good!

2. Soy contains powerful proteins, healthier fats. Soy ranks right up there with the American staples — dairy, eggs, and meat — as a rich source of protein, but without the drawbacks of these high-protein animal foods. Eggs, dairy, meat, and poultry contain mostly saturated fats, and they are high in cholesterol. Soy fat is mostly unsaturated and cholesterol free. Soy is the only plant food that is a *complete protein,* meaning that it contains all the essential amino acids that the body can't produce. (However, soy does not contain enough of the amino acid methionine for infants, so it is added to soy formulas.)

3. Soy has intestines-friendly carbs. Since soy is a plant food, it contains no lactose, which makes soy milk, soy cheese, and soy "yogurt" ideal alternatives to dairy products for persons who are sensitive to dairy. Soy contains nutritionally valuable carbs called "fructooligosaccharides" (FOS), which nourish the helpful intestinal bacteria.

4. Soy contains mood-friendly carbs. Soybeans have the lowest glycemic index of any food, so they are slow to trigger an insulin response and thereby provide a more stable blood-sugar level with fewer mood swings from high and low blood sugars. This makes soy an ideal before-school breakfast food for preventing the mid-morning low-blood-sugar crash in sugar-sensitive children.

5. Soy is a terrific source of bone- and blood-building calcium and iron. Soy gets the "Top Bean" award for the two vital minerals calcium and iron, nutritional features that make it a valuable alternative to dairy products and meat. Like other legumes, soy is a rich source of iron, in fact the richest of all the vegetables and legumes.

6. Soy is the original health food. Soy is a heart-healthy, cancer-fighting, and immune-boosting food. Let's compare the overall health of high-soy-consuming cultures, such as the Japanese, and low-soy-eating folk, like Americans. The average Japanese person eats 2 to 3 ounces (50 to 80 grams) of soy food daily in various forms, such as tofu, tempeh, and soy milk. The average American eats a scant 5 grams of soy, and that mostly in the form of oils (often hydrogenated) hidden in high-fat foods. The Japanese enjoy a longer lifespan and lower rates of cancer (especially colon, lung, breast, and prostate) and have a much lower incidence of heart disease. It will be interesting to see if a reversal in these diseases occurs as we export more beef to the Japanese and they sell us more soy. Heart and cancer doctors believe that adding as little as 2 ounces of tofu to the daily American diet could lower the risk of these deadly diseases. In Asian medicine, soybeans are valued as the tonic for long life and healthy living. In Asian countries, soy is known as the "meat without bones" and the "cow of China." While soy alone won't save your life, here's how it can help.

- *Soy reduces cholesterol.* Research has shown that replacing animal protein with 50 grams of soy protein a day can reduce cholesterol levels by 12 percent. Even better news is that soy protein lowers triglycerides, reduces LDL (bad) cholesterol, and raises HDL (good) cholesterol. In fact, soy is one of the few foods that selectively reduce LDL cholesterol. Much of the cholesterol-lowering effect of soy has been attributed not only to the soy protein, but also to the fiber and soy phytonutrients (called "isoflavones") that work along with bile acids in the intestines to escort cholesterol out of the body. Among the many health claims about soy, its cholesterol-reducing effects are the most scientifically proven. So, take your soy to heart.

- *Soy contains essential fatty acids.* Another heart-healthy feature of soy is the type of oil the soybean contains. Soybean oil is over 80 percent unsaturated fatty acids, and it contains the heart-healthy essential omega-3 and omega-6 fatty acids. (The lack of essential fatty acids in cow's milk is the reason that formula manufacturers choose soy instead of milk as a source of fat in baby formulas.)

- *Soy contains cancer-fighting phytos.* The phytonutrient most prominent in soy products is genistein, which has been shown to have anti-cancer properties. Soy also contains phytoestrogen, which has been shown to reduce the risk and spread of prostate cancer. The phytonutrient isoflavones may reduce the risk of breast cancer. The anti-cancer properties of soy seem to be associated primarily with the non-fermented soy products, such as tofu and soymilk, not with fermented soy products, such as miso and tempeh.

- *Soy is known as the "anti-aging food."* Because of the direct correlation between the longevity of a culture and the amount of soy in its diet, a wise person would, with increasing age, switch from primarily animal protein to fish, plant, and soy proteins. Osteoporosis is almost an accepted fact of getting older. The good news is this does not have to happen. Super soy to the rescue! Research has shown that the same amount of soy that can lower the risk of heart disease (40–50 grams a day) can also increase bone density and reduce the risk of osteoporosis. The anti-aging effect of soy is primarily due to its protein content.

7. Soy is a very versatile food. Now that you've been shown the joys of soy, you'll be happy to know that it comes in many forms, catering to different tastes, much like the multiple uses for wheat and dairy. There are many ways to incorporate soy into your diet.

TYPES OF SOY PRODUCTS

You can enjoy one of nature's most perfect foods in many forms and in combination with many other foods. Here's a guide to using the soy products you'll find at the supermarket or health food store.

Soy Drinks

Nutrient-rich soy beverages are made by pressing the extract, or milk, out of presoaked soybeans. Compared with cow's milk, soy beverages contain:

- less total fat
- less saturated fat
- no cholesterol
- three times as much fiber
- ten times as much iron
- ten times as much copper

NUTRITIP
Salty Soy

Before processing, soybeans are naturally low in sodium. But when those soybeans are turned into soy sauce, you can forget about the low-sodium claim. A tablespoon of soy sauce can contain around 1,200 milligrams of sodium, half the maximum recommended amount of sodium. Enjoy your Chinese food, but go light on the soy sauce, or look for the low-sodium variety.

- 75 percent less sodium
- twice the niacin
- no lactose, which may be an advantage to lactose-intolerant persons
- phytonutrients to reduce the risk of heart disease and cancer

There are some nutrients that are less abundant in soy drinks than in cow's milk. Compared with cow's milk, soy drinks contain:

- 20 percent less protein
- one-fifth as much vitamin A
- one-half as much zinc
- no vitamin B-12
- one-third as much folate
- only 3 percent of the amount of calcium (10 milligrams versus 300 milligrams in an 8-ounce glass)

Soy drinks usually contain a sweetener, such as rice syrup, and may also contain vegetable oils to improve the taste. Because of the added oils and sweeteners, current label laws prohibit soy drinks from being labeled "milk." Instead they are described either as a "drink" or "beverage." This situation is unlikely to change, since the sweeteners are usually necessary to make the soy beverage palatable. In the Sears family kitchen, we use a soy beverage as the liquid in making fruit and yogurt smoothies.

Tofu

Tofu is the curd of the soybean protein, similar to the cheese that comes from milk. The processing not only makes the soybean more useful, it makes it more nutritious. The calcium-containing ingredient that coagulates the soy protein into curds results in a cheese-like product that is high in calcium. The terrific thing about tofu is it can be consumed in many ways, such as the following:

- blended into a smoothie
- stir-fried or baked in chunks as a substitute for meat or poultry added to soup or stew
- pureed to make dips and spreads
- served raw as tiny cubes in salads

Tofu types. Firm, or Chinese-style, tofu is more nutrient dense than soft (or silken) Japanese-style tofu. It is much higher in protein, calcium, iron, and niacin, and slightly higher in fats and carbohydrates. It is also much lower in sodium. Firm tofu has the texture of most cheeses; soft tofu is more like a custard or yogurt. Firm tofu gets its texture and its calcium content from the calcium-containing coagulant used to form its more compact cakes. It has a more meaty consistency than the more delicate soft tofu.

Tofu tips. Even though firm tofu is much more nutrient dense than soft, which one you use is also a matter of taste. When making the switch to tofu as a substitute for meat and dairy, do it gradually, since to a meat-loving American palate, tofu has a relatively bland taste. After opening the container, you will notice the tofu is packed in water. To preserve its taste and texture, tofu should be kept in the refrigerator submerged in water, and the water should be changed daily. Freezing then thawing tofu gives it a firmer, more meaty texture.

Tempeh

Tempeh is a mixture of fermented soybeans (by a process similar to fermenting milk into yogurt) and grains, which results in a meat-like product that can be sliced, chopped, and made into burgers. Tempeh is higher in protein than the original soybean and is a low-fat, cholesterol-free alternative to meat. This ancient Indonesian food is also a rich source of fiber, calcium, iron, zinc, B-12, and folate. As an added perk, fermentation increases the bioavailability of isoflavones, the cholesterol-lowering and anti-cancer substances in soy products.

Miso

This Japanese favorite is made from fermented soybeans and grains and is often prepared as a soup. Miso is similar to tempeh in protein content, but it is higher than tempeh in calories and fiber. It is a very good source of zinc. Half a cup of miso contains 4.5 milligrams of zinc, nearly one-half to one-third the recommended dietary allowance. Miso's only nutritional drawback is its high sodium level. One cup of miso can contain as much as 5,000 milligrams of sodium, twice the RDA. Because of its high sodium content, miso is used more as a seasoning than as a main dish.

22

All About Oils

AS WE DISCUSSED in Part 1, a "right-fat" diet is better for you than a low-fat diet. Since most of the good fats are found in oils, it's important to know which oils contain the most nutritious fats. Also, remember that consuming too much of a healthy oil is unhealthy. Oils are high in calories and even the most nutritious oils contain some saturated fats.

OIL BASICS

Oils are liquid fats. Most commercial oils come from plant sources, such as nuts and seeds. Oils are an important part of a balanced diet because, besides being a rich source of energy, they provide essential fatty acids, which are the building blocks for cell membranes, especially cells in growing brains. Oils help the body absorb certain vitamins, such as A, D, E, and K, and contribute to healthier skin. And oils carry and intensify flavors in food and give it a pleasurable feel in the mouth.

Most oils come from the seeds of plants, which are crushed and pressed to remove the oil. Heat can damage oils and alter the fatty acids, creating harmful substances, so the best oils are produced with minimal heat. This is called "cold pressing." However, when you see the term "cold pressed" on a label, don't assume that the oil in the bottle was not heated during manufacturing. "Cold pressed" is a little fib that appeals to consumers who are savvy enough to equate heating with damage to oils. The problem is that the term has

---

HEART-HEALTHY OILS

Hydrogenated fats and oils raise the LDL (bad) cholesterol and lower the HDL (good) cholesterol. Some polyunsaturated oils tend to reduce blood levels of both HDL and LDL. Flax oil and monounsaturated oils, like olive and canola oils, reduce only the bad cholesterol without lowering the good cholesterol.

NUTRITIP
Whole-Food Oil Sources

Whenever possible, eat the food, such as fish or seeds, rather than the extracted oil. These foods contain other vital nutrients in addition to the energy-producing fats and healthy fatty acids.

no chemical, legal, or technological definition, and it means something different to a manufacturer than it does to a consumer. To a manufacturer, "cold pressed" simply means that no external heat was applied during the pressing of the oil, yet the press itself, which comes in contact with the oil, may become quite hot anyway and damage the oil. A more informative label would state the temperature at which the oil was processed, which ideally should be below 110 degrees. The words "omegaflo® process" on the label mean that the oil has been protected from reaching high temperatures during processing.

Most of the oils you'll find in the supermarket have not only been extracted with heat or solvents but have also been refined with potentially toxic substances. These processes improve shelf life and make oil cheap to produce, but they take the product further away from its natural state and leave chemical residues behind. If the label does not boast that the oil is "unrefined," you can assume that it has been through some kind of chemical process that makes it worse for your health.

COOKING WITH OILS

Cooking at high temperatures can damage oils. The more omega-3 fatty acids in the oil, the less suitable it is for cooking. The heat not only damages fatty acids, it can also change them into harmful substances called "peroxides." Hydrogenated oils are often used in cooking; because they have already been "damaged" by chemical processing, they are less likely to be further damaged by heat. The oils that are highest in saturated fats (tropical oils) or in monounsaturates (olive oil) are the most stable when heated. The more fragile oils are best used at room temperature, such as in salad dressings. To preserve the nutritious properties and the flavor of unrefined oils, pour around ¼ cup of water in the stir-fry pan

and heat just below boiling. Then add the food and cook it a bit before adding the oil. This method shortens the time the oil is in contact with a hot pan. Stir the food frequently to further reduce the time the oil is in contact with the hot metal. Never heat oils to the smoking point, as this damages not only their fatty-acid content but also their taste. The best cooking oils and fats are butter, peanut oil, high-oleic sunflower oil, high-oleic safflower oil, sesame oil, and olive oil.

STORING OILS

If you are buying oil in large quantities, it should be stored in dark bottles. Clear glass or plastic bottles allow light to penetrate the oil and oxidize the fatty acids in a chemical process similar to metal rusting. If the oil comes in a clear bottle, wrap it with a dark covering. Keep the lid on tightly between uses, as contact with air also affects the quality of the oil. Purchase oil in small quantities, and use it within a month or two. The healthier the oil, the more quickly it spoils. Store oils in a cool, dark place. Unrefined oils spoil more easily when exposed to warm temperatures, so they need to be refrigerated if you are not going to use them right away. An exception to this is olive oil, which need not be refrigerated; it is high in oleic acid and contains antioxidants, which slow spoiling. Other cooking oils, such as safflower, sunflower, and corn, are high in linolenic acid and are quick to spoil.

MORE OIL-USING TIPS

Buy organic. Oils are one kind of food that is definitely worth paying extra to get organic. Many oils come from plants that are sprayed with lots of pesticides, which are usually fat soluble and thus concentrate in the oil portion of the plant. One of the safest oils is extra virgin olive oil, which is not refined or deodorized, and may even be organically grown.

Read labels. The already lax label laws are even more slippery when it comes to oils. Avoid oil that is labeled simply "vegetable oil." A consumer has a right to know which vegetables are used in the oil. Ditto that caution for "all purpose" vegetable oils. Chances are that the manufacturer used the inexpensive, highly processed oils (e.g.,

cottonseed oil), to fill up the bottle. Labels do not usually list the types of fatty acid the oil contains, such as how much omega 3 and how much omega 6. Ideally, the label should state whether the oil was chemically extracted or mechanically pressed. Consumers have the right to know if they are possibly eating chemical residues. If the label doesn't tell you how the oil was produced, you can assume the worst.

Don't be misled into thinking there's something special about the oil that boasts "no cholesterol" on the label. No oils contain any cholesterol because they are a plant food. Avoid any oil that has the bad-fat words "partially hydrogenated" on the label.

TYPES OF OIL

The goal of a "right-fat" diet is to eat the right amount of the right kinds of oils. We have used these criteria for evaluating the various types of oil:

- the percentage of essential fatty acids in the oil
- the percentage of unsaturated versus saturated fats (i.e., how heart-healthy the oil is)
- the effect on blood cholesterol (i.e., whether the oil raises or lowers cholesterol, especially in cholesterol-sensitive persons)
- other proven health benefits of the oil
- taste
- likelihood that pesticide residues were left in the oil during processing
- how processing procedures affect the nutritional qualities of the oil

The fact that some oils rank higher than others does not mean that you should consume only the one or two at the top of the list. Balance is still the key to good nutrition, and balance depends on variety.

RANKING OILS: THE GOOD, THE BAD, AND THE IN BETWEEN

Best Oils	Comments
1. Flaxseed	Best source of omega-3 fatty acids; has heart-healthy properties; is a colon-friendly oil, lessening constipation; boosts immunity; promotes healthy skin; contains healthy phytonutrient lignan; spoils quickly without careful storage; not to be used in cooking
2. Canola	One of the oils lowest in saturated fats, making it a heart-friendly oil; a rich source of essential omega-3 and -6 fatty acids
3. Soybean	Contains both omega-3 and omega-6 fatty acids, but is often highly refined and hydrogenated
4. Olive oil (virgin or extra virgin)	Doesn't need high-temperature or chemical processing, since it is made from the flesh of the olive and not the seed; slow to spoil; okay for medium-temperature cooking; in moderation lowers LDL (bad) cholesterol without affecting HDL, thereby improving the HDL-to-LDL ratio.
5. Pumpkin seed	Low in saturated fats; rich in omega-6 fatty acids; may contain some omega 3's; refining and chemical processing lower its nutritional qualities

Medium Oils	Comments
1. Safflower	Low in saturated fats; rich in omega-6 fatty acids
2. Sunflower	Rich in omega-6 fatty acids
3. Corn	Slightly higher in saturated fats than the best oils; usually hydrogenated; rich source of omega-6 fatty acids
4. Peanut	Somewhat high in saturated fats but still less than butter, animal fat, and cottonseed oil; good for cooking at higher temperatures

Worst Oils	Comments
1. Cottonseed	High in saturated fats; likely to contain pesticide residues; frequently hydrogenated
2. Palm kernel	High in saturated fats, and therefore a potentially cholesterol-raising oil
3. Coconut	Highest in saturated fats of all popular oils; one of the most atherogenic (heart-unhealthy) oils

Flax Oil

Because, in our opinion, this is the top health oil, it merits a section of its own (see page 211).

Canola Oil

This oil is extracted from a variety of rapeseed that originated in Canada, and is known as "*Can*adian *oil low-a*cid oil," or "canola." Canola oil ranks just below flax oil and soybean oil as a high vegetable source of the essential omega-3 fatty acids. Like flax oil, it contains both omega-3 and omega-6 fatty acids, but in a different ratio. Canola oil contains an omega-6 to omega-3 ratio of 2 to 1. Flax oil is 0.3 to 1. Because canola contains one of the highest ratios of unsaturated to saturated fats, it is one of the most heart-healthy oils, reported to reduce cholesterol levels, lower serum triglyceride levels, and keep platelets from sticking together. Because of the high omega-3 content, heating canola oil may change some of the fatty acids into trans fats, which raise total cholesterol and lower the levels of good cholesterol. Be sure to buy organic canola oil, since rapeseeds are often sprayed with pesticides.

Soybean Oil

Soybean oil is extracted from beans, not seeds. Unrefined soybean oil is one of the richest sources of lecithin (2 percent). It also contains, in its unrefined state, 5 to 7 percent of the omega-3 essential fatty acids and alphalinolenic acid (ALA), in addition to being high in the omega-6 essential fatty acid, linoleic acid (LA). Unfortunately, most commercial soybean oils are refined and hydrogenated. Because it has a high boiling point, it is okay for cooking.

Olive Oil

Olive oil is made from the flesh of olives rather than the seeds. This means it requires less pressure and lower temperatures during the pressing process, which preserves the nutritional qualities of the oil. Olive oil contains 90 percent unsaturated fats, most of which are the cholesterol-lowering monounsaturates. Because it is high in oleic acid and low in linoleic fatty acid, it is slow to spoil. It has a pleasant flavor and can be used both in salad dressings and in cooking. Olive oil is a favorite in Mediterranean cuisine, since olive groves and olive presses are plentiful in that part of the world. "Virgin" olive oil means that the oil is from the first pressing, and it has not been refined or chemically processed in any way, such as being bleached or hydrogenated. "Extra virgin" is the highest-quality olive oil (for which you pay a slightly higher price). It has a richer, less acidic taste. High-temperature cooking destroys the flavor of olive oil, but it is excellent for dressings and the "sautéing with water" method described on page 206. Avoid olive oil that does not say "virgin" or "extra virgin" on the label, but instead boasts of being "refined" or "pure." "Refined" means that the oil has been chemically processed. "Pure" means nothing more than that the oil came from an olive. Even though olive oil is slow to spoil, store it in a cool, dark, place in the cupboard. Olive oil's only drawback is that it is only average in omega-6 and low in omega-3 fatty acids. A combination of flax oil and olive oil in the diet strikes a healthy balance.

Healthy (but Hard to Find) Oils

Pumpkin seed oil. This is one of the most healthful oils for several reasons. High-quality pumpkin seed oil contains over 90 percent unsaturated fats and has both omega-6 and omega-3 essential fatty acids in a 3-to-1 ratio. It contains from 0 to 15 percent linolenic acid and from 45 to 60 percent linoleic acid. Unfortunately, most commonly available pumpkin oil contains no linolenic acid.

Algae oil. Algae oil is the richest source of DHA available, with 40 percent DHA by weight. Algae are the dietary source of omega-3 fatty acids for fish, so algae represent the only vegetable source of DHA available.

Walnut oil. Another extremely healthful oil, at least on paper, walnut oil contains both omega-6 and omega-3 fatty acids in a 10-to-1 ratio. It is 84 percent unsaturated. However, most available walnut oil is sold in a refined state.

Black currant, borage, and evening primrose oils. These are popular "health oils" because they are rich sources of the essential fatty acid GLA (gammalinolenic acid), a vital ingredient for making important hormones, such as prostaglandins. Black currant oil is the richest source of GLA, followed by borage oil, and then evening primrose oil. Black currant oil has two advantages over evening primrose oil: It is less expensive, and it is one of the few oils that contain omega-3 in addition to omega-6 fatty acids. While these oils have been touted as cure-alls for many ailments, scientific evaluation of these oils yields mixed results. And the fact that they are extracted by chemical processing may render these tonics less healthy than advertised. Critics of these oils claim that since the body produces its own GLA from essential fatty acids contained in many foods, GLA supplements are not necessary. Proponents of these oils claim that some people, especially aging persons, may be unable to convert dietary essential fatty acids to GLA. GLA-containing oils, as well as the essential fatty acid DHA, are popular ingredients of a flurry of brain-boosting nutrients collectively known as "targeted nutritional intervention" (TNI) and are being studied for use in children with Down Syndrome.

Sunflower and Safflower Oils

These oils are rich in vitamin E. Because these oils are high in omega-6 fatty acids and contain no omega 3's, they are less nutritious than canola and flax oils. Even though they contain 90 percent unsaturated fats, they tend to be highly refined oils. Because of their high oleic-acid content, they are least damaged by heat and tend to be favorite cooking oils.

Corn Oil

Even though this popular oil contains mostly unsaturated fat, it is higher in saturated fats than most other oils and is usually highly refined and hydrogenated. Like other polyunsaturated oils, corn oil does lower total cholesterol. While it lowers LDL (bad) cholesterol, it also lowers the good HDL cholesterol a bit; still, the result is an improved HDL-to-LDL ratio. It is not one of the more nutritious oils.

Peanut Oil

Peanut oil is a favorite cooking oil, especially for stir-fries. Since it is relatively high in saturated fats, which do not turn into trans fatty acids when heated to normal cooking temperatures, it is more useful as a cooking oil than oils that are lower in saturates and higher in omega-3 fatty acids.

Cottonseed Oil

Cottonseed is one of the most widely used oils, added to many processed foods, such as cereals and potato chips. Relatively inexpensive and readily available, it merits its place on our "Worst Oils" list for several reasons. Cotton is a crop that is heavily sprayed with pesticides, so cottonseed oil can be loaded with pesticides. And, like tropical oils, cottonseed oil is low in monounsaturated fats and relatively high in saturated fats. Also, cottonseed oil is likely to be hydrogenated to further extend its shelf life.

Tropical Oils

Oils such as coconut, palm, and palm kernel are the least healthful naturally occurring oils. Yet because they are cheap, taste good, and have a long shelf life, they are often used in packaged foods such as cereal and cookies. Coconut oil, for example, is the ideal oil to use in chocolate candy, since it is solid at room temperature but melts in the mouth. Food processors, especially in the candy industry, separate the tropical oils so they don't have to list them collectively as "tropical oils" on the label, possibly tipping off consumers to the fact that they are eating a cholesterol-raising fat. Don't be misled by the white label lie "contains no cholesterol." Plant foods don't contain cholesterol. But coconut oil, for example, is high in the saturated fat lauric acid, one of the most heart-unhealthy fats.

FABULOUS FLAX

Flaxseed oil and flax seeds are being rediscovered as true health foods. They definitely merit being included on any "top ten" list of foods. Flax is not a new food. It is actually one of the older and, perhaps, one of the original health foods, treasured because of its healing properties throughout the Roman empire. Flax was one of the original "medicines" used by Hippocrates. Flax could be dubbed the "forgotten oil." It has fallen out of favor because oil manufacturers have found less nutritious oils to be more profitable and it has been primarily used in the chemical industry as a varnish or lacquer (flax oil is linseed oil). The very nutrients that give flax its nutritional benefits — essential fatty acids — also give it a short shelf life, making it more expensive to produce, transport, and store. Yet those who are nutritionally in the know continue to rank flax high on the list of must-have foods. Because of the flurry of scientific studies validating the health benefits of omega-3 fatty acids, flax oil has graduated from the refrigerators of "health food nuts" to gain scientific respectability.

Flax Facts

Flax oil and flax seeds are the best sources of linolenic acid (an omega-3 fatty acid). This is the precursor of DHA, a vital structural component of all the cells of the body, especially brain and eye cells (see "Smart Fats," page 9). Not only are omega-3 fatty acids vital for the health of cell membranes, hormones, and a healthy immune system, but recent research has implicated a defi-

---

NUTRITIP
Fattening Flax

Flax oil is a valuable nutritional supplement for both young and old. One tablespoon of flax oil contains 150 nutritious calories, which not only helps weight gain but also improves brain development and boosts immunity. So, infants who are failing to thrive or elderly people who are recovering from a debilitating illness such as cancer would do well on a flax oil or flaxseed supplement.

ciency of DHA in many of the degenerative diseases that afflict cultures whose diet is traditionally low in essential fatty acids.

Flax Oil

I seldom leave home in the morning without having my daily tablespoon of flax oil or 2 tablespoons of flaxseed meal. Besides being the best source of omega 3's, flax oil is a good source of omega 6, or linoleic acid (LA). It contains between 10 and 20 percent LA. This is less than sunflower, safflower, and sesame oil, but those three oils do not contain any omega-3 fatty acids. Flax oil is 45 to 60 percent the omega-3 fatty acid alphalinolenic acid (ALA).

Don't use flax oil for cooking. Oils high in omega-3 fatty acids are not good for cooking. In fact, heat can turn these healthy fats into harmful ones (see "Cooking with Oils," page 206). Add flax oil to foods after cooking and just before serving.

Flax has many virtues, but it also has one vice: It turns rancid quickly. Healthy fats spoil quickly, with olive oil being an exception to the rule. (The fats with a long shelf life are the hydrogenated shortenings, which of course are bad for you.) To prevent spoilage, follow these tips:

- Purchase only refrigerated flax oil stored in black containers.
- Keep your flax oil in the refrigerator with the lid on tight. Minimize its exposure to heat, light, and air.
- Because the oil is likely to turn rancid within six weeks of pressing, buy flax oil in small containers (8–12 ounces, depending on how fast you use it). In our family, we go through approximately 4 tablespoons of flax oil a day, using it mainly in our School-Ade smoothie (see page 309).

Flax oil taken with a meal can actually increase the nutritional value of other foods. Research shows that adding flax oil to foods rich in sulfated amino acids, such as yogurt, vegetables of the cabbage family, and animal, seafood, and soy proteins, helps the essential fatty acids become incorporated into cell membranes. Mixing flax oil with yogurt helps to emulsify the oil, improving its digestion and metabolism by the body.

Flax oil works best in the body when it is taken along with antioxidants, such as vitamin E, and other nutrients, such as vitamin B-6 and magnesium. While a tablespoon of flax oil a day might not keep the doctor away entirely, it's bound to help.

Flax Seeds

In addition to nutritious fats, flax seeds contain other nutrients that make eating the whole seed superior to consuming just the extracted oil:

- Flax seeds contain a high-quality protein.
- Flax seeds are rich in soluble fiber. The combination of the oil and the fiber makes flax seeds an ideal laxative.
- Flax seeds contain vitamins B-1, B-2, and C. They also contain iron, zinc, and trace amounts of potassium, magnesium, phosphorus, calcium, and vitamin E and carotene, two nutrients that aid the metabolism of the oil.
- Flax seeds contain over a hundred times more of a phytonutrient known as "lignan" than any of its closest competitors, such as wheat bran, buckwheat, rye, millet, oats, and soybeans. Lignans have received a lot of attention lately because of their possible anti-cancer properties, especially in relation to breast and colon cancer. Lignans seem to flush excess estrogen out of the body, thereby reducing the incidence of estrogen-linked cancers, such as breast cancer. Besides their anti-tumor properties, lignans also seem to have anti-bacterial, anti-fungal, and anti-viral properties.

Flax seeds, because they contain some protein, fiber, vitamins and minerals, and lignans, are more nutritious than their oil. Yet, for practical purposes, most consumers prefer simply using the oil for its omega-3 fatty acids and not having to bother with grinding the seeds. But nutritionally speaking, it is worth the trouble to grind fresh flax seeds (say, in a coffee grinder) and sprinkle them as a seasoning on salads or cereals or mix them into muffins. When buying seeds, be sure they are whole, not split; splitting exposes the inner seed to light and heat and decreases the nutritional value. Or, buy pre-ground flax seeds, available as flaxseed meal. One ounce of flaxseed meal (approximately 4 tbsp.) will yield about 6 grams of protein, and 8 grams of fiber.

Health-Promoting Properties of Flax

Flax oil, flax seeds, and the omega-3 fatty acids they contain are good for your health. Here are some of the ways flax helps your body.

- Flax promotes cardiovascular health. The ultra-high levels of omega-3 fatty acids lower LDL (bad) cholesterol levels. Fish oils and algae are also good sources of essential fatty acids.

- Flax promotes colon health. It has anti-cancer properties and, as a natural lubricant (and, in

---

NUTRITIP
Ketch-Oil

A trick we have used to fortify our little ketchup lovers is to mix fruit-sweetened ketchup with flax oil. Put a dollop of ketchup on a plate, make an opening in the center, pour in 1 to 3 teaspoons of flax oil, and mix together well. The oily taste is gone.

---

the case of flax seeds, a rich fiber source), it lowers the risk of constipation.

- Flax supplements can boost immunity. One study showed that schoolchildren supplemented with less than 1 teaspoon of flax oil a day had fewer and less severe respiratory infections than children not supplemented with flax oil.

- Flax provides fats that are precursors for brain building. This is especially important at the stage of life when a child's brain grows the fastest, in utero and during infancy. A prudent mom could consider supplementing her diet with a daily tablespoon of flax oil during her pregnancy and while breastfeeding.

- Flax promotes healthy skin. I recommend flax oil as a dietary supplement for my patients who have dry skin or eczema or whose skin is particularly sun sensitive.

- Flax may lessen the severity of diabetes by stabilizing blood-sugar levels.

- Flax fat can be slimming. Eating the right kind of fat gives you a better fighting chance that your body will store the right amount of fats. Fats high in essential fatty acids, such as flax, increase the body's metabolic rate, helping to burn the excess, unhealthy fats in the body. This is called "thermogenesis," a process by which specialized fat cells throughout the body (called "brown fat") click into high gear and burn more when activated by essential fatty acids. I have noticed that I crave less fat overall when I make certain I get enough of the healthy fats. A daily supplement of omega-3 fatty acids may be an important part of weight-control programs.

23

Health Nuts and Seeds

NATURE PACKS A LOT OF NUTRI-
tion into a little nut, which is why nuts
and seeds got honorable mention on our
"Top Twelve Foods" list. Nuts are the seeds
of different trees. They come in a variety of
shapes, flavors, and preparations that add to their
appeal: shelled or unshelled, raw, dry roasted, oil
roasted, sugared, salted, spiced, and honey coated.

Nuts and seeds are more nutrient dense than
most foods. They are rich sources of protein, fiber,
B vitamins, folic acid, calcium, iron, zinc, and the
antioxidants vitamin E and selenium. Do you
think nuts have too much fat to be part of a
healthy diet? Wrong! Nuts do contain a lot of fat,
but 90 percent of this fat is the heart-healthy unsaturated kind. In fact, recent studies have shown
that eating nuts may reduce a person's risk of having a heart attack. Because nuts and seeds are high
in monounsaturated fats, they have been found to
lower LDL (bad) cholesterol.

percent more fat calories to the nuts. This is no
big deal unless the nuts have been roasted in saturated or hydrogenated fats (e.g., coconut oil);
check the label. An increase in saturated fats
lessens the nut's main nutritional claim to
fame — namely, being low in saturated fats.

While heating or roasting nuts does enhance
the flavor and reduce spoilage, it also may alter
some of the essential fatty acids. This is why
processed nuts are less likely to get rancid, but the
trade-off may be a loss of healthy nutrients. Seeds
and nuts themselves are more nutritious than the
oil extracted from them, at least in theory. Seeds
and nuts contain natural vitamin E, which protects their oil from going rancid. Processing may
remove some of the natural antioxidants in the
nuts and seeds.

While nuts and seeds are a perfect snack, don't
go nutty over their nutrition. A handful of nuts or
seeds packs around 200 calories. It's best to dole

NUT KNOWLEDGE

Roasted nuts are more flavorful and spoil less
quickly than raw nuts, yet how they are roasted
makes a big nutritional difference. Dry-roasted
nuts don't have any added fat. Oil-roasted nuts
have been fried in oil, which adds around 10

NUTRITIP
Buy Organic.

When it comes to nuts, organic is better. All
nuts, and peanuts especially, pick up
pesticide residues. Ditto for nut butters.

out a small amount into a container rather than to snack right out of the bag. The good news is that the fiber in nuts and seeds fills you up quickly, making you less likely to overeat while you're snacking and at the next meal.

Sunflower and sesame seeds, along with various kinds of nuts, are a nutritious addition to salads. When used this way, a small amount goes a long way. Sprinkle on a spoonful and enjoy!

RANKING NUTS

Here's our list of favorite nuts, ranked by their nutrient density. These varieties contain the most protein, fiber, B vitamins, calcium, minerals, and vitamin E for the least amount of saturated fat:

1. Almonds
2. Filberts (hazelnuts)
3. Peanuts
4. Chestnuts
5. Pistachios
6. Walnuts
7. Cashews
8. Pecans
9. Macadamias

Our "Top Nut" award goes to the almond. Here are the main nutrients in 1 ounce of almonds (a medium-size handful):

- 166 calories
- 5 grams of protein

NUTRITIP
Soak Your Seeds.

Soaking seeds and nuts in distilled water overnight makes them easier to digest.

NUTRITIP
Nuts Are Not for Toddlers.

Because of the possibility of choking, do not give nuts to children under three years of age. Use the nut butters instead.

- 14 grams of fat (90 percent unsaturated)
- 4 grams of fiber (the highest fiber content of any nut or seed), unblanched
- 80 milligrams of calcium
- 1.4 milligrams of zinc
- 1 milligram of iron
- 6.7 milligrams of vitamin E
- some B vitamins, minerals, and selenium

Filberts (hazelnuts) because they are high in the amino acid tryptophan are a good nut for sleep. Almonds and filberts have the most vitamin E (6.7 milligrams per ounce) — nearly 25 percent of the adult recommended dietary allowance. Walnuts have the greatest concentration of omega-3 fatty acids. Chestnuts are lowest in fat, containing only about 10 percent as much fat as other nuts. What little fat is in the chestnut (1.3 grams per ounce) is nearly all the unsaturated

---

NUTRITIP
Sleep Nuts

Eating a small handful of nuts as a before-bedtime snack may help you catch some deeper winks. Some nuts and seeds, especially whole filberts and ground sesame seeds, have a high amount of the sleep-inducing amino acid tryptophan relative to the brain-stimulating amino acid tyrosine.

PRAISE FOR PEANUT BUTTER

Could life go on without peanut butter? Yes, but not as pleasurably. Not only is peanut butter a nutrient-dense food, it is one that most children enjoy. Parents like its convenience. Two tablespoons of peanut butter, the average amount in a peanut butter and jelly sandwich, contain 8.5 grams of protein, 4 milligrams of the B vitamin niacin (one-third the recommended dietary allowance for a pre-teen child), along with a touch of fiber, calcium, folic acid, zinc, and iron — all in 200 calories that provide a high source of energy for a busy child.

While peanut butter is a favorite and nutritious family food, the peanut is not without its problems:

- Children who are allergic to peanuts are *very* allergic, and, unlike many other food allergies, this is one that they do not usually outgrow. If your child is allergic to peanut butter, be sure you warn her school (children share lunches) and other adults (e.g., playmates' parents) who may be serving your child snacks. Some people are so allergic to peanuts that even a whiff can trigger an asthmatic attack. This scare has recently prompted some airlines to have "peanut-free zones" on their flights. Beware of peanuts hidden in candies and some Asian dishes. People who are allergic to peanut butter (since peanuts are not, strictly speaking, nuts) can often tolerate other nut

butters, such as almond and cashew. But try these alternatives carefully. Avoiding peanut butter during pregnancy and lactation may lower the chances of your infant being sensitized to peanut butter and later becoming allergic.

- For safety's sake spread nut butters on bread or crackers rather than allowing children to wolf down a fingerful. Globs of peanut butter and other nut butters can cause choking.

- Be careful of a toxic mold called "aflatoxin" that can grow on rancid peanut butter or spoiled peanuts. Peanut butter manufacturers are highly aware of this potentially toxic mold and take strict manufacturing precautions to eliminate it. Commercially available peanut butters are safe. If you grind your own nuts into peanut butter, take care to use roasted nuts that are fresh.

- While the fat in peanut butter is about 80 percent unsaturated, hydrogenated oils may be added to the peanut butter to increase the shelf life. If hydrogenated oil is added, it must say so on the label. You can tell whether or not peanut butter contains hydrogenated oil by checking whether it separates when it sits on the shelf. When nonhydrogenated peanut butter sits, the natural oils rise to the top, and you have to stir the oil into the peanut butter after you open it. If there is no oil floating on the top of the peanut butter when you open a new jar, check the ingredients list. It probably contains hydrogenated oils.

type. Chestnuts also contain 3 grams of fiber per ounce, but they are relatively low in protein.

Soybean nuts and peanuts are not really nuts at all. They are legumes, and they come from plants other than trees. But both are very nutritious. Soybean nuts, while less popular because of their less appealing taste, are actually the most nutri-

tious nut. One-quarter cup of soybean nuts is similar in number of calories to other nuts but packs the following nutrients:

- 17 grams of protein
- 9 grams of fat (90 percent unsaturated)
- 3.5 grams of fiber

- 138 milligrams of folic acid (33 percent of the DV)
- 116 milligrams of calcium (10 percent of the DV)
- 2 milligrams of zinc (around 15 percent of the DV)
- 1.7 milligrams of iron (10 percent of the DV)
- 19 micrograms of selenium

When purchasing soybean nuts, avoid those that are roasted in "hydrogenated" or "partially hydrogenated" oils.

COMPARING NUT BUTTERS

Peanut butter isn't the only kind of nut butter you can spread on your whole wheat bread. Try some variety. Almond butter is more nutrient dense than peanut butter, with half the amount of saturated fat, less salt (usually), and eight times as much calcium. Peanut butter, however, contains twice as much protein and four times as much niacin (20 percent of the DV). Cashew butter is less nutritious than either almond or peanut butter. It contains less protein, fiber, and niacin than peanut butter, but it still makes a tasty piece of toast. Soy butter, a healthy alternative for those allergic to other nut butters, is lower in total and saturated fats than peanut butter, but it usually has added sweeteners to make it palatable.

TOP SEEDS

Seeds have nutritional profiles similar to nuts, because, after all, seeds are nuts. One ounce of hulled sunflower seeds (one medium-size handful) offers the following:

- 165 calories
- 5.5 grams of protein
- 14 grams of fat (90 percent unsaturated)

- 3 grams of fiber
- 2 milligrams of niacin (10 percent of the DV)
- 67 milligrams of folic acid (17 percent of the DV)
- 20 milligrams of calcium
- 1.5 milligrams of zinc (10 percent of the DV)
- 1 milligram of iron
- 14 milligrams of vitamin E (50 percent of the DV)
- 78 micrograms of selenium (there is some evidence that 100 mcg. a day of selenium may reduce the risk of cancer)

Sesame seeds have a similar nutritional profile to sunflower seeds, but these tiny decorative seeds supply slightly more fiber, and twice as much calcium, zinc, and iron. Sesame seed butter (called "tahini") is a favorite of Middle Eastern cuisine. It can be mixed with ground chickpeas to make hummus or combined with eggplant and spices to make baba ghanoush, for example.

Of all the seeds and nuts, pumpkin seeds contain the most iron, packing a blood-building 4 milligrams per ounce (six times more iron than in an ounce of beef). Yet pumpkin seeds contain less vitamin E, calcium, folic acid, niacin, and fiber than sunflower or sesame seeds.

NUTRITIP
Grind Your Seeds.

Because sesame seeds are so small, you are unlikely to chew them and break down the seeds to release the nutrients. As a result, the seeds pass through the intestines undigested. To release all the good nutrients from these power-packed little seeds, first grind them into a meal, and then sprinkle them on salads.

24

Minding Your Meat and Picking Your Poultry

WHILE HAMBURGERS ARE AS AMERICAN AS THE FLAG, there are good reasons why meat didn't make it onto our "Top Twelve Foods" list. Meat is a rich source of protein, some B vitamins (including B-12), iron, and zinc, but there aren't any nutrients in meat that can't be obtained from other foods. If you skip meat, you'll miss out on a lot of things that really aren't good for you. Once you understand the nutritional benefits and risks of meat, you will see why many Americans are switching from sirloin to salmon.

WHAT'S THE BEEF WITH MEAT?

This question can be answered in two nutritional words: *fat* and *cholesterol*.

Too much fat. No matter how you slice it, meat is high in fat. Unlike milk, in which you can separate out part or all of the fat, you can never get rid of all the fat in meat, no matter how well you trim it. Even the lean parts are laced with fat. Extra-lean select-grade beef contains around 7 percent fat.

Wrong fat. Not only is there too much fat in meat, it's the wrong kind. Nearly half the fat in meat is the artery-clogging saturated type. And, of

course, meat is also high in cholesterol. Beef fat is more saturated than poultry fat because the bacteria in the ruminant stomach of cattle hydrogenate, or saturate, the fats in the plants that cows eat. It's like having a fat factory inside the food source.

Fat without fiber. Unlike meat, plant foods that are low in fat and high in fiber tend to pass through the intestines rapidly, causing less upset and fewer problems, such as gastroesophageal reflux (see "GER—the Great Masquerader," page 96, and "Indigestion," page 98). Meat has a double fault. It's high in fat and contains no fiber, so it takes longer to empty from the stomach and pass through the intestines. While most people do not experience indigestion from meat, those who suffer from reflux should not eat much meat, as it can aggravate the problem.

Problems with protein. Not only are the fats in meat unhealthy, but meat proteins have also recently come under fire. Recent evidence suggests that animal proteins increase blood-cholesterol levels, while plant proteins, especially soy, decrease them. Meats contain high levels of the amino acid lysine, which increases insulin production, prompting the liver to release fat and cholesterol into the bloodstream. If lysine is experimentally added to animal diets, blood-cholesterol levels increase by over 50 percent and the animals get plump. Studies show that substituting 30 grams of soy protein daily for a meat meal dramatically reduces cholesterol levels. So, the Japanese may have lower cholesterol levels than Americans not only because they eat less meat but also because they eat more soy. As shown in the box on page 50, the quality of meat protein ranks below that of egg white, fish, and dairy products.

Other concerns. While there is experimental evidence to implicate the meat fats and proteins in disease, the effects of muscle-building hormones and infection-killing antibiotics fed to livestock are harder to pin down. These substances do appear in the meat at the supermarket, and common sense tells us that they certainly can't contribute to our health and may harm it.

The most compelling reasons for going meatless are the undisputed studies showing that countries with a high per capita meat consumption also have high rates of heart disease and cancer. And within these countries people who eat less meat have a lower incidence of both heart disease and cancer than the general population. One of the most famous studies is the Nurses' Health Study. In this study of more than one hundred thousand female nurses, those who ate the most animal fat were twice as likely to get colon cancer as those with the lowest intake of animal fat.

Meat Tips

You may not want to completely eliminate it from your diet, but there are ways to cut back on both the meat and the fat.

Trim the fat. Trim all the fat you can see surrounding that sirloin. In addition, choose cuts of meat that are less marbled with fat, the kind of fat that not even the finest surgeon could trim. Here are some fat-trimming words to look for in reading labels on cuts of meat:*

- *Select* is the leanest cut of meat, containing around 7 percent fat by weight.
- *Choice* contains 15 to 35 percent fat by weight.
- *Prime* is the fattest grade, containing 35 to 45 percent fat by weight.

Fat content will vary with different cuts of meat, as well as with the grade. Here are different cuts of *select-grade* beef in order from lowest fat content to highest.

1. Top round	9. T-bone
2. Eye of round	10. Tenderloin
3. Round tip	11. Porterhouse
4. Bottom round	12. Brisket
5. Shank	13. Rib-eye
6. Sirloin	14. Flank
7. Arm	15. Ribs
8. Top loin	16. Blade

Drip-dry the fat. Broiling is likely to remove more fat from the meat than frying, especially if the fat drips out of the meat. Roasting or baking the meat in its own juice is certainly better than adding fat by frying, but the fat can soak back into the meat this way.

Instead of buying hamburger, choose the leanest piece of beef you can find, such as select top round (around 4 grams of fat per 3.5 ounces, compared with 18 grams of total fat for lean ground beef), and ask the butcher to grind your chosen cut into hamburger for you. (Of the popular cuts of beef, select top round has the lowest amount of total and saturated fat.)

---

* *Since there is no law requiring beef to carry these labels, you may have to ask which category of meat a particular cut is.*

Beef up the main dish without beef. Rather than making meat the centerpiece of a meal and vegetables the accent, reverse the importance of these foods. Eating 3 ounces of diced beef in a vegetable stir-fry is much healthier than sitting down to a 16-ounce sirloin. Instead of planning meals around the meat, let the meat accompany the vegetables or be part of a pasta or grain-based casserole.

Alternatives to Beef

Game meats. Game meats are the lowest in both fat and saturated fat. Some have one-fifth to one-twentieth the fat contained in domestic meats. For example, 3.5 ounces of venison contain only 3 grams of fat, 1 gram of which is saturated. Rabbit meat is higher in vitamin B-12 than any domestic meat, supplying 6 micrograms, 100 percent of the recommended dietary allowance.

Veal. Though veal is higher in cholesterol than many cuts of beef and contains about as much fat, it is much higher in niacin (a 3.5-ounce serving contains 10 milligrams, half the RDA). In addition, veal contains two to three times more calcium than most cuts of beef or pork. If possible, buy free-range veal.

Lamb. Depending on the cut, lamb is nutritionally similar to beef. It's slightly higher in cholesterol, lower in zinc, and higher in niacin than beef, except veal.

Pork. There is no nutritional advantage to eating pork over beef. It is lower than most cuts of beef in vitamin B-12, zinc, and iron. Avoid fatty processed meats, such as bacon and sausage; they not only contain lots of saturated fat but also may contain nitrates, which may cause concern.

Give your body a treat. Eat less meat.

PICKING POULTRY

Poultry holds the middle ground in the eating-of-animal-flesh debate. It's better for you than beef but not as good for you as seafood. While poultry is similar to most meats in nutrient content, there are some differences. Compared with beef, poultry is:

- slightly lower in calories, depending on the cut
- lower in fat, depending on the cut
- lower in vitamin B-12
- lower in zinc and iron (except for turkey breasts)
- higher in essential fatty acids
- easier to digest

It's easier to lower the fat level in chicken or turkey than it is in beef. To get less saturated fat from your bird, remove the skin, since most of the fat is found here rather than marbled through the bird's muscle. Removing the skin from the poultry reduces the calories by at least 20 percent and the fat by 40 to 50 percent, but it does not significantly change cholesterol levels.

Choose white meat over dark meat if avoiding fat is your goal. Compared with white meat, dark meat is approximately 25 percent higher in calories and more than twice as high in fat. Dark meat is also slightly higher in cholesterol. White meat chicken is nearly twice as high in niacin. Dark meat chicken does, however, offer two to three times as much zinc and iron.

Turkey offers certain advantages over chicken. It is around 20 percent lower in calories and 75 percent lower in fat. Three and a half ounces of turkey breast contain a paltry 1 gram of fat. Turkey is rich in niacin, with 7 milligrams in a 3.5-ounce serving (33 percent of the RDA), though this is half the amount in chicken. Turkey contains more zinc and iron and slightly more vitamin E. Ground-turkey patties are a healthier alternative to beef burgers. (But be sure to read the label on the ground-turkey package. Some ground turkey contains a lot of dark meat and a great deal of fat. Choose your cut of turkey breast and have the butcher grind it for you.)

One problem with poultry stems from the way chickens are raised and fed. At least in theory, free-roaming chickens (listed on menus and labels as "free-range" chickens) produce healthier eggs, depending on the chicken feed. If, as studies have shown, free-range chickens produce healthier eggs, perhaps we may assume the meat of free-range chickens is also more nutritious. Common sense would tell us that a chicken that is outdoors in the fresh air and sunshine would be healthier to eat than one that has spent its short, sad life penned up in a cage unable to roam and search for natural food.

EGG FACTS

Eggs are an excellent nutrient-dense food that packs 6 grams of protein, a bit of vitamin B-12, vitamin E, riboflavin, folic acid, calcium, zinc, iron, and essential fatty acids into a mere 75 calories. Except for the lactalbumin protein in human milk, eggs have the highest-quality protein of any food (for an explanation of protein quality, see page 50). In addition to being good for the body, eggs can be prepared in a variety of tasty ways.

The Cholesterol Concern

We've often heard or read that eggs are bad for the heart because they contain a lot of cholesterol. Not necessarily! The nutritional logic that gave good eggs a bad rap goes something like this: Foods high in cholesterol are bad for the heart. Eggs are high in cholesterol. Therefore, eggs are bad for the heart.

While this may meet the standards of a logical argument, it isn't altogether true. New insights into the fatty foods–heart disease connection reveal that in people with normal cholesterol metabolism, it's not cholesterol that clogs arteries but rather foods high in saturated and hydrogenated fats. There is a small proportion of people who are termed "cholesterol sensitive," because their blood-cholesterol levels rise when they eat foods high in cholesterol. But in the great majority of the population, the amount of cholesterol in the diet does not affect blood cholesterol, since cholesterol is manufactured in the liver, regardless of whether or not you eat it in a food. Saturated fats (and factory-made fats, such as hydrogenated ones) are far greater problems than dietary cholesterol, and compared with some other foods, eggs are not an especially high source of saturated fats. (Egg white is almost pure high-quality protein, so if you are a cholesterol-sensitive person, skip the yolk and eat the white.)

To show you how unfair it is to implicate the egg in cholesterol problems, consider this: An egg contains only 2 grams of saturated fat and 75 calories compared with 7 grams of saturated fat and 268 calories in a small (3.5-ounce) lean hamburger patty. Even though a hamburger may contain only 100 grams of cholesterol, compared with 210 grams in one large egg, most quarter-pound hamburgers contain four times as much saturated fat as the innocent egg. Eggs actually qualify for the "low in saturated fat" label.

If the American Heart Association is not concerned about the cholesterol in eggs, neither should you be. In light of the recent evidence clearing cholesterol as a heart-unhealthy food, the American Heart Association changed its tune and now regards an egg every other day as acceptable for people with normal cholesterol and those who are not sensitive to dietary cholesterol. Now that the egg has been found "not guilty" as a cholesterol-raising food, scramble it up and enjoy.

EAT HEALTHIER EGGS

Want more nutritious eggs for your diet? Find out what the hen was fed. Research has proven that better chicken feed results in better eggs. Free-range hens allowed to forage on barnyard plant food produce eggs that are lower in cholesterol than commercially fed caged hens. Studies comparing eggs from the average hen factory with those of free-range chickens fed diets high in essential fatty acids showed that the chickens on a healthier diet produced eggs higher in the heart-healthy omega-3 fatty acids. Studies are under way to produce what have been called "designer eggs," eggs in which the fatty-acid profile of the egg yolk has been modified by altering the hen's diet. In an interesting experiment, hens that were given feed that contained flax seed and fish oil (which are rich in omega-3 fatty acids) produced eggs with more omega-3 fatty acids; these were dubbed "omega eggs." So, even when it comes to chickens, "you are what you eat." Egg consumers are not used to asking their grocery store managers what the hens that laid their eggs were fed. But if enough consumers start asking the question, eventually egg suppliers will start putting the feed information on the cartons. The egg of the future will only be as healthy as the consumer demands.

Egg-Safety Tips

Bacteria, such as salmonella, seem to appreciate the nutrient quality of the egg inside the shell. They love to multiply in raw eggs. To protect your family from food poisoning, follow these egg-safety tips:

- Give each egg a checkup before purchasing. Examine the egg for cracks. Turn the egg over in the carton. If any eggs are stuck to the bottom of the carton, suspect cracks.

- Don't wash eggs before storing them. Washing may remove the invisible protective coating surrounding the shell, allowing bacteria to enter.

- Store eggs in the refrigerator in their original carton. They don't belong in those convenient little egg holders on the refrigerator door, because they are too warm. (It works for butter, but not for eggs.) Storing them in the carton also keeps the eggs from absorbing the aroma of other foods.

- Wash your hands (and utensils) thoroughly after handling raw eggs.

- Cook eggs thoroughly. To kill the bacteria, fry an egg for three minutes per side. Poach an egg for five minutes, and boil an egg seven minutes. Cook till both yolk and white are firm. Scramble eggs until they're no longer runny. Sunny-side-up and soft-boiled eggs with runny yolks are risky.

- Commercial egg products, such as eggnog, have been pasteurized and are therefore, at least theoretically, safe. Don't use raw eggs in recipes made at home.

- Keep eggs and egg-containing foods refrigerated and avoid letting them sit at room temperature for more than an hour.

- If you're mixing raw eggs into recipes, such as cookie dough, avoid the temptation to let your child lick the bowl.

25

Buy Organic! Yes? No? Sometimes?

ARE ORGANIC FOODS WORTH THE EXTRA MONEY and the extra shopping effort required to find them? Are there health benefits that justify the additional energy and expense? Here are some questions consumers have about organic foods.

What does the term "organic" mean?

It depends upon whom you ask. To a biochemist, "organic" means anything that contains carbon. Plastic, derived from petroleum, contains carbon; therefore, plastic is organic. Carbon is the mark of a living organism or of something that once was a living organism. When applied to food, "organic" suggests that only natural, nonsynthetic substances are involved in its production. Generally, "organic" means that the food has been grown in safe and healthy soil, using natural fertilizers and free of synthetic pesticides or additives.

Look for the words "certified organically grown" on the label. To obtain this certification, the grower submits to on-site inspections and soil and water testing by an independent organization or state agency. He keeps careful records about his farming technique, and the farmland itself must be free of agrochemical use for at least three years. The problem with the "certified organically grown" designation is that the forty-four certify-

ing agencies around the United States have different standards. So, even with all the regulations, consumers can't determine exactly what they're buying. Actually, much of the "organic" food in today's supermarket is not "certified," making it even more difficult to know what you're getting for the extra money you're paying.

The Organic Foods Production Act of 1990 required the National Organic Standards Board (an advisory board to the U.S. Department of Agriculture) to set up regulations for food labeled "organic," but the various groups involved are still haggling about a precise definition. While the USDA fiddles around with the meaning of organic certification, politics enters the food picture, as the agency tries to satisfy consumers, nutrition action groups, and the special interests of food manufacturers. In early 1998, the USDA tried to sneak a number of questionable farming practices into the definition of "organically grown food," including irradiated food, genetically engineered food (dubbed "Frankenstein foods"), and "sludge foods," those fertilized by recycling municipal waste products. The USDA also wanted to allow "organic" meat producers to use feed made from the antibiotic- and steroids-loaded remains of deceased animals. The USDA, egged on by the food industry, was trying to taint the revered word "organic," and the faithful protested. After receiving

223

LABEL BABBLE

Because "organic" is the health-food word of the decade, label makers scramble to plaster this word all over the front of packages. "Organic" has health appeal, but like the terms "all natural," "no artificial ingredients," and "pesticide free," "100 percent organic" carries no guarantee. Instead, look for the words "certified organic" or "certified organically grown." These labels have added credibility if they list the certifying agency, such as "California-certified organic."

Proposed label regulations may add to the confusion about "organic." One proposal suggests that foods containing 95 percent or more of organic ingredients should be labeled "organic," and products that contain between 50 and 95 percent of organic ingredients would be labeled "made with organic ingredients." Products with less than 50 percent of organic ingredients may use the term "organic" only in the ingredients listing. Another proposal is that the USDA organic seal should be used only on products with a minimum of 95 percent organic ingredients.

objections from two hundred thousand protesters (including the authors), in May of 1998, the USDA tabled its proposal, and the National Organic Standards Board went back to the farm to work out cleaner rules.

Until there are national rules, organic farms are not required to play by any rules. As of this writing, the organic industry polices itself with independent certifying agencies, resulting in the label "certified organic." It's not perfect, but at present it's the safest label you can buy.

Are organic foods really that much healthier?

Knowing how the organic farmer feeds the soil will tell you a lot about what "organic" really means. The basic belief of organic farming is that *healthier soil will produce healthier plants and safer food.* The organic farmer believes, and rightly so, that if you avoid treating the soil with chemicals, the food it produces will be better for humans, and the environment will benefit as well. The organic farmer begins by rotating the crops, a fine farming principle that was advised even in biblical days. Crop rotation keeps the soil from becoming depleted of nutrients. One type of plant will return nutrients to the soil that are needed by another crop. When the soil is richer, the underground creepy crawlies thrive, and earthworms and soil-dwelling bacteria feast on the rich soil. In return for a nutritious place to live, they deposit their own nutrients. Organic farmers use only natural fertilizers, such as manure and compost, and also use natural methods to control insects. This means that organically grown foods do not contain pesticide residues and other chemicals that may be harmful to human health.

Science backs up the organic farmer's beliefs. Farm workers who spray chemical pesticides have higher rates of cancer (as do their children) than organic farm workers. Yes, these workers are exposed to greater amounts of pesticides than that which is found in food, but there is a lot we don't know about the hazards of the chemicals used in modern agriculture. No one knows the long-term effects from generation to generation of consuming a tiny bit of chemicals each day over many years. Common sense tells us that if a chemical is designed to kill living pests, it can't be all that safe for living humans.

Do organic foods contain lower levels of pesticides?

Yes. In 1997, *Consumer Reports* did a study on one hundred pounds of produce, some with organic labels and some not, selected randomly from supermarkets across the country. Twenty-five percent of the organic samples had traces of pesticides compared with 77 percent of the unlabeled samples. While the tests showed that "organic" didn't necessarily mean "pesticide free," organic foods consistently had lower amounts of toxic pesticide residues. In addition, the magazine's testers couldn't detect any difference in taste between organic and unlabeled produce.

Is organic food more nutritious?

Not necessarily. The term "certified organic" means only that the food was raised without added chemicals and is not a measure of the nutritional value of that food. Many factors influence the nutritional value of a crop, including plant genetics, the weather, and how ripe the food was when harvested. But in theory, if the soil is richer in nutrients, so will be the food it yields, and there is concern that overfarmed, nutrient-depleted, pesticide-laced soil could produce less nutritious foods. If the nutrients aren't there in the soil, they won't appear in the plant. Even with chemical fertilizers, it's in the farmer's best interests to have rich soil. For practical purposes you can assume that organic and nonorganic food have about the same nutrient content. Yet no one knows if there may be subtle nutritional differences. So, it's back to common sense. Healthier soil should produce a healthier fruit.

What about organically grown livestock? Could a range-roaming, grass-eating, antibiotic- and steroids-free steer produce better beef than one fed a lot of chemical-laden feed? Experiments have shown that free-range chickens produce more nutritious eggs than cage-raised hens. Why shouldn't we expect the same results in meat? Again, back to the "unscience" of common sense. If better and safer stuff goes into the intestines of the animal, the meat should be better and safer.

Doesn't the government monitor pesticide use?

Like most government agencies, the U.S. Department of Agriculture (USDA) and the Environmental Protection Agency (EPA) try to balance what is good for the economy with what is good for people's health. Laws require that pesticides in food not exceed certain minimal levels, while acknowledging that pesticides are necessary to produce an "adequate, wholesome, and economical food supply." In plain language, the government accepts a bit of a risk as long as a pesticide keeps the price of food down and the supply up. However, there's always controversy about what should be "minimal allowable levels"; scientists and government officials cannot agree on what level of risk is acceptable. Logically, pesticides should be treated like drugs, which must be proven safe before being approved for widespread use. However, with the current laws, pesticides must be proven harmful before they are banned.

NUTRITIP
Pesticide-Free Fats

Chemical pesticides, because they are fat soluble, are likely to accumulate in fatty or oily foods. So, it's more critical to look for the "certified organic" label on foods high in fats, such as salad oils, cooking oils, butter, and nuts, especially peanuts. "Certified organic" peanut butter with a spread of organic grape jam is a healthy treat your child deserves.

Don't expect the government to make your food safe on its own. New pesticides are being developed faster than government agencies can monitor them. Although the Government Accounting Agency (GAA), Congress's watchdog, has gotten after the FDA to clean up the mess, government agencies haven't been able to stunt the growth of pesticide use. Consumer groups such as the Natural Resources Defense Council (NRDC) try to expose the ways in which these agencies are not doing their jobs, but consumers do not wield the power of the food-industry lobby. The bottom line is that the government really doesn't know and the food industry won't tell what pesticides get into the food supply. And consider this: Whoever's in charge now — in Congress or the various administrative agencies — won't be around decades from now when the consequences of current pesticide use show up in the cancer rates of the U.S. population.

Understanding more about how the testing is done reveals the magnitude of this problem. The FDA and EPA actually test only a fraction of the pesticides used in food production, and even the results of those tests are of questionable value. Testing is done with animals that are given various amounts of these chemicals and then examined for ill effects. Besides obvious problems, such as death, paralysis, tumors, and growth retardation, the tissues are examined for microscopic evidence of cell damage. Once a level is found that causes no identifiable damage, a fraction of that level is extrapolated to humans as the "maximum acceptable level" — the level of pesticide residue in a food that is legally acceptable. But what is legal may not be completely safe for the following reasons:

- Levels of pesticides that cause no apparent effects in the animal and satisfy a committee are not necessarily safe for humans. The process of extrapolating results from animal studies to humans is plagued with errors. How do you measure subtle IQ changes in a rat?

- These studies measure short-term effects, not long-term damage. This concern is especially important in children who consume small amounts of pesticide residue accumulating over a long period of time, possibly causing damage years later, perhaps even in the next generation.

- How animals are tested does not reflect how humans eat. Usually one or a few chemicals are tested on an animal. In reality, we may eat a hundred different pesticides. Chemicals have a *synergistic effect,* meaning that two plus two sometimes adds up to five or more. When you put a bunch of chemicals together, all of them combined may produce more harm than each one separately.

- The EPA does batch testing. If you lump one hundred pounds of potatoes together and test the batch, you get an average pesticide level. But what if the chemicals are actually concentrated in a few potatoes, and your child eats one of these "hot" potatoes?

- There are facts the government doesn't know and that the industry won't tell. Ingredients are labeled "inert" because they have no known pest-killing action, not because they are harmless to humans. Even though the EPA has recently identified 110 inert ingredients as hazardous, there are no food standards or tolerance limits for inerts. Also, the FDA does not monitor foods for inert ingredients, and pesticide manufacturers consider inerts trade secrets and seldom list them on package labels.

Could pesticides be more harmful to children than to adults?

Absolutely. In 1989 the Natural Resources Defense Council released results of the most comprehensive analysis ever conducted on pesticide residues in foods commonly eaten by children. This study, called *Intolerable Risk: Pesticides in Our Children's Foods,* identified sixty-six potentially carcinogenic pesticides in foods that a child might eat. The researchers in this report estimated that children have four times as much exposure as adults to eight of these carcinogenic pesticides. These are some reasons why kids and pest killers don't mix:

- The "maximum acceptable levels" allowed by government agencies are based upon estimates of the harm in adults, using adult eating habits and adult weights. Children's eating habits are different from those of adults. They eat proportionally more contaminated food on a volume-per-weight basis than adults do. Infants and children consume much more fruit and juice than do adults. They also do not eat the variety of foods that adults do, often bingeing on applesauce, for example, three days in a row.

- Cancer researchers believe that prolonged exposure to a toxic chemical may have a cumulative effect. You don't all of a sudden "get cancer." You get cancer one pesticide-polluted cell at a time. Today's children will be exposed to toxic chemicals over a longer time, so they face greater health risks as adults.

- Another cancer fact is that rapidly dividing cells (like those of growing infants and children) are more susceptible to damage from carcinogens, such as pesticides.

NUTRITIP
Risky Foods

Foods such as strawberries and raspberries that don't contain peels, have rough, difficult-to-clean surfaces, and are heavily sprayed are likely to contain more pesticides in their flesh. For these risky foods, it's better to buy organic.

- Some pesticides have been implicated as being neurotoxic, or brain damaging. It's possible that the brain is most susceptible to damage when it is growing the fastest, that is, during the first years of life.

- Children swim in rivers and lakes and drink a lot of municipal water, which brings up concerns about secondhand pollution. Not only do pesticides pollute the farms, but they pollute the water that drains those farms. The brain-toxic chemicals that are sprayed on strawberries miles away may someday come out the family faucet.

- In 1998 a private organization called the Environmental Working Group analyzed USDA, FDA, and EPA data on current pesticides in food and concluded that over one million children consume more than the "safe" adult dose of potentially brain-damaging poisons daily. Since children are more vulnerable than adults to the effects of chemicals, this is an alarming situation. However, the toxic effects may not show up in standard animal testing, and measuring the effects in groups of kids would be nearly impossible. Again, we go back to the drawing board of common sense: Any chemical that kills the body of a pest can't be good for the brain of a child.

- The liver has the job of breaking down chemical toxins so that they can be eliminated from the body. An infant's liver is less mature and may have less capacity to detoxify chemicals.

- Pesticides are stored in fat. Children, especially infants, have proportionally more body fat than adults do.

So, an apple a day may not keep the doctor away. After researching the pesticide issue, we felt like moving our family to some unpolluted area (if there are any left), planting our own garden, milking our own cows, and drilling for clean water. In reality, we realized we had two alternatives. One would simply be to resign ourselves to a world in which we coexist with pesticides, realizing that the hazards of pesticides are a trade-off that goes along with convenient and lower-priced food. The better alternative would be to do what we could to clean up the food we feed to our children. The information presented in this chapter is not meant to scare you; it is meant to motivate you to take action about a potentially serious problem that affects you, your children, and your grandchildren. Here's how you can protect your children against pesticides.

Just say no. Don't buy poisonous food. Parents control the top of the food chain. Suppose one hundred parents on a given day went into their local supermarket and asked, "Where is your organic foods section?" It wouldn't take long before that store had organic produce on the shelf. Grocers purchase what consumers ask for; wholesalers supply what grocers ask for; and farmers grow what wholesalers buy. If you buy it, farmers will grow it. The law of supply and demand starts with you.

You can control the top of the food chain when it comes to food prices. Since price is based on supply and demand, the more pesticide-free food you demand, the greater will be the supply, which will bring prices of organic food down to near the level of chemical food.

Lobby for safe food laws. The government is not going to make food safe for you and your children just because it's the right thing to do. Parents and consumers must take the initiative. Why? Because your motive is pure: to protect the health of yourselves and your children. Any government motive is laced with residues of trying to please various powerful lobbies. Allow a little bit of cancer in return for a little bit of pesticides in the food supply if this means you have a happier food grower more likely to make campaign contributions to influential representatives in Congress. Put the right spin on it, and most voters don't know what's really going on. Of course, the people most at risk, babies and children, don't even have a vote. To get your views heard, support organizations interested in a safe food supply, such as the Natural Resources Defense Council (NRDC), 40 West 20th Street, New York, NY 10011 (or http://www.nrdc.org).

Another way you can influence the food chain is to write to your local congressional representatives and ask them to support laws that ban chemical farming. This will also prompt manufacturers to produce safer pesticides. Farmers will use what manufacturers produce; and eventually the price of organic food will go down and the safety of food will go up. Everyone wins.

Pay a price. Many consumers pay more attention to price than product, at least when it comes to food. We may be willing to pay a bit more for gas that makes our car run better, clothing that looks, feels, and wears better, or even for shoes that display a designer trademark, yet we quibble about paying a few cents more for a safer apple. Meanwhile, the organic-produce salesman is warning, "Pay me now, or pay the doctor later." Until the food chain changes, expect to pay more for pesticide-free food. At present, only around 2 percent of the food produced by U.S. farms is organic, hardly worth the fuss and expense to the rest of the food industry to make changes in how food is grown.

Buying organic is especially important when it comes to baby foods. There seems to be an ongoing label war on the jars of commercial baby food: "no salt," "no sugar," and "no preservatives," yet an important "no" is missing from the popular brands — namely, "no pesticides." Manufacturers claim that they have reduced pesticides far below the legal limit, and that's commendable — but not enough. Don't accept what's legal as being safe for you or your children. It makes no sense to eat cheap foods when you're young and pay high prices for medical problems when you're older. That's a bad investment. But isn't organic food so much more expensive? It depends upon what you mean by expensive. Yes, organic food costs more, primarily because the demand is so much less than for chemically treated food. Yet in the long run, it's a great bargain. Suppose someone were to tell you that for a couple of extra bucks a day you could lower your child's risk of getting cancer or losing a few brain cells, and that he might even live to see his own great-grandchildren. Think of the extra expense as just a bit more health insurance.

Buy American. Imported produce may contain more pesticides than domestically grown food and may also contain pesticides that are banned from use in the United States. American chemical manufacturers export pesticides that cannot be used in this country, but the laws don't protect us if the toxic stuff comes back to U.S. markets in imported produce. Interrupt the cycle of poison. Require your supermarket to label produce with its country of origin and buy only U.S.-grown food.

Wash, scrub, and peel. Studies have shown that washing fruits and vegetables in a dilute solution of water and dish detergent (¼ tsp. to 1 pint of water) can remove most of the surface pesticides, even though it can't remove the pesticide residues that remain inside the produce. Peeling fruits and vegetables also removes some of the pesticide residue but also much of the fiber.

Grow your own. If you really want to eat produce you can trust, plant your own garden. (See "Growing Your Own Garden," page 163.)

Eat variety. Play the numbers game. If you and your children eat a variety of foods, you lower the risk of overdosing on foods that are raised with lots of chemicals. This nutritional trick is especially important for children who tend to eat only a few kinds of food over several days. Children who happen to binge on a bad bunch of produce could be exposed to a higher dose of pesticides.

While we urge you to buy organic foods whenever possible, the fear of pesticides should not keep you from serving lots of fruits and vegetables to your family, even if they are nonorganic.

We hope that this chapter about organic food will motivate you to keep the momentum of the healthy food chain going. Putting pesticide-free food into your mouth is one of the best long-term investments you can make in your health.

III

OPTIMAL FEEDING OF INFANTS AND CHILDREN

New research is proving what wise parents have long suspected: There is a relationship between what children eat and how they behave and learn. In my pediatrics practice, I have noticed that in general the children with the most nutritious diets have the fewest illnesses. Children's nutritional needs change from birth through adolescence, and knowing about these changing needs will not only help you help your children grow but also help them develop to their fullest potential. An important part of feeding children is teaching them healthy eating habits. The eating patterns children grow up with are the ones they are most likely to carry with them into adulthood. Children who grow up with a steady diet of nutritious foods eventually learn to make the connection "I eat right; therefore, I feel right." As those children programmed to be healthy eaters venture from your "pure" home kitchen into the world of junk food, they may experiment with junk foods but will not overdose on them. Serving nutritious foods to your children is a healthy, long-term investment. As parents of eight, we realize that preparing good food takes time and energy, both of which are at a premium in most families. But the time you spend is well worth it.

26

Breastfeeding — The Best Feeding

BABY WHALES DRINK WHALE MILK. Baby chimps drink chimpanzee milk. Baby cows drink cow milk. What's the natural food for baby humans? Human milk — their own mother's milk.

Human milk is best for every part of baby's body — for the digestive system, the immune system, the nervous system, the endocrine system. Breastfeeding builds brains as well as brawn and helps baby's body develop exactly as nature intended. Many of the benefits are immediate, appreciable to parents and pediatricians from the first day of life. Other benefits are life-long.

HUMAN MILK: THE GOLD STANDARD FOR INFANT NUTRITION

Human milk truly is the gold standard when it comes to infant nutrition. Artificial baby milks are just what the name suggests — something less than the real thing. So it's ironic that the nutritional benefits of breastfeeding are often explained by comparing human milk and formula. It's not a fair contest, because the artificial product will always fall short of the real thing.

The Changing Composition of Milk

Human milk is a living fluid, more like blood than like a product from the supermarket shelf, and its composition is constantly changing to meet the changing needs of the baby — from the beginning to the end of a feeding, throughout the day, and over the weeks and months of lactation.

Early Milk — Liquid Gold

The first milk a mother produces is called "colostrum," a yellowish, thick fluid present in her breasts late in pregnancy and in the first days postpartum. Colostrum is produced in small amounts, and people who are not well informed about breastfeeding might suggest that the first day or two of nursing are not important, telling a mother that, after all, her milk "hasn't come in yet." But these first colostrum feedings are very valuable — the equivalent of nutritional gold. They're exactly the kind of nutrition that gets newborns off to a healthy start.

A baby fresh from his mother's womb does not yet have any experience fighting germs, and his intestinal tract has never encountered food before. Colostrum is power packed with immunities, especially an immunoglobulin called "secretory IgA." Secretory IgA coats the lining of baby's im-

BREASTFEEDING RESOURCES

Breastfeeding is meant to be a pleasurable experience. Otherwise, the human race would not have survived. How the breastfeeding mother and baby get started with one another determines whether this is a pleasurable relationship or a nutritional duty. Here are some resources to help mother and baby get the right start.

- *The Baby Book* (William and Martha Sears [Little Brown, 1993]) includes two comprehensive chapters, written mainly by Martha, who has logged sixteen years of breastfeeding our eight children, including Stephen, with Down Syndrome, and Lauren, who came into our family by adoption. The step-by-step illustrated positioning and latch-on section is particularly helpful.

- La Leche League International (800-LALECHE or http://www.lalecheleague.org) is another source of information about breastfeeding. La Leche League Leaders can help solve breastfeeding problems, and monthly LLL meetings give women a chance to share breastfeeding challenges and insights with other mothers. La Leche League also offers information for mothers who want to continue breastfeeding while working outside the home.

- For a certified lactation consultant in your area, contact the International Lactation Consultant Association (ILCA), 4101 Lake Boone Trail, Suite 201, Raleigh, NC 27607. You can reach them at 919-787-5181 (tel.), 919-787-4916 (fax), or ilca@erols.com (e-mail).

---

mature digestive system and prevents germs from getting through. It may also help prepare a baby's stomach and intestines for the milk feedings coming soon.

Shortly after birth a baby's intestines become populated with bacteria — good and bad bacteria. The best is *Lactobacillus bifidus,* similar to the bacterial culture found in yogurt. In return for a warm place to live, these healthy bacteria produce nutrients and perform other healthy functions in the gut. Colostrum creates an environment in baby's intestines that allows *Lactobacillus bifidus* to thrive. When good gut bacteria take over the intestines, it's much harder for bad bacteria and viruses to cause trouble. *Bifidus* bacteria in the intestines have another benefit, one you can smell. An exclusively breastfed baby's diaper may smell a bit cheesy, but it's not an offensive odor.

Live factors also contribute to the immunological defense system packed into colostrum. White blood cells gobble up germs. The super-milk

colostrum is rich in bacteria-eating lysozyme. The concentrations of these immune factors are highest in the early days after birth, but immunities continue to be present in mother's milk throughout lactation. In fact, when babies begin to wean and a mother's milk supply decreases, the levels of immunities rise again. It's as if mother's body says, "Oh, taking less milk? Better make sure every drop is packed with goodness."

Mature Milk

As hormone levels change in the days after birth, the mother's body starts to make more plentiful amounts of milk. Colostrum gradually changes into mature milk — the stuff babies have been thriving on for thousands of years. Milk's basic ingredients are fats, proteins, lactose, vitamins, minerals, and water. This is true of all kinds of milk from all kinds of mammals. Yet, the proportions of the ingredients differ, as do the kinds of protein and fat. This is what makes each species' milk

WHAT THE EXPERTS ADVISE

In the last twenty-five years of the infant feeding debate, science has come out overwhelmingly in favor of human milk. Former surgeon general Dr. Antonia Novello was publicly quoted as saying, "It's the lucky baby, I feel, who continues to nurse until he's two." Breastfeeding is better for babies in every way, and better for their mothers' health, too. That's why the American Academy of Pediatrics, always an official advocate of breastfeeding, used stronger language than ever before in a December 1997 statement recommending that human babies receive human milk. Specifically, the new breastfeeding policies advised by AAP were:

- For healthy newborns, breastfeeding should begin as soon as possible after birth, usually within the first hour.
- Newborns should be nursed whenever they show signs of hunger, such as mouthing, rooting, or whatever feeding cues the mother has learned to recognize. It is not advisable for a mother to always wait for a newborn to cry to signal hunger, since crying is a late indicator of hunger.
- Newborns should be nursed approximately eight to twelve times every twenty-four hours, or until satisfied.
- No supplements (water, glucose, or formula) should be given to breastfeeding newborns unless medically indicated. Supplements and pacifiers should be avoided whenever possible and, if used at all, only after breastfeeding is well established.
- Supplements of water, juice, or other foods are generally unnecessary for breastfeeding infants for the first six months. Fluoride supplements should not be administered to infants during the first six months after birth, whether they are breastfed or formula fed. Fluoride supplements may be given after six months of age if recommended by baby's doctor.
- Exclusive breastfeeding is ideal nutrition and sufficient to support optimal growth and development for approximately the first six months. It is recommended that breastfeeding continue for at least twelve months and thereafter for as long as is mutually desired.

The statement made front-page headlines and nightly newscasts in many cities across the United States. Also making headlines were reactions to the Academy's recommendations, especially the ones that advised that infants receive their mother's milk exclusively for the first six months and that breastfeeding continue for at least the first year. Commentators felt that this placed an unrealistic burden on mothers, especially those who work outside the home.

Is there a conflict between good nutrition for babies and the realities of modern mothering? The Academy was careful to include recommendations that employers provide time and facilities for mothers working outside the home to pump milk for their babies, along with other suggestions for making American culture more breastfeeding-friendly. We have a long way to go, but the benefits of breastfeeding as outlined by modern science should compel us to make modern society more supportive of nursing mothers and babies.

MAKING ENOUGH MILK?

"Is my baby getting enough milk?"

Many mothers experience this worry, especially in the early weeks of breastfeeding. You can't measure the milk as it's going in, and sometimes women find it hard to trust their own bodies to deliver enough of a high-quality product.

The biggest influence on how much milk a mother makes is how much the baby nurses. When a baby removes milk from the breasts, the nerves send a signal to the brain to secrete the hormone prolactin, which stimulates the glands in the breast to make more milk. Frequent nursing keeps prolactin levels high and ensures that mother will have an ample supply of milk.

There's a simple way to know if baby is getting the nutrition he needs. In the early weeks, a baby who is breastfeeding well will have six to eight wet cloth diapers each day (four to six disposable) and two to three substantial stools. If there's enough stuff being deposited in baby's diaper, there must be enough going in the other end.

---

uniquely suited to its young. It's also why cow's milk and cow's milk–based formulas are an inferior food for human infants.

Breast milk contains high-quality protein. Protein is a prime example of how human milk is unique nutrition for human babies. Human milk is low in protein, at least when compared with the milk of other species, especially cow's milk. There are good reasons for this. Human infants are designed to grow slowly. While it's important for humans to develop strong bodies, even more important is brain development and the learning of social skills. The experiences that shape the brain come from close contact between mother and baby when baby is held and carried. If human infants doubled their birth weight in less than fifty days the way calves do and then continued growing, how could their mothers carry them and talk to them and keep them close? Baby cows need to learn where to find the best grass in the meadow; baby humans need to learn how to work with others so that everyone's needs get met.

HUMAN MILK — THE ULTIMATE COMFORT FOOD

Babies nurse for reasons beyond hunger. Sucking comforts them and helps them adjust to a big scary world. Babies nurse to go to sleep, and they nurse when waking up. Breastfeeding eases the transition from one state to another. As breastfeeding babies grow into nursing toddlers, mothers use the breast to make "ouchies" go away and to forestall temper tantrums.

Does this set a baby up to use food for comfort and gratification later in life? We don't think so. Remember that with breastfeeding, the food delivery system is always attached to a person. Babies whose needs are met at the breast learn to seek comfort from people — not things.

Breastfed babies also learn to trust themselves. They're the ones who decide how long they are going to nurse and when their tummies are full. This sensitivity carries over into later life. Children with high self-esteem are less likely to have eating problems or to experiment with drugs and alcohol.

Though the protein content of human milk is generally low, the types of amino acids that make up these proteins are important. One particular amino acid, taurine, is found in large amounts in human milk. Studies show that taurine has an important role in the development of the brain and the eye. Infants can't change other kinds of amino acids into taurine, so its presence in human milk is significant — so significant that some formula manufacturers have begun adding it to artificial baby milks.

If you let milk stand out of the refrigerator and sour, you will see that milk proteins fall into two categories, curds and whey. (Remember Miss Muffet?) The curd portion, the casein proteins, are the white clots; the liquid is the whey. Cow's milk is mostly casein protein, which forms a rubbery, hard-to-digest curd in babies' tummies. Human milk has more whey than curd, and the curds that are formed are softer and more quickly digested. Breastfed babies get hungry again sooner than babies who are formula fed, because human milk proteins are digested so efficiently. It doesn't take as much energy to digest human milk as it does to digest cow's milk–based formulas. Frequent feedings also ensure that human babies get lots of attention from their mothers.

Breast milk contains self-digesting fats. There's another reason why babies digest human milk so quickly: The fat in human milk comes with an enzyme, lipase, that breaks the fat down into smaller globules so this important nutrient can be better absorbed into the bloodstream. Fat is a valuable source of energy for babies, so the presence of lipase makes the fat in human milk more available. This is one of the reasons human milk is so good for premature babies, who need lots of energy to grow but whose digestive systems are very immature.

The fat in breast milk is a changing nutrient for changing needs. The fat content of human milk changes constantly. Typically, fat levels are low at the beginning of a feeding and high at the end. Babies nurse eagerly to get the low-fat, thirst-quenching foremilk, then slow down and linger over the high-fat dessert at the end of their meal. Babies who nurse again soon after the end of their last feeding get more high-fat milk, so babies who breastfeed more frequently during a growing spurt get more calories. Longer intervals between feedings bring down the fat content of the milk stored in the breast. This nutritional fact of human milk is one of the many reasons why the rigid three-to-four-hour scheduled style of feeding is biologically incorrect.

The fats in breast milk are smarter fats. The special kind of fat in human milk is important to brain development. As newborn babies grow, the nerves are covered with a substance called "myelin," which helps the nerves transmit messages to other nerves throughout the brain and body. To develop high-quality myelin, the body needs certain types of fatty acids — linoleic and linolenic — which are found in large amounts in human milk.

As Dr. Michael Schmidt in his book *Smart Fats* points out, the fats needed to make a large brain are different from those needed to make a large body. Cows, for example, provide milk to their calves that is high in saturated fatty acids, fats that provide for rapid body growth, but the milk is low in fats that provide for rapid brain growth. A calf's body grows fast in the first six months, but the brain grows very slowly. And in the adult cow, which isn't a whole lot smarter than a calf, the brain is small compared with the body. In human infants, on the other hand, the brain and the overall neurological development progress quickly. To provide for faster brain growth, human milk is rich in unsaturated fatty acids and, unlike cow's milk, low in saturated fats. Even though a baby's body grows relatively slowly (tripling in weight, but not in size), a baby's brain triples in size during the first year.

Breast milk is packed with vitamins and minerals. The vitamins and minerals listed on the formula can are no match for those in the milk made by mom. When formula researchers want to know how much of a particular vitamin or mineral babies need each day, they look first at how much of that nutrient is present in human milk and how much milk a baby of a given age takes in a day. But just doing the math doesn't tell the whole story. More important than the amounts of nutrients in the milk is the amount that is available for the infant to use, a nutrient principle called "bioavailability." This is a more complex issue, since the bioavailability of a nutrient is influenced by many factors, including its chemical form and the presence of other substances.

Tracing the history of iron supplementation in breastfed babies is a good way to explain the concept of bioavailability. Twenty years ago, many doctors routinely prescribed iron supplements for breastfed babies since human milk, like other animal milks, is (at least on paper) "low in iron." They assumed that babies would need an additional iron source once the iron stored while in the womb was used up.

But more research showed that "the real thing" had again outsmarted the scientists. Breastfed babies do not routinely become anemic. Studies that took a closer look at iron nutrition in breastfed babies found that at least 50 percent of the iron in human milk could be absorbed by babies, compared to 10 percent of the iron in cow's milk, and only 4 percent of the iron in iron-fortified infant formulas. The vitamin C in human milk promotes iron absorption, as does the higher level of lactose. Moreover, when it comes to iron, more is not better. Many bacteria need iron to thrive. Human milk contains a protein called "lactoferrin" that binds up extra iron in the stomach, preventing harmful bacteria in the gut from multiplying. When lactoferrin is kept busy binding up extra iron from supplements, it can't do its job properly and the baby loses one line of defense against infection. So, in the case of iron, less is more.

Breast milk contains important hormones and enzymes. Several times a year, I pick up a medical journal article describing yet another valuable substance discovered in human milk. And scientists are only beginning to write the story on factors in human milk that may be important to baby's growth and development. For example, other enzymes besides lipase are available to aid infant digestion. Epidermal growth factor, present in human milk in significant amounts, may promote the development of tissues in the digestive tract and elsewhere. Other hormones in milk will influence a baby's metabolism, growth, and physiology. The effects may be subtle, but they will also have implications that reach into adulthood. The late Dr. Frank Oski, world-renowned pediatrician, former professor of pediatrics at Johns Hopkins School of Medicine, and my friend, once told me, "When researching the difference between human milk and formulas, I discovered that there are over four hundred nutrients in breast milk that aren't in formula."

ADVANTAGES OF BREASTFEEDING — THE LONG AND THE SHORT OF IT

Looking at what's in the milk tells only half the story about how breastfeeding is better for babies. The rest of the proof is in the babies and the children and adults they become. Here are some short- and long-term advantages to breastfeeding that can't necessarily be traced to a specific nutrient but are nevertheless very real and important.

Short-Term Advantages

Immunological Defenses

Human milk is more than food. It's a complex living substance, like blood, with a long list of active

BREASTFEEDING BENEFITS FROM TOP TO BOTTOM

Breastfeeding is good for every part of baby's body — from the brain to the diaper area. Here's a list of benefits, all backed up by research:

- *Brain.* Breastfed children have higher IQs. Cholesterol and other types of fat in human milk support the growth of nerve tissue.
- *Eyes.* Visual acuity is higher in babies fed human milk.
- *Ears.* Breastfed babies get fewer ear infections.
- *Mouth.* There is less need for orthodontia in children who were breastfed for more than a year. Sucking at the breast leads to improved muscle development of the face. Subtle changes in the taste of human milk prepare babies to accept a variety of solid foods.
- *Throat.* Children who were breastfed are less likely to require tonsillectomies. Breastfeeding also offers protection against the effects of hypothyroidism.
- *Respiratory system.* Breastfed babies have fewer and less severe upper-respiratory infections, less wheezing, less pneumonia, and less influenza.
- *Heart and circulatory system.* Breastfed children may have lower cholesterol levels as adults. Heart rates are lower in breastfed infants.

- *Digestive system.* Babies who are breastfeeding have less diarrhea and fewer gastrointestinal infections. Six months or more of exclusive breastfeeding reduces the risk of food allergies. In adulthood there is less risk of Crohn's disease and ulcerative colitis. Breastfeeding can continue during gastrointestinal illness.
- *Immune system.* Breastfed babies respond better to vaccinations. Human milk helps to mature baby's immune system. Breastfeeding decreases the risk of childhood cancer and diabetes.
- *Kidneys.* With less salt and less protein, human milk is easier on a baby's kidneys.
- *Appendix.* Children who were breastfed are unlikely to develop acute appendicitis.
- *Urinary tract.* Breastfed infants have fewer infections.
- *Joints and muscles.* Juvenile rheumatoid arthritis is less common in children who were breastfed.
- *Skin.* There is less incidence of allergic eczema among breastfed infants.
- *Growth.* Breastfed babies are leaner at one year of age and less likely to be obese later in life.
- *Diapers.* Breastfed babies are less constipated and their stools have an inoffensive odor.

germ-fighting ingredients. These help protect babies against all kinds of infections, including ear infections, respiratory illnesses, and diarrhea.

Breastfeeding is friend to little ears. Ear infections are a childhood nuisance, often following on the heels of stuffy noses and colds. The middle ear fills with fluid, and eventually that fluid becomes infected, causing pain, especially in the middle of the night. Repeated ear infections or those that go untreated can lead to hearing problems. This is an important concern in young children, since hear-

ing difficulties can interfere with language learning, and language problems can later affect reading skills.

Breastfeeding protects against ear infections in four possible ways. First, the many germ-fighting ingredients in human milk keep harmful bacteria from bothering baby, so that stuffed-up noses and ears are less likely to become infected middle ears. Second, because breastfed babies are fed in a more upright position, they're less likely to experience milk backing up through the eustachian tubes into their ears; if this does happen during a breastfeeding session, human milk is less irritating to the tissues of the middle ear than infant formula is. Third, breastfed babies have fewer, or at least less severe, colds than formula-fed babies. Fewer colds may lead to fewer problems with ear infections. Finally, breastfed babies have fewer respiratory allergies, another cause of fluid building up in the middle ear, setting the stage for bacteria to grow.

Breastfeeding protects tiny tummies. Human milk excels at protecting babies from diarrhea and tummy upsets. This is important not only for individual babies but also on a global scale. Diarrhea is a major cause of infant mortality worldwide, and breastfeeding is the simplest, most cost-effective way to protect babies from repeated bouts of gastrointestinal illness.

The secretory IgA fights germs in the stomach of a breastfed baby and also works to prevent food allergies. By coating the intestinal lining like a protective paint, it prevents molecules of foreign foods from getting into the bloodstream to set up an allergic reaction.

Breastfeeding protects against a wide variety of other diseases. Here's a partial list: *Haemophilus influenzae* type b, pneumonia caused by *Streptococcus pneumoniae,* infant botulism, urinary tract infections, cholera, salmonella, *E. coli* infections, respiratory syncytial virus, Sudden Infant Death Syndrome (SIDS), and necrotizing enterocolitis, a serious threat to premature infants in neonatal intensive care units. Newborns face a scary world full of germs. How fortunate that mother's milk is there to protect them.

In fact, each mother's milk provides custom-designed protection for her infant. When a baby is exposed to a new germ, mother is likely to be exposed, too. So she manufactures antibodies to that germ. The antibodies show up in her milk and are passed to the baby. Many a nursing mother can tell the story of the entire family —

dad, mom, baby's siblings — coming down with flu, and the nursing baby having the mildest case, or not getting sick at all. When mother comes down with a bug, the best thing she can do for her baby is to keep breastfeeding.

Long-Term Advantages

The advantages of breastfeeding reach into childhood and even adulthood. Children who were breastfed are less likely to become diabetic; research indicates that early exposure to cow's-milk protein triggers the autoimmune response that causes diabetes. There is some evidence that breastfeeding protects against childhood cancer, obesity, and high cholesterol levels.

Breastfeeding's role in myelin production may have far-reaching effects. Multiple sclerosis, a muscle disease that strikes adults, may be caused in part by myelin breakdown. Multiple sclerosis is less common in places where breastfeeding rates are high, so human milk's contribution to the myelin formation may help to prevent multiple sclerosis in later life.

Sucking at the breast uses more muscles than sucking on a bottle nipple. This leads to better development of the face, the mouth, and the

---

THE BENEFITS OF SNACKING

Babies who are breastfed spend more time grazing rather than eating a set amount according to a rigid schedule. Having small, frequent feedings translates into more time spent interacting closely with mom. This is probably one of the reasons breastfed babies have improved intelligence and better social skills than formula-fed babies. Babies who are bottlefed will benefit if they switch to the smaller, nonscheduled feeding style enjoyed by breastfed babies.

tongue, which gives teeth a better chance to grow in straight. A study of ten thousand children found that those who were breastfed for a year or more were 40 percent less likely to require orthodontic treatment. Those parents saved some money!

Better Brains

Impressive studies published during the 1990s have shown that breastfeeding makes a measurable difference in babies' brains. Breastfed children actually turn out to be smarter. As a result of these studies, in 1995 the World Health Organization recommended that all infant formulas contain the brain fat, DHA, at the same level as mother's milk. Unfortunately, you still cannot get a formula that contains DHA in the United States.

Intelligence depends on a number of factors: heredity, environment, education, and what kind of stimulation a child receives in the first years of life. This can make it difficult for researchers to separate the effects of receiving human milk from other influences. Parents who conscientiously choose breastfeeding because they want the very best for their baby probably also provide caring, stimulating surroundings. Breastfeeding rates are in direct proportion to the education level of the mother, so it used to be thought that breastfed babies are smarter because their mothers are smarter. Yet, carefully designed studies suggest that something in mother's milk contributes to better brain development.

"MOTHER'S MILK: FOOD FOR SMARTER KIDS." This was the headline in the February 2, 1992, issue of *USA Today*. This study suggested that something in mother's milk, rather than (or in addition to) the extra nurturing of breastfeeding, gives babies a developmental advantage. Researchers in England divided three hundred premature infants into two groups: those who received their mother's milk and those who didn't. Prematures who got their mother's milk during the first four to five weeks of life averaged

8.3 points higher on IQ tests at age seven and a half to eight years. And the research suggested a dose-response relationship: The more mother's milk they got, the better these children scored.

In 1993, Dr. Frank Oski, chairman of the Department of Pediatrics at Johns Hopkins University School of Medicine, reviewed the numerous studies on infant feeding and later outcome and concluded, "Infants who receive human milk have higher scores on tests of intelligence, even after controlling for confounding variables."

In another study, researchers were gathering data on nine hundred infants to determine whether PCB's in human milk were harmful. ("PCB" stands for "polychlorinated biphenyl," a common environmental pollutant that babies may be exposed to in the womb and through their mother's milk.) They found, first of all, no harmful effects from PCB's in human milk. But they also found that the babies in the study who were breastfed scored higher on developmental tests and IQ tests than formula-fed infants. Even their fourth-grade report cards were better.

The intellectual advantage given breastfed babies used to be attributed to the increased nurturing (being held and being given a nurturant response to their cues) that breastfed babies often receive. New studies and new insights suggest that there could also be some brain-building substances in mother's milk that contribute to this intellectual advantage.

Many researchers now believe that a particular fatty acid, DHA, which is present in human milk in large amounts, may explain the differences in intelligence between breastfed and formula-fed babies. DHA is needed by the light-processing cells in the eye and neurons in the brain. In a fascinating postmortem study, Australian researchers compared the DHA composition of the brain, retina, and red blood cells of breastfed and formula-fed infants who died of SIDS within the first year. They discovered that breastfed infants had a greater proportion of DHA in their red blood cells and brain relative to formula-fed babies. (No differences were found in the retinas.) The longer the infants were breastfed, the higher was the content of DHA in their brains. These researchers went on to suggest that infants fed artificial baby milk have a DHA-deficient brain.

Since infants have no reserve pool of DHA fatty acids and have a limited ability to synthesize DHA from other fatty acids, DHA should be considered an essential fatty acid for the first year of life, or at least during the period of rapid brain growth. Otherwise, DHA deficiency during this critical period of rapid brain growth may delay the formation of connections between growing nerve cells. In essence, human milk helps a baby's developing brain make the right connections. Some researchers even go one step further and speculate that DHA deficiency during infancy

DOES BREAST MILK BUILD BETTER BRAINS?

New research is proving what mothers have long suspected: Breast milk does build better brains. Recent studies show that breastfed infants who were studied later in childhood tended to have higher IQs and better academic skills. This observation used to be attributed solely to the increased holding and interaction with mother associated with breastfeeding (with the implication that formula-feeding parents could make up for this by simply holding and interacting with their baby as much as a breastfeeding family). However, new evidence suggests that it is also the milk itself that enhances brain growth.

Human milk contains higher levels of DHA, and autopsy analysis of brain tissue shows that the cerebral cortex of a breastfed baby has a higher level of DHA than that of a formula-fed baby. *The longer the infant was breastfed, the higher the concentration of DHA in the brain.* In formula-fed infants, DHA levels were lower and the brain cells contained more omega-6 fatty acids. While adults can make DHA from other fats, albeit poorly, infants have an extremely limited ability to do so. Thus, formula-fed infants actually have a DHA deficiency compared to breastfed infants. Studies have also shown that preterm infants fed standard formulas score lower on visual-acuity tests than infants fed human milk or infants given formula with supplemental DHA. DHA-supplemented infants also performed significantly better than controls on standardized tests of mental development. This leaves companies scrambling to figure out how much DHA to add to infant formulas. (As of this writing, most formulas made in America are not supplemented with DHA.)

The presence of DHA in human milk may even have long-term implications. Some researchers speculate that a DHA deficiency during infancy might predispose the adult brain to neuro-degenerative diseases, such as multiple sclerosis, as well as depression, A.D.H.D., and schizophrenia. In fact, a study in the *British Medical Journal* showed that patients with multiple sclerosis were less likely than controls to have been breastfed for a prolonged period of time. One possible explanation for this is that the lower concentration of DHA in the brain cell membranes of formula-fed infants could make it easier for infectious or toxic agents to cross the blood/brain barrier. Moreover, recent data has shown that DHA levels in the brain are correlated to levels of certain neurotransmitters, such as serotonin. DHA deficiency may also contribute to degeneration of the myelin sheath itself.

Breastfeeding, the longer the better, is a great long-term investment in your child's academic future.

might predispose adults to degenerative diseases of the central nervous system, such as multiple sclerosis. As mentioned above, there is evidence that people with multiple sclerosis are less likely than controls to have been breastfed for prolonged periods of time. Researchers speculate that the lower concentration of DHA in the brain cell membranes of formula-fed infants could over time lead to defective cell membranes and easier entry of infectious or toxic agents into the brain cell or lead to degeneration of the myelin sheath that insulates nerve fibers.

A number of other studies have also shown that breastfeeding is associated with better scores on intelligence tests and other measures of development. The differences between breastfed children and those who were artificially fed are small, eight points or less, and it's important to remember that these numbers represent *averages* for hundreds of children, not the effect of breastfeeding on a specific individual. But if you wanted to raise

---

DO AMERICAN MOTHERS HAVE AN ELSIE-POOFA DEFICIENCY?*

Not only are American babies DHA deficient, but new studies suggest that American mothers could use a DHA boost. The growing fetal nervous system uses up a lot of the DHA in the mother's bloodstream. The diet of most American women is low in DHA. Also, since studies have shown that the breast milk of American women tends to be lower in DHA than the breast milk of women in many other countries, it would be wise to have a diet adequate in DHA (especially seafood) throughout pregnancy and lactation.

* LCPUFA. (DHA is a long-chain polyunsaturated fatty acid.)

---

the intelligence level of an entire generation of children, breastfeeding would be a simple and cost-effective way to do it. Or think of it this way: Artificial feeding is actually compromising children's intelligence. Other factors that can affect children's development (e.g., lead poisoning) receive plenty of attention from public health officials. Shouldn't they be encouraging mothers to breastfeed with the same energy and resources they devote to removing lead from the environment? In Quebec, Canada, mothers who receive government assistance are given a bonus if they breastfeed their babies.

Even seventy years ago, scientists showed that breastfed babies developed better and smarter than their formula-fed mates. A 1929 study showed that children aged seven to thirteen years who had been breastfed for four to nine months had higher intelligence scores and talked earlier than their bottlefed mates. A 1950 study of more than two thousand two-year-olds showed that the age when children walked was inversely related to the length of breastfeeding. Other studies have shown improved speech and reading abilities in breastfed children.

How breastfeeding benefits baby's brain is a complex process. It involves many nutrients and other factors that work together in complex ways, and it may never be possible to completely separate the effects of what's in mother's milk from the overall benefits of the close contact with mother and the way breastfeeding mothers learn to understand their babies. This means that manufacturers can't simply add whatever magical ingredients are in human milk to infant formula and expect the same results.

Better Eyes

Studies in both premature and full-term infants have shown better vision in breastfed children, as babies and at three years of age. Researchers found that preterm babies fed their mother's milk showed better visual acuity and development of the retina than formula-fed preterm babies. Another study compared the visual acuity of three groups of infants between four and seven months of age: breastfed infants, infants fed a formula supplemented with DHA, and infants receiving standard formula that was not fortified with DHA. The visual acuity of breastfed and DHA-fortified-formula-fed infants was better than the visual acuity of infants fed a formula deficient in DHA. Formula manufacturers are now experimenting with adding DHA to the formula. Some are fortifying their formula with only percursor essential fatty acids, such as linoleic and alpha-linolenic acids, in the hope that babies will be able to metabolize these essential fatty acids into DHA. But there is evidence that some formula-fed infants aren't able to change these essential

fatty acids into DHA. Again, attempts to duplicate mom's milk with factory-made formulas are failing. The best brain fats are those made by mom.

Better Hearts

Formula is cholesterol free, but this is nothing to boast about, because human milk actually does contain cholesterol. Heart researchers theorize that it's because human milk contains cholesterol that a baby's liver develops the mechanisms needed to metabolize cholesterol in the diet. A formula-fed baby, on the other hand, does not get a chance to develop the mechanism at a critical period of growth. As a result, the formula-fed infant grows up at a disadvantage, being less able to metabolize dietary cholesterol. This can lead to higher blood cholesterol and subsequent cardiovascular disease. Furthermore, human milk contains the natural fat DHA, which has been shown to have a rhythm-stabilizing effect on the heart rate. Heart rates are lower in breastfed babies.

Another heart-healthy benefit of human milk is the scientifically validated observation that breastfed babies are leaner than their formula-fed friends. Studies comparing the growth of breastfed and formula-fed babies showed that both groups have comparable growth in height and head circumference, but the breastfed babies tend to be lighter in weight, at least during the first eighteen months. This finding suggests that breastfed babies are leaner, and leanness is now known to be an important factor in lowering the risk of many illnesses, especially adult cardiovascular disease.

WHAT'S IN IT FOR MOTHERS

Lactation is part of a woman's reproductive cycle, like menstruation, ovulation, pregnancy, and childbirth. Nourishing a baby at the breast is as natural as growing a baby inside the womb. Completing that reproductive cycle by nursing a baby for several months, or years, allows a mother's body to do what it was designed to do, and this has benefits for her.

In the days immediately after birth, breastfeeding helps the uterus contract and return to its prepregnant size. Breastfeeding mothers can lose extra pounds put on during pregnancy without dieting (although a steady diet of high-fat junk foods will keep those pounds from coming off).

Most women do not menstruate or ovulate during the time their baby is receiving all his nourishment at the breast. Fertility returns as the baby starts solid food, but depending on how much the baby is nursing, a woman may go for a year or more without a period and without being able to get pregnant. This is nature's way of spac-

---

HOW BREASTFEEDING BENEFITS MOTHER

Most people are aware that there are many ways that breastfeeding benefits babies. What is not fully appreciated are all the good things that happen to moms.

It reduces the risk of breast cancer. Women who breastfeed can reduce their risk of developing breast cancer by as much as 25 percent. The reduction in cancer risk comes in proportion to the cumulative lifetime duration of breastfeeding. That is, the more months or years a mother breastfeeds, the lower her risk of breast cancer.

It reduces the risk of uterine and ovarian cancers. One of the reasons for the cancer-fighting effects of breastfeeding is that estrogen levels are lower during lactation. It is thought that the less estrogen available to stimulate the lining of the uterus, ovaries, and breast, the less risk there is of these tissues becoming cancerous.

It lessens the incidence of osteoporosis. Nonbreastfeeding women have a four-times-greater chance of developing osteoporosis than breastfeeding women do. They are less likely to suffer hip fractures in the postmenopausal years.

It benefits child spacing. Since breastfeeding delays ovulation, the longer a mother breastfeeds, the longer she is able to practice natural child spacing if she desires. How long breastfeeding delays ovulation depends on the baby's nursing pattern and the mother's individual fertility.

It promotes emotional health. Not only is breastfeeding good for mother's body, it's good for mother's mind. Studies indicate that breastfeeding mothers show less postpartum anxiety and depression than do formula-feeding mothers.

It promotes postpartum weight loss. In studies breastfeeding mothers showed significantly larger reductions in hip circumference and more fat loss by one month postpartum when compared with formula-feeding moms. Breastfeeding mothers tend to have an earlier return to their prepregnant weight.

It costs less to breastfeed. It costs around $1,200 a year to formula-feed your baby. Even taking into consideration the slight increase in food costs, a breastfeeding mother will save a lot of money during the first year of breastfeeding in addition to having fewer medical bills.

BREASTFEEDING WHILE WORKING

There was a time when mothers automatically thought they had to wean their babies when they returned to work. New insights and methods of collection, transport, and storage of milk now make breastfeeding and employment outside the home a compatible and advisable combination, one that benefits mother, baby, and their relationship.

Working and parenting is the juggling act of the nineties. And part of this juggling act is that more and more mothers are finding that working and breastfeeding are compatible. Most of the mothers in our practice who return to full- or part-time work outside the home still continue many months of at least part-time breastfeeding. In fact, working outside the home and breastfeeding isn't all that new. Thirty-two years ago, when our first baby, Jim, was born, because we couldn't live on an intern's meager salary Martha returned to part-time work as a nurse a few weeks after Jim's birth. Motivated by an intuitive desire to give Jim her milk, despite facing the financial realities of life, Martha knew she'd be able to continue. Doctor and nurse would shuttle their precious baby to work, home, and substitute caregiver. Some folks would say this wasn't ideal parenting, but at the time, we could not achieve the ideal. We did the best we could under less-than-perfect circumstances.

The first ingredient in the recipe for successful breastfeeding while working is commitment. Once you are convinced of the emotional, physical, and intellectual advantages of continuing to give your baby nature's perfect milk, you will find a way to do it. Here are some ways that worked for us:

- **Pump your milk.** Set up a breastfeeding pumping system at work, along with a bag full of bottles that you can tote your pumped milk in. (Medela makes an excellent portable double-pump and milk-transport system.) Expect to develop a love-hate relationship with your breast pump. It helps to look at a picture of your baby and imagine you are nursing your baby while pumping. Make time for three pumpings while you are at work. Put your liquid gold in cooled containers in a tote bag, and take it home as the next day's supply for the caregiver.

- **Store milk while at work.** While a refrigerator for storing milk is ideal, new studies have shown that it is not absolutely necessary. Pumped breast milk stays fresh for up to eight hours (a typical workday) in a small cooler with ice packs. Milk can be safely kept at room temperature in the typical office for up to four hours.

- **Begin a milk bank** if you haven't already done so. Pump as much milk as you can and store 6-ounce portions in bottle bags in the coldest part of your freezer. This will keep as long as you need it.

- **Breastfeed during breaks.** If your baby is being cared for close to your workplace, have your caregiver bring baby to you for a feeding or go to your baby for a feeding once or twice during the day. With on-site day-care centers, some working mothers are able to breastfeed their babies during lunch and coffee breaks.

- **Enjoy a happy departure and happy reunion.** Breastfeed your baby right before leaving for work and as soon as you return. Instruct your caregiver not to feed your baby within an hour before you return home. An eager baby and a full mother make for a happy reunion. As an added perk, the relaxing effects from the hormones of breastfeeding will help you unwind from a busy day. You can usually get in at least four feedings within twenty-four hours: one before you leave for work, one as soon as you get home, an evening feeding, and a before-bed feeding.

BREASTFEEDING WHILE WORKING (CONTINUED)

- **Breastfeed full-time during off-time.** Periodic full-time breastfeeding on weekends, holidays, and days off is necessary to keep up your milk production.

- **Sleep with your baby.** Expect baby to wake up and want to breastfeed more often at night after you return to work. Sleeping with your baby allows you and your baby to reconnect at night and make up for missed touch time during the day. Since baby will probably wake up more once you return to work, you will lose less sleep if you

let baby sleep right next to you. You simply roll over and nurse your baby once or twice during the night, and eventually you will find that neither member of the nursing pair awakens fully. Mothers in our practice who have achieved this nighttime harmony with their baby report they sleep better.

Continuing to breastfeed when you return to work is a wonderful way to stay connected with your baby, even while you're apart.

---

ing babies.* Evidence is growing that extended breastfeeding offers protection against breast, ovarian, and uterine cancers, especially in pre-menopausal women.

Breastfeeding has practical benefits for mothers, too. It saves money. Milk for the baby is always available, making it easier to travel the world with a breastfed baby or even just complete a morning's worth of errands. And the hormones that regulate the production and delivery of breast milk, namely, prolactin and oxytocin, have a natural calming effect on mothers. Breastfeeding soothes both mother and baby.

Many mothers worry that if their own eating habits are less than perfect, their milk won't be good for their babies. In reality, even undernourished mothers living in poverty produce good-quality milk, milk far superior to any artificial substitute. Mothers who have read about the calcium demands of lactation may worry that breastfeeding will increase their chances of having osteoporosis later in life. However, studies show that although there is some bone loss while a

mother is making milk for her baby, the bone is replaced after weaning, and in fact, women who breastfeed may actually lower their risk of osteoporosis.

Nevertheless, it is important to eat well while nursing a baby. Good nutrition helps mothers cope with the stresses of adding a baby to the family. Eating well doesn't have to mean eating fancy meals. Nutritious snacks throughout the day will keep energy high and nerves calmed.

To some in this modern world, it seems that breastfeeding asks a lot of mothers. Mother has to be with the baby to feed the baby, and since newborn breastfed infants nurse ten to twelve times a day, this means breastfeeding mothers are with their babies pretty much all the time. As a mother we know described it, "Breastfeeding is one big give-a-thon." The early days and weeks of breastfeeding can be challenging, so information and support are critical to get a mother through the days when it seems that all the baby wants to do is nurse. (See "Breastfeeding Resources," page 233.)

Fortunately, breastfeeding has its rewards. Mothers treasure the sense of closeness they experience with their baby. They feel that breastfeeding helps them know their child deeply, and this sense of knowing their child well helps them be

---

* *If you're interested in knowing more about breastfeeding and fertility, read* Your Fertility Signals *by Merryl Winstein (Smooth Stone Press, 1991) or* Breastfeeding and Natural Child Spacing *by Sheila Kippley (Couple to Couple League, 1989).*

better parents as their child grows. The more immediate rewards — a happy, healthy, smiling baby at the breast, the woman's pride in the nurturing power of her body — are empowering. Giving a baby the best nutritional start in life pays off for the entire family.

THE STATE OF THE (LOST) ART!

Below is a 1992 chart comparing the percentage of infants in the United States receiving different types of milk or formula from birth to one year of age. As you can see, current practice is far from ideal (although more babies are breastfed now and for longer periods of time than babies in the 1970s). By ten months of age, more than 90 percent of infants receive more than 90 percent of their milk from either prepared formula or cow's milk instead of from human milk.

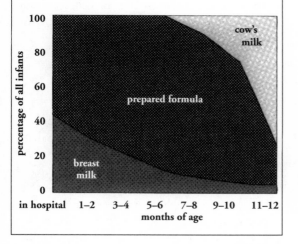

27

Choosing and Comparing Infant Formulas

I N THE PAST twenty-five years, thanks to support groups such as La Leche League International, there has been a return to breastfeeding, with more and more new mothers now leaving the hospital breastfeeding their babies. Even formula manufacturers acknowledge publicly that breastfeeding is best, yet sometimes substitutes are necessary. In fact, in recent years there has been a strong underground anti-formula movement. This was brought home to me recently in my office, when I received a letter from a new patient that began, "I'm not going to be bringing my baby back to your practice because you have SIN in your office." This concerned mother went on to explain that in my office she had noticed cases of formula (left at the front desk by a formula-company rep), which she dubbed "SIN" for "synthetic infant nutrition." This mother believed in the cause of being not only pro-breastfeeding but also anti-formula.

The new term coined by breastfeeding advocates for formulas is "artificial baby milk" (ABM), a reminder that infant formula, despite its widespread use, is still only a substitute for nature's food for babies, human milk. But children aren't raised in an ideal world and infants aren't always fed the ideal milk. Even though breast milk is best, for a variety of reasons you may choose to give your baby formula, and if you are going to do this, you need to make an informed choice about infant formula. This chapter contains information you must know.

HOW FORMULAS ARE MADE

Using human milk as the nutritional standard, formula manufacturers follow a basic recipe that includes proteins, fats, carbohydrates, vitamins, minerals, and water. They combine various ingredients so that the nutrients in artificial baby milks follow the same rough proportions as human milk. The big difference between formulas is the different sources of these elements — cow's milk, soybeans, or something else. Most formulas are cow's-milk based, meaning, the basic nutritional building blocks of proteins, fats, and carbohydrates are taken from this nutritional source. Cow's milk contains most of the nutrients necessary for adequate infant nutrition, although not in the appropriate proportions. Soybeans are also a ready source of certain nutrients necessary for human nutrition. Formula manufacturers start with the basic nutritional elements in cow's milk or soy beans and add ingredients until the mixture approximates human milk as closely as possible. They adjust levels of carbohydrates, proteins, and fat and add vitamins and minerals.

FORMULA FIGHTS

The principles of free enterprise suggest that competition among the big three formula makers, Carnation (maker of Good Start®), Ross Laboratories (maker of Similac®), and Mead Johnson (maker of Enfamil®), should improve the quality of artificial baby milks, and it has. Today's formulas are better than the ones made a decade ago. This is commendable, but it's not enough. Research must continue to be a priority. My concern is that formula companies are spending more on advertising and packaging than on improving the product, and they have begun competing on price rather than quality. The fact is that formula is already too expensive. Formula prices have skyrocketed 800 percent over the past ten years, boosted in part by government subsidies for formula purchased by low-income families. Meanwhile, European formula making is far ahead of ours, with the addition of probiotics, *Lactobacillus bifidus,* DHA, and other nutrients — improvements that are being held up in the United States by a formula-company committee awaiting government approval or by the economics of adding these costly nutrients. Parents can affect capitalism's food chain by comparison shopping, becoming savvy label readers, insisting on quality formula for their baby, and giving formula makers the message that nutritional value, not just price, is important.

NUTRIMYTH

New and Improved. When formula manufacturers claim that their product is closest to mother's milk, don't believe it. None of the formulas are close to human milk, even though they are closer today than they were ten years ago. When I see the word "improved" on a formula can I have mixed feelings. On the one hand, I'm glad for the babies who receive the "improved formula." I'm sad for the babies who had the misfortune of receiving the less improved one.

To be fair, formula companies have produced milk for babies which, at least on paper, seems to resemble the real thing. Formula is definitely better than it used to be. But on close inspection, what the factories make doesn't quite measure up to what mom makes. It is nearly impossible for artificial baby milk manufacturers to make a milk with nutrients even close to what mothers' bodies can make. And these companies' primary goal is to make a profit, so marketing and manufacturing issues influence what finally gets into that can.

One of our concerns is that even though formula-fed infants appear to grow normally, are they really thriving? "Thriving" means more than just getting bigger. It means developing to the child's fullest physical, emotional, and intellectual potential. We just don't know about the long-term effects of improvising on what to feed babies, though we do know that there are significant health differences between formula-fed and breastfed infants. Human milk is a live substance containing live white blood cells and immune-fighting substances. It is a living, dynamic, changing nutritional source, which daily (sometimes hourly) adjusts to meet the individual needs of a growing baby. Formulas are a collection of dead nutrients. They do not contain living white cells, digestive enzymes, or immune factors. In terms of human history, they are a new experiment.

Even though the Infant Formula Act passed by Congress in 1985 mandates the Food and Drug Administration to see that formulas contain all the nutrients that babies need, we don't really know everything there is to know about what babies need. The good news is that formula companies are constantly updating their recipes in order to keep up with new research into infant nutrition. The bad news is that each change in formula is really just a new experiment.

HOW TO CHOOSE A FORMULA

There are some subtle but important differences among the major brands of infant formulas. Reading the labels may leave you feeling like you need a Ph.D. in biochemistry to make an intelligent deci-sion. This chapter is designed to help you with an analysis of the big three nutrients: proteins, fats, and carbohydrates. The vitamins and minerals in all formulas are similar, since these are governed by strict regulations. However, the nutritional fine points of the fats, carbohydrates, and proteins differ from one brand to another.

Standard Formulas

Standard formulas are those that are tolerated by most infants. Infants with special digestive needs require special formulas (see page 256). Here are some details on how the standard formulas differ

DON'T KNOW!

Thoroughly researching the nutritional content of the formulas listed in the chart on page 257 was an experience. I spent over a hundred hours studying scientific articles and interviewing the chief biochemists and head nutritionists at each of the big three formula companies. At the end of my research, I had mixed feelings. On the positive side, I was impressed both by how thoroughly the formula companies investigate their products and by how much money they spend in order to turn out the best formula.

I was most impressed with the honesty of the chief nutritionist of Ross Laboratories, who shared with me that eight years ago the company made a philosophical change. They undertook an expensive project to try to come up with the best infant formula and realized that trying to duplicate the human milk recipe was not only biochemically impossible, it was misleading to the public. Instead, they studied the composition of the baby's blood in response to various formulas and compared that with the nutrients in the blood of breastfed infants. In other words, they compared babies rather than

the contents on the can. Ross Laboratories is the first formula company to come out and admit that no formula company can even come close to duplicating mother's milk.

I am also impressed by the fact that the older and more reputable formula companies, such as Ross Laboratories and Mead Johnson, continue to avoid advertising formula on TV or in parents' magazines. I was gratified to learn that the formulas that today's babies are receiving are nutritionally superior to those of the past. I was also impressed with the extent of government regulation, such as the fact that manufacturers must batch test their formula every thirty minutes.

After my research, I also had some misgivings. Many times, in answer to a query these nutritionists would reply, "Good question. We don't know." There are so many important facts that formula makers really don't know about the short- and the long-term effects of artificial baby milks on infants. As a pediatrician, I feel uneasy about prescribing a can full of "don't knows" for the babies I care for.

and guidelines on how to match a formula to your baby's needs.

Comparing Proteins

In looking at the protein content of Similac, Enfamil, and Carnation's Good Start (see page 257), you will notice the main difference is in the whey-to-casein ratio. In recent years there seems to be a whey war going on among formula makers, and each company has its own semi-scientific rationale as to why its product is best. Carnation contains 100 percent whey instead of the cow's-milk casein used by other brands, which, unlike the casein in human milk, forms difficult-to-digest curds that contribute to constipation. As an added perk, Carnation predigests the whey, breaking the protein up into smaller particles that are supposed to be easier for a baby to digest.

Enfamil promotes a 60-to-40-percent whey-to-casein ratio similar to human milk. Actually, a 70-to-30-percent whey-to-casein ratio is more typical of human milk, and the whey content of some human milk can be as high as 80 percent. Similac had always claimed that casein was the best protein, and for many years Similac formulas were 82 percent casein and 18 percent whey. In recent years, Similac has "improved" on this, and now boasts 48 percent whey and 52 percent casein. How much of this is science, how much is market pressure, and to what degree other factors are involved is hard to say. A consumer might interpret that Similac wasn't or isn't quite sure about the optimal protein composition and seems to be going along with the whey crowd, but not as far as Carnation. Similac backs up its protein choice with studies showing the amino-acid profile in the blood of Similac-fed infants is similar to the amino-acid profile in the blood of breastfed infants. Unlike the manufacturers of Carnation and Enfamil, who claim their formulas are most like human milk "on paper," Ross Laboratories, the maker of Similac, has taken a more scientific approach and formulates its protein based on what

actually gets into baby's blood, not what is listed on the can. Until this whey war is settled, let your baby's own digestion be the guide.

Comparing Fats

The label tells you that the fat in all artificial baby milks comes from vegetable oils. There is no acceptable alternative source, though long ago some infant formulas were made with lard. The five types of vegetable oils that are used are palm olein (not to be confused with saturated palm or palm kernel oil), soy, coconut, safflower, and sunflower. The different blends of these oils used in different formulas all have percentages of saturated, monounsaturated, and polyunsaturated fatty acids similar to breast milk, though some rely more on one oil than another. Enfamil, for example, has less polyunsaturated fats than Isomil or Carnation. When it comes to saturated fats, Carnation has the most, Similac the least. Formula companies claim that regardless of the source of the fat, as long as the final blend yields a fatty-acid profile similar to human milk's, then it's okay for babies. Actually, comparing the fat profile of human milk with the fat blends of formulas is more difficult than it seems because the fat content of human milk changes with the age of the baby and from feeding to feeding. The fat blend of formulas tries to match an "average" fat profile for human milk (whatever that means).

Of all the nutrients in formulas in the United States, the fatty-acid profile is the most concerning. While formula fat does contain the two essential omega acids, linoleic and linolenic, it does not have any docosahexaenoic acid (DHA), the fatty acid vital for brain development. Up until recently, researchers believed that infants could make DHA from these essential fatty acids as adults do, but recent studies have shown that formula-fed infants don't have the same high DHA levels that breastfed infants do. Babies may need a supply of DHA ready-made. This biochemical infant quirk has caused a lot of controversy among formula manufacturers as to whether or not to add DHA. As it stands now, the DHA precursors, linoleic and linolenic acid, are there, but they are not sufficient. In Europe, additional DHA fatty acids are added to artificial baby milks, and some nutritionists believe that American babies are currently being fed formulas that have a fatty-acid deficiency. Many researchers attribute the intellectual advantages of breastfeeding that are showing up in new studies to DHA. But formula makers are doubtful, maybe because of the cost of adding DHA to the formula.

Another problem with the current fat blends is that they contain no cholesterol. This may sound like a nutriperk, but we are tampering now with a proven recipe. Human milk is sort of a medium-cholesterol diet, like all animal milks. (For concerns about cholesterol, see page 243.)

Comparing Carbohydrates

Similac and Enfamil are practically the same in carbohydrate content, both containing only lactose. Carnation, on the other hand, contains 70 percent lactose and 30 percent maltodextrin, a table sugar–like carbohydrate that is, according to the manufacturers, necessary to balance the biochemical properties of the whey.

Iron-Fortified Formulas

You will notice at the store that both Enfamil and Similac produce both iron-fortified formulas and formulas that are lower in iron. In our opinion, and that of the Committee on Nutrition of the American Academy of Pediatrics, low-iron formulas have no place in infant nutrition. Carnation does not make a low-iron formula; it has only one formulation, which contains the recommended amount of iron, similar to that in the other two iron-fortified formulas.

Our conclusion: With current knowledge, it's impossible to rate one formula higher than another. And they're all likely to change with time. While the three main brands seem to be nutritionally similar, choose which formula is most friendly to your baby's intestines. Let the baby be the judge. (See signs on page 267.)

Follow-Up Formulas

A new trend in artificial baby milk, popular in Europe and now on the shelves in U.S. supermarkets, is formula designed for the infant older than six months. These formulas are meant to be a bridge between regular formula and cow's milk, which should not be introduced until sometime after age one. Two questions arise about follow-up formulas: Are they nutritious and are they necessary? The rationale for follow-up formulas is that the nutritional needs of infants greatly increase after the age of six months (especially for calcium, iron, and protein), and some infants may have difficulty meeting these increased requirements with greater volumes of standard formula plus solid foods. The following discussion concerns Carnation's Follow-Up™ formula, which, at this writing, is the most popular brand used in the United States.

NUTRIWORRY
Could American Infants Have Elsie-Poofa Deficiency?

There is concern that unlike some formulas made in Europe, as of 1999 American formulas do not contain some important long-chain polyunsaturated fatty acids (LCPUFA's). These long-chain fatty acids (specifically DHA) are thought to be an important constituent of vital organs such as the brain and eyes. Babies fed formulas without supplemental DHA have lower brain levels of DHA than breastfed babies.

SAFE FORMULA FEEDING

Always be sure to do the following:

- Use formula before the expiration date on the label.
- Use refrigerated, opened, ready-to-feed, and prepared formula within forty-eight hours.
- Don't leave bottles of formula out of the refrigerator for more than two hours.
- Throw away the formula left in the bottle after a feeding, since germs from baby's saliva will multiply in the warm formula.
- Refrigerate any formula saved from one day to the next.
- It's better not to heat formula in a microwave. Because of uneven heating, hot spots develop. If you do use the microwave, shake the bottle well before testing the temperature on your wrist; or place the bottle inside a mug filled with microwave-heated water and swirl the bottle often to even the heat.
- Avoid bottle propping, and don't let a baby fall asleep holding his own bottle. He could choke or aspirate the formula into his lungs. Falling asleep with a bottle allows the sugary formula to pool in the mouth, in contact with teeth, causing tooth decay. When a baby feeds from a bottle in the lying-down position, formula may travel from the back of the baby's throat up through the eustachian tube into the middle ear, causing ear infections.
- Remember that bottlefeeding, like breastfeeding, is a social interaction, in addition to a method of delivering nutrition. There should always be a person at both ends of the bottle, and babies should go to sleep attached to a person, not a bottle.

Advantages

Here are the advantages of follow-up formula:

It contains more calcium. From six months to a year the recommended dietary allowance for calcium in infants increases by 50 percent, from 400 milligrams to 600 milligrams. Carnation Follow-Up formula contains 600 milligrams of calcium in 24 ounces. It would take 39 ounces a day of standard formula to meet these calcium requirements.

It contains more iron. From six to twelve months a baby's daily iron requirements increase from 6 milligrams to 10 milligrams. This extra iron is supplied in 26 ounces of follow-up formula compared with 27 to 33 ounces of standard formula. This is not a significant difference, so there isn't a great advantage to the follow-up formula here.

It contains more protein. From six to twelve months an infant requires an extra 3 to 4 milligrams of daily protein. Follow-up formula contains from 10 to 25 percent more protein than standard formula. A baby would need an extra 3 to 8 ounces of standard formula per day to get this extra protein.

It costs less. Carnation Follow-Up formula costs around 20 percent less than regular formula.

It may taste better. Because it is basically milk, it tastes more like milk.

Disadvantages

Here are the disadvantages of follow-up formula:

The casein-to-whey ratio is different from that found in human milk. Basically, unlike Carnation's standard formula, which is 100 percent whey, Carnation Follow-Up is like the older version of Similac: 82 percent casein and 18 percent whey, plus calcium and a newer fat blend.

It is sweetened with corn syrup. The rationale for replacing lactose with corn syrup is to get it to taste sweeter. In our opinion, using corn syrup as the prime milk-carbohydrate source in an infant under a year is unwise nutrition. Besides ensuring proper nutrition, one of the main goals in feeding an infant over six months is to shape young tastes toward the normal taste of fresh foods. Corn syrup is too sweet to accomplish this and certainly shouldn't be part of a food babies eat several times each day.

Our conclusion: We do not recommend follow-up formulas that contain corn syrup. They are nutritionally unwise and unnecessary. You are better off giving your baby a higher volume of standard formula (growing babies need more fluid anyway), plus calcium- and iron-containing solid foods.

Soy Formulas

Even though around 25 percent of formula-fed American babies take some form of soy formula, we recommend that parents, with their doctor's advice, begin their baby on a standard cow's milk–based formula. Soy formulas became popular as an alternative formula in infants who are allergic to cow's milk. Some babies are less allergic to the soy protein than to cow's-milk protein. We have several reservations about soy formulas, including the following:

- Even though soy-based artificial baby milks may be less allergenic for some babies, between 30 and 50 percent of infants who are allergic to cow's milk are also allergic to soy.

- There is no precedent in nature to feeding young mammals a plant-based protein. In the early 1970s it was discovered that soy proteins

---

> ## HOW MUCH? HOW OFTEN?
>
> As you develop a bottlefeeding routine for yourself and your baby, the two of you will work out which formula is best, how much, and how often. This routine may change as your baby grows. Here is a general guide:
>
> Between birth and six months of age, your baby will need an average of 2 to 2.5 ounces of formula per pound per day. So, if your baby weighs 10 pounds, she will need 20 to 25 ounces per day.
>
> - newborns: 1 or 2 ounces at each feeding
> - one to two months: 3 to 4 ounces per feeding
> - two to six months: 4 to 6 ounces per feeding
> - six months to a year: up to 8 ounces per feeding
>
> Small, more frequent feedings work better than larger ones spaced farther apart. Your baby's tummy is about the size of his fist. Take a full bottle and place it next to your baby's fist and you'll see why tiny tummies often spit the milk back up when they're given too much at one time.

---

are deficient in some amino acids that babies need. For this reason, methionine, carnitine, and taurine have to be added from other sources. Current soy formulas only list methionine. According to the amino-acid profile, at least in Carnation Alsoy®, there is no carnitine or taurine. Even though current biochemical knowledge has fixed some of the previous problems with soy protein for babies, formula manufacturers are still just improvising on a proven recipe, leading us to conclude that feeding soy protein to growing babies is still experimental. Plant protein is a good protein for older infants and adults, but the protein that mother makes is ideal.

- To prevent calcium deficiencies and consequent deficiencies in bone mineralization, the calcium content of soy formulas is generally 20 to 30 percent higher than the calcium content of milk-based formulas. However, the protein in the soy contains phytates, substances that bind calcium and phosphorus.

- The phytates in soy's protein also bind iron and zinc. As a result of this finding, artificial soy baby milks, such as Carnation's Alsoy and Mead Johnson's ProSobee®, have extra added iron and zinc. Isomil® (made by Ross Laboratories) does not have more zinc or iron than the company's cow's milk–based formulas. Studies done by Ross Laboratories show that the blood-mineral profile of babies on cow's-milk and soy formulas are no different.

- In 1996 the Committee on Nutrition of the American Academy of Pediatrics voiced some concern about the relatively high content of aluminum in soy-based formulas and the possible toxicity to infants. Although the American Academy of Pediatrics concluded that the elevated aluminum levels in some soy formulas do not seem to be harmful for term infants, the fact is no one really knows. Because of this worry and because of studies showing less bone mineralization in preterm infants on soy formula, the Committee on Nutrition of the American Academy of Pediatrics recommended that soy formula be reserved for term infants and not be used for preterm or small-for-date infants.

- Soy formula was once routinely recommended for infants with a family history of milk allergy in hopes of preventing allergies from developing. Research has failed to support the idea that starting a newborn on soy formula will decrease the later incidence of allergy.

- Recent research has disproven the belief that babies who drink soy formulas are less colicky. For this reason, the Committee on Nutrition of the American Academy of Pediatrics recommends against the use of soy formulas in the routine management of colic or in infants who are potentially allergic to cow's milk. Instead of soy, hypoallergenic formulas (see page 258) are recommended.

- Giving an infant soy in the early months before intestinal closure (for an explanation of closure, see page 260) may predispose the infant to soy allergies later on. Since soy is used as a filler in so many foods in the American diet, this is a serious concern.

- Soy formulas contain around 33 percent more sodium than standard cow's milk–based formulas, and formulas in general are saltier than human milk. It is nutritionally unwise to accustom young palates to salty tastes.

- Carbohydrate sources in soy formulas are a serious concern. Just as there is a whey war going on between formula companies, there is now a sugar war, too. Enfamil now advertises "no table sugar" in their soy formula, ProSobee, so they use corn syrup instead of sucrose. Does this make a big difference? Some nutritionists might prefer plain old table sugar to corn syrup. Corn itself is an allergen, and corn syrup is very sweet.

- Because soy formulas are made with bean "milk" and not cow's milk, they are naturally lactose-free. The problem is that lactose is the sugar in human milk, as in the milk of all other mammals, and there is no basis in nature for feeding mammals lactose-free milk. Lactose is an intestines-friendly sugar, enhancing calcium absorption and helping to colonize those little intestines with favorable bacteria. While the "lactose-free" nature of soy formulas benefits infants who are congenitally lactose intolerant (which is really quite rare in the first year of life), omitting the lactose is really tampering

with nature's ideal. Soy formulas are often recommended for infants who develop a temporary lactase deficiency following an intestinal
infection. Research on whether or not this helps
shows mixed results. The American Academy of
Pediatrics does not recommend the *routine* use
of soy formulas in infants recovering from diarrhea but suggests they be used only in babies
shown to be temporarily intolerant of cow's
milk–based formulas.

Our conclusion: Unless recommended otherwise
by your baby's doctor, soy formulas:

- should not be used in infants with a family history of milk allergy in hopes of preventing later
  allergy;
- should not be used as a substitute for cow's
  milk–based formulas unless baby has been
  proven to be allergic to cow's milk–based formulas;
- should not be used to prevent or treat colic unless advised by your doctor;
- should not be used in preterm or small-for-date
  babies.

Even though we discourage the use of soy formula as a first-choice artificial baby milk, in
some babies it is a necessary alternative to cow's
milk–based formulas. Many of our objections to
soy formula may be more theoretical than practical (since studies have shown that healthy term
babies grow just as well on soy as they do on
cow's milk–based formulas). It's what we do not
know about soy that concerns us. The soybean
protein brings along with it a lot of other phytochemicals (plant nutrients), some of which may
be healthful for the baby, but the effects of others
we just don't know about. Cow's milk–based formulas have been around for nearly a century. We
don't have that much experience with soy. So be
cautious.

NUTRITIP
Choosing Formulas

Be sure to consult your doctor when
choosing a formula for your baby, as one
brand may be better suited to your baby's
individual needs than others. This book will
help you make an informed nutritional
decision, but your baby may have individual
nutritional needs that must be discussed
with your doctor.

Special Formulas for Special Problems

Special formulas are those in which one of the basic nutrients (usually the protein and/or carbohydrate) has been changed to an alternative nutrient
that an individual baby may better tolerate. When
formula shopping, be sure not to make a change
to any of these specialty formulas without your
doctor's advice. Specialty formulas:

- are usually much more expensive;
- usually taste bitter to downright bad because
  the technology required to predigest (hydrolyze)
  the protein into more easily digestible units results in a more bitter-tasting protein;
- may be lower in nutritional quality than standard formulas due to the changed or absent nutrient;
- are even more experimental than other
  formulas — that is, even less is known about
  the long-term effects of feeding babies these
  special formulas.

The following are the most popular specialty formulas at this writing.

Lactose-Free Formulas

Lactose-free formulas (e.g., Mead Johnson's
Lactofree®) are an example of new formula prod-

COMPARING FORMULA CONTENTS

Formula Name	Protein Source	Fat Source	Carb Source
Enfamil® (Mead Johnson)	whey 60 percent, casein 40 percent, from nonfat milk	palm olein, 45 percent soy, 20 percent coconut, 20 percent sunflower (high oleic), 15 percent	lactose
Similac® (Ross Laboratories)	whey 48 percent, casein 52 percent, from nonfat milk	safflower (high oleic), 42 percent coconut, 30 percent soy, 28 percent	lactose
Carnation® Good Start® (Nestle)	whey (predigested) 100 percent, nonfat milk	palm olein, 47 percent soy, 26 percent coconut, 21 percent safflower (high oleic), 6 percent	lactose, 70 percent maltodextrine, 30 percent
Carnation® Follow-Up™ (Nestle)	whey 18 percent, casein 82 percent, from nonfat milk	same as Carnation Good Start	corn syrup, 63 percent lactose, 37 percent
Isomil® (Ross Laboratories)	soy	corn, 50 percent coconut, 38 percent soy, 12 percent	corn syrup solids, sucrose
Enfamil® ProSobee® (Mead Johnson)	soy	same as Enfamil	corn syrup solids
Carnation® Alsoy® (Nestle)	soy	same as Carnation Good Start	corn maltodextrine, sucrose
Enfamil® LactoFree® (Mead Johnson)	same as Enfamil	same as Enfamil	corn syrup, sucrose
Alimentum® (Ross Laboratories)	hydrolyzed casein from nonfat milk	same as Enfamil	sucrose, modified tapioca starch
Enfamil® Nutramigen® (Mead Johnson)	hydrolyzed casein from nonfat milk	same as Similac	corn syrup, modified corn starch
Enfamil® Pregestimil® (Mead Johnson)	hydrolyzed casein from nonfat milk	MCT (medium-chain triglyceride) corn, 20 percent soy, 12.5 percent safflower (high oleic), 12.5 percent	corn syrup, dextrose, modified corn starch

ucts that are driven more by market demand than scientific sense. Many formula-fed babies (and breastfed babies, too) get fussy, resulting in what we call the formula parade: switching from one formula to another until either something works or the baby's intestines mature and he outgrows the problem. Whatever formula you're using at the time gets the credit. The fact is that oftentimes baby's fussiness is not due to the formula but to other unrelated causes. Nevertheless, formula gets the blame, so factories step up with new varieties to keep up with the demand. Hence lactose-free formulas.

Lactose-free formulas (including soy formulas) are often tried when a baby has symptoms of lactose intolerance, such as excessive bloating, gas, diarrhea, a red burnlike rash around the anus, and abdominal cramping. They are useful in babies who have a rare metabolic disease in which they are missing the enzyme that metabolizes lactose. (This disease occurs in only around one of sixty-five thousand babies.) Lactose-free formulas can also be tried in babies recovering from a diarrhea-producing illness and who suffer from a temporary lactase deficiency while the intestinal lining is healing.

Lactose intolerance is overdiagnosed in babies (as it is in adults). It's easy to blame formula, and specifically lactose, for baby's fussiness. Think for a moment. If so many babies are lactose intolerant, why would lactose be the sugar in human milk? True, human milk also contains the enzyme lactase that helps babies absorb the lactose, whereas formula does not, but milk lactase doesn't do the whole job. It seems reasonable that nature provides the intestines of nearly all babies with enough lactase to get through at least a year or so of milk feeding (lactose is present only in milk products and not in other foods).

In lactose-free formula, the lactose sugar has been replaced by other sugars, usually corn syrup and sucrose (table sugar). The protein-and-fat blend is the same as in cow's milk–based formulas.

No doubt the biochemist who dreamt up the formula thought that sugar is sugar, so substituting corn syrup and sucrose for lactose was no big deal. Lactose is eventually broken down into glucose, as are corn syrup and sucrose, so it shouldn't matter. In fact, the intestines break the lactose down into two sugars — galactose and glucose — and both of these sugars are absorbed into the bloodstream. No one really knows what galactose does or why it's beneficial, just as no one knows the whole story about how the body reacts to sugars from corn syrup and sucrose. So we're back to the non-science of common sense. If the human baby (like all mammals) didn't do better with galactose, it wouldn't be there in the first place. The milk sugar would have been pure glucose.

We also know that lactose does more than just supply energy. The lactose that doesn't get digested in the upper intestine contributes to what is called the "friendly ecology of the gut." Lactose helps healthful bacteria thrive. Lactose-free formulas may deprive baby not only of lactose but also of those trillions of friendly bugs that live in the intestines and do good things for the body. Lactose also facilitates calcium absorption in the gut, so babies on lactose-free formulas may run the risk of not getting enough calcium. To compensate for this theoretical problem, manufacturers add a bit more calcium.

Our conclusion: As with so many other nutrients in formula, there is one big WE DON'T KNOW about lactose-free formulas.

Hypoallergenic Formulas (Alimentum®, Nutramigen®, Pregestimil®)

If you see the term "hypoallergenic" on the label, it means that the formula has been proven to cause fewer allergies in babies than standard formulas. Since, by definition, the term "allergy" implies a sensitivity to a protein, the term "hypoallergenic" means that the protein in the formula is even less likely to cause allergic reactions. The protein has been "hydrolyzed" or "predigested," broken down into tinier proteins. Consider the following potential problems inherent in hydrolyzed protein formulas:

The taste problem. Unlike formulas that advertise "partially hydrolyzed protein," hypoallergenic formulas contain proteins that have been completely hydrolyzed or broken down into smaller parts. This requires intense processing that results in a bitter, almost unpalatable flavor, despite the high content of sweeteners. Tasting one of these formulas is enough to make any mother want to relactate.

The carbohydrate problem. When the protein is hydrolyzed, the lactose is also taken out of the milk, so the manufacturer has to add carbohydrates — usually corn syrup, sucrose, corn starch, or even tapioca. As we discussed above, substituting other sugars for lactose may not be a good idea. Nor is it necessarily true that a baby with protein allergies will also be lactose intolerant.

The salt problem. Hypoallergenic formulas are 30 to 90 percent higher in salt content.

The fat problem. The fat blend of Alimentum or Nutramigen is the same as that found in each manufacturer's cow's milk–based formulas, Similac and Enfamil, respectively. The primary fats in Pregestimil are medium-chain triglycerides (MCT's), intestines-friendly fats that are used in children with fat-malabsorption disorders. MCT's are factory-made fats. They provide no essential fatty acids — essential for a baby's growing brain and body. MCT's can be used as an energy supplement to boost weight gain in infants growing slowly. Yet, they should not be a baby's main fat source unless advised by your doctor. Pregestimil should not be given to healthy babies with no proven fat-malabsorption disorder or to infants with impaired liver function.

The price problem. The infant pays a high nutritional price for these formulas, and parents discover that hypoallergenic formulas are four to five times more expensive than standard formulas.

Our conclusion: Hypoallergenic formulas should not be used without a doctor's recommendation, and then only if there is a definite medical reason. Don't switch to one of these formulas just because baby is "fussy," not without trying different standard formulas first and learning other ways to help baby with his discomfort.

28

Beginning Solid Foods: When? What? And How?

READY TO OPEN your baby's mouth to a whole new world of textures and tastes? Is baby ready to open her mouth? Get ready for the joys — and the mess — of eating solid foods. *When* you begin feeding your baby solid foods and *how* you go about it set baby up for healthy eating habits. You are not only putting food into your baby's tummy, you are introducing lifelong attitudes about nutrition. Consider for a moment that during the first year or two you will spend more time feeding your baby than in any other single interaction. You both might as well enjoy it.

WHY WAIT?

Gone are the days when pressured mothers stuffed globs of cereal into the tight mouths of reluctant six-week-olds. Nowadays parents feed their baby on the timetable that is developmentally and nutritionally correct — as determined by their baby. Don't be in a rush to start solids. Here are some good reasons for waiting.

Baby's intestines need to mature. The intestines are the body's filtering system, screening out potentially harmful substances and letting in healthy nutrients. In the early months, this filtering system is immature. Between four and seven months, a baby's intestinal lining goes through a developmental growth spurt called "closure," meaning the intestinal lining becomes more selective about what to let through. To prevent potentially allergenic foods from entering the bloodstream, the maturing intestines secrete IgA, a protein immunoglobulin that acts like a protective paint, coating the intestines and preventing the passage of harmful allergens. In the early months, infant IgA production is low (although there is lots of IgA in human milk), and it is easier for potentially allergenic food molecules to enter the baby's system. Once food molecules are in the blood, the immune system may produce antibodies to that food, creating a food allergy. By six to seven months of age the intestines are more mature and able to filter out more of the offending allergens. This is why it's particularly important to delay solids in general if there is a family history of food allergy and especially to delay the introduction of foods to which other family members are allergic.

Young babies have a tongue-thrust reflex. Not only is the lower end of baby's digestive tract not ready for early solids, but neither is the mouth end. In the first four months a tongue-thrust reflex protects the infant against choking. When

MAKING YOUR OWN BABY FOOD

Baby food doesn't have to come in jars. You can make your own at home, and it's not difficult. Baby food is simply strained, pureed, or mashed adult food, just a different version of the food you prepare for yourself. Here are three good reasons for making your own baby food:

- You know what's in it.
- You can custom-tailor the texture to your baby's preference.
- You can shape your baby's tastes and help her learn what fresh foods taste like (see "Shaping Young Tastes," page 277).

Tips for Making Your Own Baby Food

- Buy organic fruits and vegetables. Your baby deserves pesticide-free foods. Scrub fruits and vegetables extra well with a vegetable brush. Trim stringy parts and remove any part of the food that could cause choking, such as pits, peels, and seeds. Trim excess fat off poultry and meat.
- Steam vegetables. This softens them, makes them easier to puree, mash, strain, and chew, and preserves more of the vitamins and minerals than boiling.
- There's no need to add salt or sugar. Try a bit of lemon juice as both a preservative and a natural flavor enhancer.
- Avoid deep-frying, which adds unhealthy fats to foods.
- Don't feel you have to prepare separate meals for your baby. You can simply take portions of your adult food (before you add any strong seasonings) and puree or mash to a stage appropriate for your baby.
- Make several meals' worth at a time and pour the freshly cooked and pureed food into an ice cube tray. Cover with cellophane wrap and freeze. Then, remove the frozen food cubes from the tray and store in air-tight freezer bags. Remove one serving-size cube at a time when needed.
- When baby graduates from cube-size portions, store the homemade food in recycled commercial baby food jars or small, plastic freezer containers. Be sure not to fill the jars to the brim, as food expands as it freezes.
- Label all your freezer packages with contents and date and rotate stock like the supermarket does — putting the most recently frozen foods behind the previously frozen ones. Homemade baby foods can be safely kept frozen for three months.
- For slow thawing, place a day's worth of baby food in the refrigerator. It will thaw in about four hours. For fast thawing, use an electric warming dish or place a heat-safe dish over water in a small saucepan and heat gently. If you use a microwave to thaw or warm baby food, be sure to stir the food well to avoid hot pockets.
- No matter what method of heating and thawing you use, stir the food well and test it with your finger to be sure it's not too hot.
- To avoid wasting your carefully prepared cuisine, dole out small portions. Gradually add more, using a clean spoon as needed.

any unusual substance is placed on the tongue, it automatically protrudes outward. Between four and six months this reflex gradually diminishes, giving the glob of cereal a fighting chance of making it from the tongue to the tummy.

Baby's swallowing mechanism is immature. Another reason not to rush solids is that the tongue and the swallowing mechanisms may not yet be ready to work together. Give a spoonful of food to an infant less than four months old and she will move it around randomly in her mouth, pushing some of it back into the pharynx where it is swallowed, some of it into the large spaces between the cheeks and gums, and some forward between the lips and out onto her chin. Between four and six months of age, most infants develop the ability to move the food from the front of the mouth to the back instead of letting it wallow around in the mouth and get spit out. Prior to four months of age, a baby's swallowing mechanism is designed to work with sucking, but not with eating.

Baby needs to be able to sit up. In the early months, babies associate feeding with cuddling. Feeding is an intimate interaction, and babies often associate the feeding ritual with falling asleep in arms or at the breast. The change from a soft, warm breast to a cold, hard spoon may not be welcomed with an open mouth. Feeding solid foods is a less intimate and more mechanical way of delivering food. It requires baby to sit up in a high chair — a skill that most babies develop between five and seven months. Holding a breastfed baby in the usual breastfeeding position may not be the best way to start introducing solids, as your baby expects to be breastfed and clicks into a "what's wrong with this picture?" mode of food rejection.

Young infants are not equipped to chew. Teeth seldom appear until six or seven months, giving further evidence that the young infant is designed to suck rather than to chew. In the pre-teething

stage, between four and six months, babies tend to drool, and the drool that you are always wiping off baby's face is rich in enzymes, which will help digest the solid foods that are soon to come.

Older babies like to imitate caregivers. Around six months of age, babies like to imitate what they see, so they are more receptive to trying something new. They see you spear a veggie and enjoy chewing it. They want to grab a spoon and do likewise.

COMMON QUESTIONS NEW PARENTS ASK

How will I know when my baby is ready for solids?

As with all aspects of parenting, watch your child, not the calendar. Besides the developmental milestones discussed above, watch for these ready-to-eat cues in your baby:

- Baby is able to sit with support, reaches and grabs, and mouths hands and toys.
- Baby watches you eat, following your fork as it moves from the plate to your mouth.

RESOURCES FOR MAKING YOUR OWN BABY FOOD

Here are some useful resources for making your own baby food:

Mommy Made and Daddy Too: Home Cooking for a Healthy Baby and Toddler, Martha and David Kimmel (Bantam Doubleday Dell, 1998)
The Natural Baby Food Cookbook, Margaret Elizabeth Kenda and Phyllis S. Williams (Avon, 1988)
Baby Let's Eat, Rena Coyle (Workman, 1987)

NUTRITIP
Milk Plus

Consider solid foods to be an addition to, not a substitute for, breast milk or formula, which are more nutritionally balanced than any solid food. This food fact is especially important for breastfeeding babies. For a breastfeeding baby, it's best to start solids slowly, so that they don't become a substitute for the more nutritious breast milk. Also, solids fed at an early age can interrupt the supply-and-demand routine, with the result that milk production dwindles.

- Baby "mooches," reaching for food on your plate.

- Baby mimics your eating behaviors, such as opening her mouth wide when you open your mouth to eat. (Grabbing your spoon is not a reliable sign of feeding readiness, since baby may be more interested in the noise, shape, and feel of your utensils than the foodstuff on them.)

- Baby can show and tell. Around six months of age, babies have the ability to say yes to food by reaching or leaning toward it, and no by pushing it or turning away. Expect mixed messages as your baby learns to communicate. When in doubt, offer, but never force.

- Baby seems unsatisfied after a feeding or is shortening the intervals between feedings, and several days of more frequent feedings don't change this.

I'm not sure if my baby is ready. Should I try offering solids anyway?

Is your baby both ready and willing to try solid foods? Here's how to tell. If your baby eagerly opens his mouth when he sees a spoonful of food coming toward him, he is probably both ready and willing. If he turns away, he's not. Or, give him a spoon to play with to see if it quickly ends up in his mouth. (Feeding tip: Use plastic spoons with smooth, rounded edges. They do not get too cold or hot, and they are quiet when banged or dropped.) Remember, your immediate goal is to *introduce* your baby to solid foods, not to fill him up on solids. Milk feedings will continue to be a major part of his diet for the next several months. Gradually introduce baby to a different texture, taste, and way of swallowing. Overwhelming your child with big globs of too many new foods all at once invites rejection. At this point, solids are add-ons, not substitutes for feedings from breast or bottle. However, if you have a six-to-nine-month-old formula-fed baby who is taking in 40 ounces a day, you may consider substituting a solid-food feeding for a bottle.

Which foods are best to begin with?

Begin with foods that are not likely to cause allergies and that are most like the milk that baby is used to. If your baby is used to the sweet taste of human milk, start with mashed bananas. If baby is used to the more bland flavor of formula, try rice cereal mixed with formula (or with your milk if your breastfed baby prefers rice cereal to bananas). Rice is the most intestines-friendly grain because it is gluten free, low in protein, and high in carbohydrates. Mix the cereal to a soupy consistency and add less liquid as baby gets better at eating.

How do I start?

Use your finger as baby's first "spoon." It's soft and the right temperature, and baby is familiar with it. Encourage baby to open her mouth wide. Place a fingertipful of this glorious glob on baby's lips while letting her suck on the tip of your finger. Next, advance the fingertipful of food to the tip of your baby's tongue (where there are taste buds receptive to sweetness). If the food gets swallowed, or at least is not spit back at you, try placing the next glob toward the middle of baby's tongue.

Watch baby's reaction to this new experience. If the food goes in with an approving smile, baby is ready and willing. If the food comes back at you, accompanied by a disapproving grimace, baby may not be ready. But some babies make funny faces because this is all so new to them. What happens in the mouth may be a more accurate indicator of whether a baby is ready to eat solids. If the mouth opens for a second helping, give it another try — you may have a winner. Even if the food comes back out, this baby may just need to learn to seal his mouth shut when he moves the food from the front to the back. Rejection of the food could also indicate that the tongue-thrust reflex is not yet gone, so baby can't move the food backward in the mouth and swallow it. If your baby just sits there with an open mouth, confused by the glob of food perched on her tongue, she's probably having difficulty with the tongue-thrust reflex. Let her practice a while. If she still doesn't seem to know what to do, wait a week or two before you try again.

How much food should I offer?

If your baby eagerly accepts the first fingertipful of food, offer a little more the next time. At these first feedings, baby may actually swallow only a teaspoon or two of food. Increase the amount gradually until you are offering a quarter cup or more at a time. Remember, your initial goal is to introduce your baby to the new tastes and textures of solid foods, not to stuff him. As with all areas of development, babies take two steps forward and one step back. Expect erratic eating patterns. Baby may take a couple of tablespoons one day and only a teaspoon the next. Baby may devour pears and refuse bananas one day, then the next

day ignore the pears and gobble down the banana. That's all part of the feeding game. Relax and realize now that you can't control your child's every mouthful. Don't force-feed a baby. Know when enough is enough. (Your baby knows.) *Observe these stop signs:*

- Baby purses her lips, closes her mouth, and turns her head away from the approaching spoon.

- Baby leans away from the advancing spoon, uninterested or wanting to avoid the food entirely. Leaning toward the food or grabbing the spoon or hand of the feeder indicates a desire for more.

What time of the day is best for feeding solid foods?

Offer *new* foods in the morning. If by some chance your baby is allergic to a particular food, the intestinal upsets should wear off by the end of the day. Beginning a new food in the evening puts baby at risk for painful night waking. Otherwise, offer solids at the time of the day when your baby seems hungriest, is bored, or you both need a snack and something interesting to do. Mornings are usually the time when babies are hungriest and in the best mood for social interactions, including feeding.

If breastfeeding, try offering solid foods toward the end of the day, when your milk supply is likely to be the lowest and baby will be more eager to eat. Feed baby solids between breastfeedings, not right after, since solid foods may interfere with the absorption of some of the nutrients in your milk.

Choose a time of the day when you are not in a hurry, since dawdling, dabbling, spewing, spattering, smearing, and dropping are all part of the feeding game. Forget fast feeding. Remember, meals are both a food-delivery system and a social experience. Take your time, and enjoy this new nutritional stage.

My baby enjoys rice cereal and bananas. What foods should I feed her next?

Work your way from soupy to lumpy as you also increase how often and how much baby eats. At first, you'll offer food only once a day; but within a few months, you'll be feeding whenever you sit down to a meal. Babies differ so much in their preferences and their readiness for solids that it's difficult to make hard-and-fast rules about the consistency, amount, and type of solid foods to offer. But here are some suggestions from our family and from our pediatrics practice for babies aged from five to eight months:

Bananas. Because of their sweetness and smooth consistency, ripe bananas closely resemble mother's milk, which makes them an ideal starter food. They are one of the few fruits that can be served uncooked. Let the banana get very ripe before serving it to baby (the skin should be covered with brown spots). After peeling it, cut and mash it with a fork, and serve it either straight or mixed with formula or breastmilk for a more soupy consistency. Bananas are a great quick meal for par-

ents and babies on the go — mash a few slices and eat the rest yourself.

Cereal. Begin with rice or barley cereal, the least allergenic. Don't serve a mixed cereal until you've tried each of the components separately to be sure baby is not allergic to any of them. Rice is approximately 75 percent carbohydrates and 7 percent protein. High-protein cereals, made primarily with soybeans, may contain as much as 35 percent protein. Cereals made especially for infants are fortified with minerals, such as calcium and phosphorus, along with B vitamins and iron. Begin with ¼ teaspoon of cereal and advance to 1 tablespoon, and so on. Mix it with breastmilk or formula to the desired consistency. Cereal alone is very bland and may be refused by your baby. Once you know your baby is not allergic to different fruits and cereals, you can experiment by combining various fruits with cereal in various consistencies. Cereals are often suggested as a way to fill baby up, so that she'll lengthen the interval between feedings and even sleep through the night. This "filler fallacy" is an unwise feeding pattern. Cereal is not nearly as nutritious as human milk or formula. Besides, this practice rarely works.

Pears. Pears are easy to digest and have a mild flavor perfect for babies. As with all fruits, they are mostly carbohydrates and a good source of potassium and vitamins A and C. Try pear sauce instead of applesauce.

Applesauce. Applesauce is an ideal first fruit. It is low in citric acid, which can cause allergic reactions in some infants. Cook a cored and peeled apple with 2 tablespoons of water over medium heat until fork tender. Blend or whip until smooth. Applesauce can be combined with a variety of foods, including cereal, or use it as a "sauce" to disguise less palatable, but more nutritious, foods. Uncooked apples are difficult for babies

NUTRITIP
Don't Sweat the Small Feedings.

Take it from the Sears family: Relax and have fun with this new stage. By four months of age babies are very astute at reading parents' facial expressions. If you're anxious about getting solid food into your baby, expect baby also to be anxious. Approach the feeding game as just another social interaction that you will both enjoy.

under one year of age to gum and chew, and they are a choking hazard.

Carrots. Cooked carrots are a very good source of vitamin A and beta carotene, and, as mom always said, carrots improve night vision. Peel, slice, and steam carrots until tender without spices, salt, sugar, or butter. Small blobs of mashed, cooked carrots are usually well accepted and enjoyed by babies. Bite-sized cooked carrots or a pile of steamed, grated carrots are good finger foods beginning at eight months. Avoid raw carrots, which can cause choking.

Sweet potatoes and winter squash. Babies enjoy sweet potatoes and winter squash for their flavor, texture, and color. They are both high in beta carotene. Sweet potatoes contain vitamin B-6, which helps the body use carbohydrates, protein, and fat needed for healthy skin, nerves, and circulation. Winter squash supplies potassium and other nutrients. Carrots, sweet potatoes, and squash can all be cooked quickly in the microwave, with minimum nutrient loss. Sweet potatoes are like convenience foods in the microwave: Wash, cook for seven or eight minutes, open, and serve. You don't even need a plate. Be sure to stir the warm potato and test for hot spots, since microwaved food may heat unevenly. Alternatively, wash and peel sweet potatoes before cooking in a small amount of water, or steam over medium heat until fork tender. Blend with a small amount of liquid. For variety, mix sweet potatoes with peas, carrots, or squash. For squash, cut it in half, remove the seeds, and bake it. Or, you can peel it and steam the pieces. Blend until smooth and add water to reach the desired consistency.

Avocados. Avocados are an ideal food for babies. The avocado's smooth, creamy consistency makes it a fresh fruit even a baby can enjoy. Low in sodium and cholesterol free, avocados contain such valuable nutrients as vitamins A and B-6, folic acid, niacin, phosphorus, magnesium, and iron. Ounce for ounce, avocados contain more potassium than forty-five other fruits, juices, or vegetables, including bananas, peaches, carrots, and green beans; and they are the only fruit or vegetable that contains monounsaturated fats, essential for your baby's development. Avocados are higher in calories than any other fruit or vegetable. This is a plus for babies, since feeding infants calls for nutrient-dense foods, foods that contain a lot of nutrition per unit of weight and volume. Ripe avocados can be served without any cooking — a time-saver for mom and dad. To prepare, cut in half around the entire circumference of the seed. Grab a half in each hand and twist to remove the seed. Scoop out the meat inside and mash it with a fork, or simply spoon-feed it directly from the shell. For variety, avocados can be mixed with apple or pear sauce, cooked squash, or sweet potatoes. One of the reasons avocados are one of the Sears family's favorite foods for babies, infants, and children is their versatility. Avocados can be spread, scooped, mashed, or made into children's guacamole (avocado dip without the strong spices).

I've heard that it's better to start vegetables before fruits. Is this true?

Purists recommend that vegetables be introduced before fruits so that infants don't learn to expect that food should always taste sweet. This is one of those nutritional directives that sound great in theory but, as many of us who have fed lots of babies have found, are hard to put into practice. First of all, babies are born with a sweet tooth. Their tiny tongues are more richly supplied with sweet taste buds than with any others. This makes sense, because human milk is sweet, and breastfed babies are less likely to willingly accept the bland taste of vegetables than formula-fed babies. While there is no doubt that vegetables are nutritionally superior to fruits, most parents find that babies will happily eat fruits, making them hassle-free first foods. The nutritional content of starter foods is of secondary importance; the main goal of these early solid-food feedings is for the baby to learn how to swallow foods of different textures. You're likely to have more success with fruits than with vegetables. When introducing veggies, try the sweet ones first: carrots and sweet potatoes. If you have a baby who loves vegetables, lucky you! But don't worry if your baby views veggies with less enthusiasm than fruit. He'll learn to like them eventually if you keep offering them.

How will I know if a food is upsetting my baby?

Begin with single-ingredient foods and space the introduction of each new food at least one week apart. If your baby has a reaction, you'll know what to blame. Here are the most usual beginning signs of food allergy:

- bloating and gassiness
- a sandpaper-like raised red rash on the face
- runny nose and watery eyes
- diarrhea or stools with mucus
- a red rash around the anus (we call this the "target sign")

- generally cranky behavior
- vomiting or increased spitting up

If you have a family history of food allergies or are particularly worried about them, keep a food diary (see below), which not only helps you learn your baby's preferences but helps you be more objective about which symptoms are caused by which foods. As you change the foods that go in one end, expect a change in the color, consistency, and frequency of the waste that comes out the other. This is normal, and not a sign of food intolerance. You may notice bits of food in baby's stools, or the color may change — red stools with red vegetables, such as beets, and yellow stools with carrots. *Babies who overdose on bananas and/or rice products may become constipated.* As your baby's intestines mature enough to digest the food more thoroughly, the stools will not take on so many characteristics of yesterday's meals.

What foods should I serve for breakfast, lunch, and dinner?

It makes no nutritional difference to your baby when you serve what, since babies have no concept of breakfast, lunch, and dinner. What you

Foods Baby Likes	Foods Baby Doesn't Like	Symptoms/ Possible Food Sensitivities

serve has more to do with your time and energy and baby's mood and willingness than with any traditional ideas about what to eat when. Whatever schedule you and your baby work out is the best one for you. Be prepared for the fact that babies have erratic feeding patterns and some babies do better eating small amounts throughout the day rather than three larger meals. (See the related discussions "Tips for Feeding the Picky Eater," in Chapter 29, and "Grazing for Good Digestion," page 97.)

Feeding time is such a mess, I dread it. How can I make feeding times easier on my baby and myself?

We have logged many hours in feeding eight babies, and we know that babies spit, fling, smear, and drop their food. One mother of a messy eater in our pediatrics practice told us, "Our floor has a more balanced diet than my baby does." Here are some tips that we have learned for getting more food into our babies with fewer hassles for ourselves:

Show and tell. To entice the reluctant eater to eat, model enjoyment. Capitalizing on baby's newly developing social skill — mimicking her caregivers' actions — feed yourself in front of baby, but in an exaggerated way, slowly putting a spoonful of baby's food into your mouth. With big, wide eyes showing how much you enjoy it, overreact, saying "Mmmmm, good!" Let baby catch the spirit and want to do likewise.

Open mouth, insert spoon. Wait for a time when baby is hungry and in a mood for facial gestures and interaction. As you engage your baby face-to-face, open your mouth wide and say, "Open mouth!" Once your baby opens the door, put the food in.

Use lip service. Try the "upper lip sweep." As you place a spoonful of solids in your baby's mouth, gently lift the spoon upward, allowing the upper lip to sweep off the food.

Dress for the occasion. As you and your baby are working out a feeding routine, expect a lot of the food to wind up in the laundry rather than in baby's tummy. While some of our babies were neat eaters, others were total-body feeders. With these messy eaters, we found it easier to simply undress them for a meal and hose them off afterward. Don't forget the bib. Best bibs are large ones with an easy-to-clean surface and a bottom pocket to catch the spills. One of our babies equated eating with body painting. To keep him clean, we clad him in a total-body bib, a long-sleeved gown-type nylon bib that rinsed and dried quickly.

Try gadgets from the baby store. If baby keeps pushing her plate or tray off the high chair, find a way to attach it more firmly. Look for baby bowls and plates with suction-cup bottoms. If she keeps batting at the food with her hands, put toys with suction cups on the high-chair tray to occupy baby's hands while you sneak in the solid food. If baby grabs the spoon in your hand, give her one (or two) to hold on her own, so you get to keep yours.

Rotate the menu. Babies become bored with foods just as they do with toys. If your baby refuses a previous favorite, put more variety in what you serve and the way in which you serve it.

Avoid food fights. Your baby will not go hungry if he misses a day of solids or is simply not ready. If your child fights feedings, take that as a signal to change the food and/or the method. Sometimes you may just have to skip solid foods for a day or two and then try again.

FEEDING THE SEVEN- TO NINE-MONTH-OLD

As with other developmental skills, babies' feeding skills and food preferences go through stages, and other areas of development influence how babies accept their food. First came the introducing solids stage, when parents' main goal was to get baby through the transition from liquids to solids and from sucking to mouthing and chewing. During this stage, baby got used to mouthing and swallowing different tastes and textures. Many beginning eaters just dabble in solid foods, taking only a couple of spoonfuls of a few select solids.

Feeding should match baby's developmental stage. From seven to nine months, babies develop the following skills that make mealtimes more interesting:

- They begin to pick up objects with the thumb and forefinger.
- They develop a fascination with tiny objects, such as morsels of food.
- They want to "do it myself."

You can capitalize on a baby's developing fine-motor abilities and growing curiosity by adding

---

NUTRITIP
Substitute Feedings

For mothers who are away from their babies while working, it often helps to have the substitute caregiver do the solid-food feeding so that mom can concentrate on breastfeeding when she returns. Baby can fill up on solids during the day but will want to nurse more in the evening. This helps keep up mother's milk supply and simplifies busy mealtimes.

NUTRITIP
Pasta Picking

Place a pile of spaghetti or a few pasta squares or shells on baby's tray and sit back and enjoy the show. To minimize problems with allergies, begin with rice pasta before introducing wheat. Wait till around one year of age to add tomato sauce, as tomatoes are one of the more common allergens.

---

new tastes and textures to baby's diet that give him an outlet for these skills. By nine months, it's time for finger foods. Try these:

- cooked carrots tidbits
- rice cake pieces
- O-shaped cereals
- pasta/spaghetti pieces (see box, above)
- mashed potatoes
- teething biscuits
- tofu cubes
- avocado wedges
- peas
- egg yolk crumbles
- more cereals: barley, oatmeal
- cubes of cheese (1/4-inch)
- cubes of cooked fruit (1/4-inch)

Baby's growing ability to pick things up and put them in her mouth also means parents need to be more vigilant about foods that can cause choking. As a precaution, emphasize melt-in-the-mouth finger foods, such as rice cakes, pasta, pear, and cooked carrots. Stay away from crunchy, raw fruits and vegetables. Raw carrots, nuts, and seeds can wait until your child is at least three years old.

FEEDING THE NINE- TO TWELVE-MONTH-OLD

By baby's first birthday, solid foods can make up around 50 percent of baby's nutrition. Try to continue to feed most solid foods to your baby by spoon, since you are likely to get more food into baby's mouth than on the floor. If your baby is the "do it myself" type, though, finger foods may be the main fare by this time.

Here are some tips gleaned from the Sears family feeding experiences, as well as shared by patients in our pediatrics practice.

Keep feeding times short. Remember, babies have tiny tummies. Small helpings and frequent feedings are still the best. Many babies seldom take more than 1 or 2 tablespoons of a food at any one meal. Don't overwhelm baby with a whole pile of food on her plate. Begin with a small dollop and add more as baby wants more.

Give your baby a bone. Our babies have enjoyed a chicken leg bone with all the tiny bone slivers removed and a small amount of cooked meat remaining. Beginning around nine months, babies love to hold this bone like a rattle, gnaw on it, bang it, transfer it from hand to hand, teethe on it, and play with it. They even, occasionally, eat a little chicken.

Pressure tactics make feeding harder, not easier. Never force-feed a child, as this can create long-term unhealthy attitudes about eating. The parent's role is to select the nutritious food, prepare it well, and serve it creatively, matched to baby's individual capabilities and preferences. Baby's role is to eat the amount he wants at the time, according to his needs, moods, capabilities, and preferences. We have taught all of our children to swim, and we think of feeding our children as similar to teaching them to swim — we are neither overprotective nor overrestrictive. Allow a child to explore and experiment. Allow a certain amount of mess, but not when it gets out of control. Above all, teach your child that food is to be enjoyed.

Expect erratic feeding habits. There may be days when your baby eats solids six times, or she may refuse solids three days in a row and only want to breastfeed or take a bottle.

Understand that food fears are normal. To help your baby overcome these fears, you eat a bit of an unfamiliar food first and let your baby catch the spirit of your enjoyment. Expect baby to explore a new food before she eats it (just like adults want

---

NUTRIMYTH

Putting cereal in baby's bottle will help her sleep longer. Adding cereal to a bottle of formula to get baby to sleep through the night or space feedings further apart is an old strategy that seldom works and is generally not recommended by pediatricians with a respect for good nutrition. Adding cereal to baby's formula bottle usually requires significantly enlarging the nipple hole. Suddenly having to deal with a thicker, fast-flowing substance may confuse baby at a time when you are trying to teach her the difference between swallowing liquid and swallowing solids. Thickening formula with cereal is recommended only for babies who have regurgitation problems, such as gastroesophageal reflux, and only if advised by your baby's doctor.

to know what they're eating). One way to encourage the cautious feeder is to take a bite of the new food yourself and then place some food on his index finger and guide his own fingerful of food into his mouth.

Gradually increase variety and texture. For the youngest eaters, fruits and vegetables should be strained. (If you wait until six months to start solids, you'll probably skip this stage.) As babies gain eating experience, they can advance to pureed foods, then foods that are finely minced. Most babies can begin to accept chopped foods by one year of age.

Settle the squirmer. Here is a toy trick that worked for one of our babies who would constantly windmill her arms during feeding. Use three plastic spoons — one spoon for each of her hands to occupy them and one for you to feed her. Also, try this toy trick. Put toys with suction cups on a high-chair tray so baby can play with them with her hands while you sneak food into her mouth. Sometimes when babies open their mouths to suck on toys, this primes them to open their mouths to receive food.

Use camouflage. Cover more nutritious but less favorite foods with one of baby's favorites. Try dabbing a thin layer of applesauce (or other favorite) over the vegetables or meat. Baby gets the applesauce on his tongue first and then gets a scoop of the more nutritious but less liked food on top of it. If he still hates it, lay off.

Let baby eat off your plate. Sometimes babies just don't want to eat like a baby; they reject both baby food and baby plates. Around one year of age, babies enjoy sitting on parents' laps and picking food off their plate, especially mashed potatoes and cooked soft vegetables. Try putting baby's food on your plate and trick the little gourmet into eating his own food.

Let baby enjoy the lap of luxury. If your child refuses to get in or stay in his high chair, let him sit on your lap and eat off your plate. If baby begins messing with your food, place a few morsels of food on the table between baby and your plate to direct his attention away from your dinner.

Overcome lip lock. To relax tight lips from refusing a feeding, back off and overenjoy the food yourself. Model the excitement by replaying the old reliable "Mmmmm, good!" As your baby watches you open your mouth and savor the food, he may catch the spirit and relax his mouth and his attitude. And, use one of your child's favorite foods as a teaser. As he opens his mouth for his favorite, quickly follow with the food you wanted him to try.

Minimize the mess. Too much food on a baby's dish leads to two-fisted eating and major mess making. Encourage neatness by scattering only a few morsels of finger foods on baby's tray at one time and refill as necessary.

Each new developmental skill has its nutritional benefits and humorous nuisances. Baby's newly developing thumb-and-forefinger grasp stimulates him to want to pick up tiny morsels of food and feed himself, but it also creates an opportunity for more messes. Allow baby the luxury of messing around a bit with his newly discovered utensils. Believe it or not, baby is actually learning from this mess. While some food makes its way into the mouth, other pieces scatter. Food flinging, dropping, and smearing are usual mealtime antics parents can expect to deal with. To discourage flinging and give more of the food a fighting chance to make it into baby's mouth, put on baby's plate *a few* pieces of O-cereals, cooked carrots, pieces of rice cakes, and any other bite-sized pieces of fruits and vegetables that baby likes. Then refill as needed. Placing a whole pile of food in front of baby is inviting a mess. We noticed that our babies were fascinated with pieces of cooked spaghetti placed within easy reach. The ability to pick up with thumb and forefinger enables baby to pick up one strand at a time. Spaghetti-picking holds baby's mealtime attention longer than most foods.

Picking up, banging, dropping, and flinging are all part of baby's natural desire to explore. Teaching your baby manners is also important. Show him how to be a polite explorer.

CUP FEEDING

You can save yourself a lot of spills by not being in a hurry to introduce the cup. Most babies can't master drinking from a cup independently until around one year of age. Expect a lot of liquid to dribble out the sides of baby's mouth until she learns to form a tight seal between lip and cup. Try these cup strategies:

- Wait till baby is able to sit up and hold an object with both hands before trying cup feedings.

- Use a trainer cup that has two easy-to-grasp handles, a tight lid with a small spout, and a weighted bottom on a wide base to prevent tipping.

- Market the cup first as a toy rather than a feeding utensil. Place an empty cup within grabbing distance of baby. As you drink from your cup, baby is likely to try to drink from hers.

- The less you put in the cup, the less mess there will be to wipe up when it all spills. Begin by filling the cup only a quarter full and increase the amount as baby's cup skills mature.

> ### NUTRITIP
> #### Tricking Tiny Taste Buds
>
> As the figure on page 101 shows, the taste buds for sweet flavors are found toward the tip of the tongue; the taste buds for salt are on the sides of the tongue; the taste buds for bitter are at the back of the tongue. In the middle of the tongue, the taste buds are more neutral. So it would be wise to place a new sweet food on the tip of the tongue, but a new less sweet food on the neutral area in the middle in order to give the food a fighting chance of going into baby instead of coming back out. Veggies, for example, have a better chance of being willingly swallowed if placed on the middle of the tongue rather than on the tip of the tongue, except perhaps for sweet ones, like sweet potatoes.

- Offer water, diluted juice, or infant formula in the cup. Water is a good training cup beverage, since it doesn't leave a sticky mess.

SELF-FEEDING

Around one year of age babies enter the "do it myself" stage and may want to feed themselves with a spoon. Most parents find it much easier to feed a baby themselves than to let baby take over the job with her own utensils. Compromise is needed here. A trick we have used with the determined self-feeder is to do the job together. The parent holds the spoonful of food and when baby grabs the spoon, mom or dad continues to hold on and helps baby guide the spoon into her mouth. Take advantage of baby's desire to mimic you at this stage. When he sees you using a spoon properly, baby is more likely to want to copy you.

Now is the time to offer baby thicker food that will stick to the spoon and have a better chance of making it into baby's mouth. Spearing is also fun at this age. Give baby a safe child's fork with sturdy, blunt tines and a few cubes of fruit (melon is a terrific target). After a bit of target practice, the little hunter will actually get most of his catch into his mouth. Now that your baby has acquired a taste for new foods and developed new feeding skills, both of you are ready to move on to the challenge of toddler feeding.

Feeding Toddlers: Seventeen Tips for Pleasing the Picky Eater

WHEN OUR FIRST few children were toddlers, we dreaded mealtime. Martha would prepare all kinds of sensible meals composed of what she thought were healthy, appealing foods. Most of these offerings would end up piled up on a high-chair tray or handed to the dog. To make matters worse, she took our kids' "rejection" of her cuisine very personally, sure that this was a sign of some parental lapse on her part. What was wrong? Why were these kids such picky eaters?

We didn't get it. We didn't understand that being a picky eater is part of what it means to be a toddler. We have since learned that there are developmental reasons why kids between one and three years of age pick and poke at their food.

After a year of rapid growth (the average one-year-old has tripled her birth weight), toddlers gain weight more slowly. So, of course, they need less food. The fact that these little ones are always on the go also affects their eating patterns. They don't sit still for anything, even food. Snacking their way through the day is more compatible with these busy explorers' lifestyle than sitting down to a full-fledged feast.

Learning this helped us relax. We now realize that our job is simply to buy the right food, prepare it nutritiously (e.g., steamed rather than boiled, baked rather than fried), and serve it creatively. We leave the rest up to the kids. How much they eat, when they eat, and if they eat is mostly their responsibility; we've learned to take neither the credit nor the blame.

Toddlers like to binge on one food at a time. They may eat only fruits one day and vegetables the next. Since erratic eating habits are as normal as toddler mood swings, expect your child to eat well one day and eat practically nothing the next. Toddlers from one to three years need between 1,000 and 1,300 calories a day, but they may not eat this amount every day. Aim for a nutritionally balanced week, not a balanced day.

All this is not to say that parents shouldn't encourage their toddlers to eat well and develop healthy food habits. Based on our hands-on experience with eight children, we've developed seventeen tactics to tempt little taste buds and minimize mealtime hassles.

1. Offer a nibble tray. Toddlers like to graze their way through a variety of foods, so why not offer them a customized smorgasbord? The first tip from the Sears kitchen is to offer toddlers a nibble tray. Use an ice-cube tray, a muffin tin, or a compartmentalized dish, and put bite-sized portions of colorful and nutritious foods in each section. Call these finger foods playful names that a two-year-old can appreciate, such as:

FEEDING AS THEY GROW			
4–7 months			
breast milk/formula	bananas	rice cereal	sweet potatoes
7–9 months			
breast milk/formula	mashed potatoes	avocados	peaches
carrots	pears	teething biscuits	prunes
squash	applesauce	barley cereal	
9–12 months			
breast milk/formula	tofu	pasta, non-wheat first	lamb
papaya	cheese	rice cakes	veal
peas	yogurt	egg yolk	poultry
refried beans	oatmeal	ripe apricot	
12–18 months			
breast milk/ whole cow's milk	fish: tuna, salmon	steamed spinach	blueberries
cottage cheese	peanut butter	steamed broccoli	oranges
frozen yogurt	bread, bagels	wheat cereals	strawberries (organic)
whole egg	melon	cherries	grape halves
healthy cookies	mango	apple slices	honey
	kiwi	whole-grain crackers	dips: avocados, yogurt

- apple moons (thinly sliced)
- avocado boats (a quarter of an avocado)
- banana wheels
- broccoli trees (steamed broccoli florets)
- carrot swords (cooked and thinly sliced)
- cheese building blocks
- egg canoes (hard-boiled egg wedges)
- little O's (O-shaped cereal)

Place the food on an easy-to-reach table. As your toddler makes his rounds through the house, he can stop, sit down, nibble a bit, and, when he is done, continue on his way. Expect an empty tray by the end of the day.

2. Dip it. Reserve two compartments in the nibble tray for dips. Young children think that immersing foods in a tasty dip is pure fun (and delightfully messy). Here are some possibilities to dip into:

- cottage cheese or tofu dip
- cream cheese, thinned with juice or milk
- fruit juice–sweetened preserves, thinned
- guacamole (without the strong spices)
- healthy salad dressing/ketchup
- pureed fruits or vegetables, refried bean dip
- yogurt, plain or sweetened with juice concentrate

These dips serve equally well as spreads on apple or pear slices, bell-pepper strips, rice cakes, bagels, toast, or other nutritious platforms.

3. Spread it. Toddlers like spreading, or, more accurately, smearing. Show them how to use a

FOODS BABIES CAN CHOKE ON

To minimize the risks of a baby or toddler choking, follow these safe feeding tips:

- Be careful of big globs of food, such as golf ball–sized, pasty globs of white bread or spoonfuls of peanut butter. Even though these foods are soft, babies can choke on them. Don't spread peanut butter too thick, and monitor how quickly the bread gets packed into the mouth. The more whole grains in a bread, the less likely it is to form a pasty glob.
- Check the chunks. Once baby's molars appear (usually around the middle of the second year), chunky soft fruits (e.g., size and texture of fruit cocktail) are safe.
- Allow toddlers finger foods under supervision only. Be sure toddlers stay seated as they eat and are not lying down or running around. Choose snacks for the backseat of the car carefully, or don't eat in the car.
- Hold the hot dogs. Since hot dogs are neither nutritious nor safe for baby, you can scratch them from the diet. If you are fortunate enough to find a healthy hot dog (nitrite free, low in salt) or veggie dog, slice it lengthwise in thin, noodle-like strips. Don't let your toddler bite chunks off a hot dog, since a hot dog chunk is about the size of a baby's windpipe.
- Avoid whole raw vegetables and fruits that snap into hard chunks, such as carrots and celery stalks and firm apples. Use thin sticks or slices or grate the food.
- Peel and slice grapes. Whole grapes can cause choking.

Chokable Foods

cherries with pits	whole grapes	raw apple
candy, hard	meat chunks	raw pears
hot dog, whole chunks	nuts	raw carrots
raisins in a glob	nut-butter globs	raw green beans
stringy foods	popcorn	whole olives

small blunt butter knife to spread cheese spread, peanut butter, and fruit concentrate onto crackers, toast, or rice cakes.

4. Top it. Toddlers are into toppings. Putting nutritious familiar favorites on top of new and less desirable foods is a way to broaden the finicky toddler's menu. Top toppings are yogurt, light cream cheese, melted cheese, guacamole, tomato sauce, applesauce, and peanut butter.

5. Drink it. If your youngster would rather drink than eat, don't despair. Make a smoothie — *together*. Milk or juice and fruit — along with supplements such as egg protein powder, wheat germ, yogurt, honey, and peanut butter — can be the basis of very healthy meals. So what if they are consumed through a straw? One note of caution: Avoid drinks with raw eggs or you'll risk salmonella poisoning.

6. Cut it up. How much a child will eat often depends on how you cut it. Cut sandwiches into four small squares. Or cut sandwiches, pancakes, waffles, and pizza into various shapes using a cookie cutter.

7. Package it. Appearance is important. For something new and different, why not use your

SHAPING YOUNG TASTES

The first three years of a child's life are a window of opportunity for forming lifelong healthy eating habits. Just as you teach proper behavior to a child, you also want to teach a child what good food is supposed to taste like. If baby begins solid food life from the can or jar, baby concludes that this is what food is supposed to taste like. The taste of this food and the way his body feels when he eats it become the child's norms. And, for better or worse, the child's eating habits and desire for packaged and fast foods become the norm. He is likely to crave this taste — because that's what his body has been used to — and shun the fresh taste of healthy foods.

To get your child on the right track, teach him to enjoy the flavor of fresh food before he gets hooked on canned, artificial tastes. If your baby and toddler eats only homemade, freshly prepared, unsalted, unsweetened foods, this becomes the standard to which other foods are compared. The canned and packaged stuff then tastes foreign to his selective taste buds. While babies are born with a natural preference for sweets (breast milk is very sweet), the rest of their taste preferences are learned.

Many kids ago we had a theory that if we exposed young taste buds and developing intestines *only* to healthy foods during the first three years, when the child was older, these healthy eating habits would be likely to continue and the child would have a greater chance of shunning junk foods. We have tested this theory with our own children, as have other parents in our pediatrics practice. For the first three years we gave our infants and toddlers only healthy foods. We made homemade baby food and used few jars, cans, or packaged foods. We shopped for farm-to-market-type produce. In essence, relative to their peers, our kids were really junk-food deprived.

What happened when these "pure" children got out into the sugar-coated, fat-filled world of birthday parties and fast-food outlets? Yes, they tried these foods. They ate french fries and licked icing from their fingers, *but they did not overdose on junk food.* That's the difference. Halfway through the mound of icing-filled birthday cake, they would slow down or stop. They certainly would not ask for a second helping as they began to recognize the signs of "yuck tummy." One day we watched them go through the line at a local salad bar restaurant. Like most kids, they bypassed the fresh greens in the adult salad bar and headed for the kiddie salad bar, filled with fatty, breaded chicken, artificially colored and heavily sugared cereal, and dye-colored gelatins. But after a few bites, much of the junk food remained on their plates and they gravitated back to the adult salad bar. Eventually, they bypassed the kiddie bar altogether. Our preschoolers Hayden and Peter proudly wore T-shirts displaying, "If you love me, don't feed me junk." Even children as young as three years old can make the connection between good food and feeling good. Health food–primed children seldom overindulge, and that's the best we can hope for in raising a healthy body — a child and an adult who avoid excesses. (See the related discussion "Pure Moms," page 306.)

"GROW FOOD" — FUN FOOD

Between three and four years of age, children can begin to comprehend which foods are the most nutritious and why. We would often say to our children, "Eat the food that makes you grow first and then you can have your fun food." "Grow foods" would be veggies, grains, fish, fruit, salads, and cereals. While wise parents make sure that "grow foods" can still be fun, the fun category can also include a little cake, ice cream, and apple pie. One of the moms in our pediatrics practice, a believer in "pure" eating, trained her child to eat almost all healthy food, to the extent that when a piece of junk food found its way into their home, the child saw this food as a foreign intruder. Since the mom, Kathy, called the healthy food "grow food," her son Matthew learned to think of it as "grow food" also. One day four-year-old Matthew found some white bread in their otherwise whole wheat home (a sandwich left by one of his friends). Matthew asked his mom why his friend ate white bread: "Doesn't she need to grow anymore?"

---

child's own toy plates for dishing out a snack? Our kids enjoy the unexpected and fanciful when it comes to serving dishes — anything from plastic measuring cups to ice-cream cones.

You can also try the scaled-down approach. Either serve pint-sized portions or, when they're available, buy munchkin-sized foodstuffs, such as mini bagels, mini quiches, chicken drumettes (the meat part of the wing), and tiny muffins.

8. Become a veggie vendor. I must have heard "Doctor, he won't eat his vegetables" a thousand times. This is a challenge, but don't give up. Vegetables require some creative marketing, as they seem to be the most contested food in households with young children. Although kids should be offered three to five servings of veggies a day, for children under five each serving need be only a tablespoon for each year of age. In other words, a two-year-old should ideally consume 2 tablespoons of vegetables three to five times a day. So if you aren't the proud parent of a veggie lover, try the following tricks:

- Plant a garden with your child. Let her help care for the plants, harvest the ripe vegetables, and wash and prepare them. She will probably be much more interested in eating what she has helped to grow.

- Slip grated or diced vegetables into favorite foods. Try adding them to rice, cottage cheese, cream cheese, guacamole, or even macaroni and cheese. Zucchini pancakes are a big hit at our house (see recipe, page 399).

- Cover the vegetables with a favorite sauce.

- Use vegetables as finger foods and dip them in a favorite sauce or dip.

- Using a small cookie cutter, cut bread into interesting shapes and make veggie sandwiches.

- Steam your greens. They are much more flavorful and usually sweeter than when raw.

- Make veggie art. Create colorful plate faces with olive-slice eyes, tomato ears, mushroom noses, bell-pepper mustaches, and any other playful features you can think of. Our eighth child, Lauren, loved to put an olive slice on the tip of each finger and nibble this nutritious and nutrient-dense food off her fingertips. Zucchini pancakes make a terrific head to which you can add pea eyes, carrot nose, shredded cheese hair, and a green bean smile.

IS YOUR CHILD EATING ENOUGH? HOW TO TELL

Most mothers and all grandmothers worry that children don't eat enough. While few infants and children pack in enough food to satisfy their parents, the more important question is whether your child is eating enough of the right kind of foods to meet his or her individual nutritional needs. It's not just the quantity of food that's important, it's the quality and whether or not your child has a balanced diet. Here's how to tell if the eating habits of your toddler and young child are supplying optimal nutrition:

Step 1: Check your child's growth pattern.
Using a growth chart, plot your child's height and weight. Ask your doctor for a copy of your infant's or child's growth records from past office visits. If your child is at the fiftieth percentile or higher in both height and weight, chances are she is getting enough calories, if not a balanced diet. Significant drops in the percentile ranking on the growth chart suggest there may be a problem with undernourishment. The percentile where your child now plots is not as informative as the *degree of change* from the percentiles in previous months. For example, if your child has consistently been around the fiftieth percentile in weight and then there is a gradual fall to a lower percentile, say the twenty-fifth percentile, over several months, take this as a clue that your child may be undernourished. Undernourishment shows up first in a slowing of weight gain. Tapering off in height reflects a more severe, prolonged nutritional deficiency. Remember, however, there are two normal reasons why a baby's weight can taper off on the growth chart: First, previously plump babies, when they begin burning more energy by crawling, walking, and running, will often taper

off in their weight gain and drop a bit on growth chart percentiles between nine months and two years. Second, children with ectomorph body builds (tall and lanky) will also normally show a drop in weight percentile while going up in height; they may wind up around the seventy-fifth percentile for height and the twenty-fifth percentile for weight. While growth charts are not infallible as indicators of optimal growth, at least they provide clues as to whether or not your child is getting proper nutrition.

Step 2: Examine your child for signs of nutritional deficiency. In consultation with your child's physician, do a head-to-toe examination of your child for signs of possible nutritional deficiency:*

- *Hair:* sparse, brittle, dry, and easily plucked
- *Skin:* pale, dry, flaky, wrinkled, and loosely attached to muscle, easily bruised in areas not usually exposed to falls; spiders (broken blood vessels in the skin), delayed healing of wounds
- *Eyes:* dull, dark circles underneath
- *Lips:* cracking and fissures at the corners of the mouth that are slow to heal, pale
- *Gums:* soft and bleeding
- *Teeth:* brittle with many cavities
- *Tongue:* pale and smooth
- *Nails:* brittle, thin, concave
- *Bones:* bowed legs, prominent ribs

Step 3: Do a nutritional analysis. The first two steps will give you an indication of whether your child has a moderate-to-severe nutritional deficiency, but they do not tell you if your child is getting optimal nutrition for optimal growth.

---

* Most of these signs indicate severe nutritional deficiencies of vitamins and minerals, as well as overall undernutrition. If a child is only slightly undernourished, you may see only a few or none of these signs.

IS YOUR CHILD EATING ENOUGH? HOW TO TELL (CONTINUED)

The only way you can be absolutely certain of that is to do a detailed nutritional analysis. Here's how:

- Record everything your child eats for a week. Because children have such erratic eating habits, a week-long record is more informative than a daily one. Record the type of food, the brand, and the amount eaten (e.g., ounces, cups, tablespoons, pieces).
- Next set up an appointment with a nutritionist who is knowledgeable and equipped to do nutritional analyses. The nutritionist will take your food record and, using a computer program, analyze the nutrient content of what your child has eaten and print out the child's daily average intake of calories, proteins, carbohydrates, fats, vitamins, minerals, and fiber. The nutritionist will then compare these values with the recommended dietary allowance or optimal values for your child's age. If deficiencies are identified, you and the nutritionist will work out a plan to remedy the problems. This will include changes in the child's diet and possibly some supplements to make up for any vitamin and mineral deficiencies.

This is a time-consuming process for you and the nutritionist. (It can be expensive, too, though some health-insurance plans cover the cost.) But in my own pediatrics practice, where

I've struggled with finding an accurate way of determining if a child is getting enough to eat, I have found that the nutritional analysis is the only way to get the answers that parents want and the child deserves. Of course, the nutritional analysis is only as accurate as the data you put into it. Be a keen observer and an accurate recorder.

You may be surprised at the results of your child's weekly nutritional analysis. When I do these in my pediatrics practice, parents often exclaim, "I didn't know he was eating that much junk," or "I felt sure he was getting enough protein," or "I really was being careful about how much sugar she ate. I didn't realize how many foods contained so much sugar."

If you want to bypass the nutritionist and the computer program, you can do a nutritional analysis on your own (and learn a lot about nutrition in general). Here is the resource you will need: *Bowes and Church's Food Values of Portions Commonly Used,* 17th ed., by Jean A. T. Pennington (Lippincott, 1998). Using this reference and a calculator, you can add up the nutrients in all the foods your child has eaten in a week and compare the daily averages with the RDA's. This will probably take you a couple of days and a lot of paper. Putting the same data into a nutritional-analysis computer program will produce results within a couple of hours.

- Concoct creative camouflages. There are all kinds of possible variations on the old standby "cheese in the trees" (cheese melted on steamed broccoli florets). Try, for example, veggies topped with peanut-butter sauce, a specialty of several Asian cuisines.

9. Share it. If your child is going through a picky-eater stage, invite over a same-age or slightly

older friend who you know likes to eat. Your child will catch on. Group feeding lets the other kids set examples.

10. Respect tiny tummies. Keep food servings small. Wondering how much to offer? Here's a rule of thumb — or, rather, of hand. A young child's stomach is approximately the size of his fist. So dole out small portions at first and refill

---

NUTRITIP
Stretching Nutritional Truths

By two years of age many children have learned to regard certain foods as treats. Sometimes it helps to call more nutritious but less favorite foods by "treat" names, such as calling fish "chicken." Crackers are "cookies," and low-fat frozen yogurt is "ice cream."

---

the plate when your child asks for more. This less-is-more meal plan is not only more successful with picky eaters, but it also has the added benefit of stabilizing blood-sugar levels, which in turn minimizes mood swings. As most parents know, a hungry kid is generally not a happy kid.

Use what we call the "bite rule" to encourage the reluctant eater: "Take one bite, two bites . . ." (however far you think you can push it without force-feeding). The bite rule at least gets your child to taste a new food, while giving her some control over the feeding. As much as you possibly can, let your child — and his appetite — set the pace for these meals. But if you want your child to eat dinner at the same time you do, try to time his snack-meals so that they are at least two hours before dinner.

11. Make it accessible. Give your toddler shelf space. Reserve a low shelf in the refrigerator for a variety of your toddler's favorite (nutritious) foods and drinks. Whenever she wants a snack, open the door for her and let her choose one. This tactic also enables children to eat when *they* are hungry, an important step in acquiring a healthy attitude about food.

12. Use sit-still strategies. One reason that toddlers don't like to sit still at the family table is that their feet dangle. (Try sitting on a stool while eating — you'll naturally begin to squirm and want to get up and move around.) Children are likely to sit and eat longer at a child-sized table in a chair in which their feet touch the floor. When they are eating at the family table, place a small stool under their feet.

13. Turn meals upside down. The distinctions between breakfast, lunch, and dinner have little meaning to a child. If your youngster insists on eating pizza in the morning and fruit and cereal in the evening, go with it — it's better than her not eating at all. This is not to say that you should become a short-order cook, filling lots of special requests. But why not let your toddler set the menu sometimes? Other family members will probably enjoy the novelty of waffles and hash browns for dinner.

14. Let them cook. Children are more likely to eat their own creations, so, whenever appropriate, let your child help prepare the food. Let your child use cookie cutters to create edible designs out of foods like cheese, bread, thin meat slices, or cooked lasagne noodles. Or, give your assistant such jobs as tearing and washing lettuce, scrubbing potatoes, or stirring batter. Put pancake batter in a squeeze bottle and let your child supervise as you squeeze the batter onto the hot griddle in fun shapes, such as hearts, numbers, letters, or even your child's name.

15. Make every calorie count. Offer your child foods that pack lots of nutrition in small doses. This is particularly important for toddlers who are often as active as rabbits but who seem to eat like mice.

Nutrient-dense foods that most children are willing to eat include these:

- avocados
- broccoli
- brown rice and other whole grains
- cheese
- eggs

NUTRITIP
Filler Food

We found a classic collection of junk food at the kids' salad bar at a popular family-restaurant chain. The selection was obviously put together by marketing types with zero nutritional knowledge or no regard for the health of children. Nearly every food was in the junk-food category, and many were on our "worst foods" list, including colored O-cereals, red dye–filled gelatins, and other nutritionally unmentionable items. Don't give this cheap stuff to your baby or toddler. It's filler, not food.

- fish
- kidney beans
- yogurt
- pasta
- peanut butter
- potatoes
- poultry
- squash
- sweet potatoes
- tofu

16. Count on inconsistency. For young children, what and how much they are willing to eat may vary daily. This capriciousness is due in large part to their ambivalence about independence, and eating is an area where they can act out this confusion. So don't be surprised if your child eats a heaping plateful of food one day and practically nothing the next, adores broccoli on Tuesday and refuses it on Thursday, wants to feed herself at one meal and be totally catered to at another. As a parent in our practice said, "The only thing consis-

tent about toddler feeding is inconsistency." Try to simply roll with these mood swings, and don't take them personally.

17. Relax. Sometime between her second and third birthday, you can expect your child to become very set in her ideas on just about everything — including the way food is prepared. Expect food fixations. If the peanut butter must be on top of the jelly and you put the jelly on top of the peanut butter, be prepared for a protest. It's not easy to reason with an opinionated two-year-old. It's better to learn to make the sandwich the child's way. Don't interpret this as being stubborn. Toddlers have a mind-set about the order of things in their world, and any alternative is unacceptable. This is a passing stage.

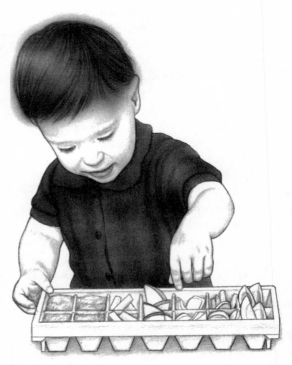

Toddler Nibble Tray

30

The ABC's of Teaching Nutrition to Your Kids

DO YOU HAVE MEMORIES of your parents trying to get you to eat nutritious food as a child? I do! My mother's lecture about the starving children in the world who would be happy to have my food didn't do much to motivate me. In fact, I offered to pack it up and share it with those poor children! Maybe your first nutrition lesson was watching Popeye gulp down a can of spinach and then flex his iron biceps. How effective was that in getting you to eat more vegetables? How do we as parents get our children to choose healthy foods?

The best kind of learning happens in a positive atmosphere, often as part of everyday life, and it's reinforced in different situations. Don't relegate nutrition learning to a dinnertime lecture about the virtues of vegetables. Make it a part of your family's lifestyle.

Here are twenty-six A to Z artistic, interactive, musical, problem-solving, and even tasty ways to get the "good nutrition" message across to your children. Some of these are fun activities (you don't have to tell the kids they're also educational). Some can be easily incorporated into your family's lifestyle. Choose the ones that work for you, that you and your children enjoy, and give your children a head start on a lifetime of healthy, happy eating.

A IS FOR ACCESSIBILITY

> **NUTRITIP**
> *You* control the food that comes into the house. Make sure the good food you want your children to appreciate is child accessible.

The saying "caught, not taught" certainly applies to teaching nutrition to kids. More powerful than any amount of talking about nutrition is the example you set in your home. Give new meaning to "fast foods." Make the best foods for your children readily available. Plan to have fresh foods that are good for them within easy reach, so that when they're hungry and foraging for something to eat, it's easy for them to help themselves! If you want to control the serving sizes, consider prepackaging healthy snacks in plastic sandwich bags. Here are some ideas for accessible snacks.

- a raw-vegetable tray kept in the refrigerator at children's eye level (see "Nibble Tray," page 274)
- a tempting assortment of fresh fruits washed and ready to eat in a fruit bowl — or cut up in bite-sized pieces in the refrigerator, ready to eat

- a special place in your cupboard or pantry for "kids' snack attacks." It may include popcorn, whole-grain crackers, bread sticks, rice cakes, and raisins
- a premixed snack that includes a variety of cereal pieces, pretzels, and dried fruit

A IS ALSO FOR AMBIANCE

NUTRITIP
Create a positive environment for eating at the breakfast, lunch, and dinner table!

Create a pleasant, supportive, and unhurried environment in which your children can enjoy healthy foods. Meal and snack times should be happy times. If there is enjoyable, light conversation and relaxing background music playing, it is more likely that appetites and dispositions will be good. To lighten moods and facilitate pleasant conversation, ask each family member to share one positive thing that happened that day. Appetites are likely to be poor if parents are impatient with children's behavior, if mealtime is a platform for discipline or criticism, or if the TV is on. So create the mood — and set your kids up to enjoy their mealtimes. And, by all means, enlist their help!

- Pick kid-friendly ethnic meal themes, such as Mexican or Italian.
- Make special place cards or table decorations.
- Pick some flowers from the garden (or purchase at the florist or grocery store) for the dinner table or light candles.
- Use special dishes — paper plates for a picnic atmosphere, the best china for mom's birthday. When you involve your children in the meal planning and give them choices, they are more likely to have a good attitude toward eating and to eat the foods that are best for them.

B IS FOR BOOKS

NUTRITIP
Read picture books about nutrition and then discuss them.

Choose books at the library or bookstore that weave a message about good nutrition or adventuresome eating into the story line. Discuss what you read. Ask questions along the way. Did the characters learn to eat the food that was good for them? What foods are good for you? Try these favorites:

Bread and Jam for Frances, by Russell Hoban (HarperCollins, 1993)
Bread Is for Eating, by David and Phillis Gershator (Holt, 1995)
Green Eggs and Ham, by Dr. Seuss (Random House, 1960)
Picky Nicky, by Cathy East and Mark Dubowski (Grosset & Dunlap, 1996)
The Berenstain Bears and Too Much Junk Food, by Stan and Jan Berenstain (Turtleback, 1985)
The Carrot Seed, by Ruth Krauss (HarperTrophy, 1989)
The Very Hungry Caterpillar, by Eric Carle (Philomel, 1994)
What Happens to Your Food? by Alastair Smith (EDC Publications, 1997)
D. W. the Picky Eater, by Marc Brown (Little, Brown, 1995)

A useful and fun workbook for kids aged six to ten is *How to Teach Nutrition to Kids,* by Connie L. Evers (24 Carrot Press, 1995).

C IS FOR COPYCAT!

> ## NUTRITIP
> You are your child's first nutrition teacher. Would you want your kids to copy your eating habits?

Kids will copy your food habits. Do you eat nutritious foods? Set an example by being a good role model. If children see their parents enjoying nutritious food, they are more likely to do so, too, as children and as adults. Kids will pick up on your habits at an early age. If what you do does not mirror what you say, you will likely hear little voices asking, "Mommy, why are you eating that when you said I couldn't have it?" If a family member such as grandma or uncle is on a special diet for health reasons, talk with your children about why this person eats certain foods and not others, and how the diet helps this special someone stay healthy. Model the positive value of good nutrition, and children will eventually begin to see that consistent daily choices translate into health and happiness.

Don't expect your child to like a food just because you do. Use a small helping of peer pressure to get your child to eat. If your child is going through a food-refusal stage, invite over peers with adventuresome palates, kids who like to eat new and wholesome foods. Monkey does what monkey sees.

D IS FOR DISCOVERY ON A FIELD TRIP

> ## NUTRITIP
> Make learning nutrition fun by packing up the kids and discovering good food on a field trip!

There are many places to learn about good food right in your own community. Try one of these ideas when you need to get out of the house:

- Visit a grocery store and have your child help pick out produce and other items on your grocery list. Talk about the nutritious and not so nutritious foods you see. (Hints: Feed your child and yourself before you go! Also, lay out some ground rules so that your child knows what to expect, such as the need to stay by the cart, what snacks are acceptable, and no begging for toys or candy.)

- Take a behind-the-scenes tour of a grocery store. Many stores will arrange a tour for children of the different areas of the store, including delivery docks, meat counter, bakery, and produce department.

- Visit an orchard or farm where fruits and/or vegetables are grown. Perhaps the children can pick fresh strawberries or apples. They'll have fun eating the fruit they pick.

- Visit a nursery and look at the different fruit trees and vegetable plants.

- If you're planning a garden, let your children choose the plants or seeds (once you've decided on what is appropriate given your climate and soil conditions).

- Visit a farmer's market. Many cities have scheduled times when local farmers come to town to sell their produce, plants, and flowers. Ask the farmers questions about what they're selling, such as, How long did it take to grow? When was this fruit or vegetable picked? What's a good way to cook and eat it?

- Visit an animal farm or zoo. Milking and feeding time can be particularly educational. Have the guide explain what the animals eat and why.

- Visit a bakery or food-processing plant and observe how bread is made or other foods are produced.

- Visit a restaurant or food establishment to view cooking and food preparation. Watch how pretzels are formed, how pies are made, how pasta is cooked, how omelets or waffles are prepared, how pizza is put together.

- Visit a museum with exhibits on nutrition and health. Children's museums especially may have "hands-on" exhibits about food.

E IS FOR EDIBLE ART

NUTRITIP
Children love to create. Make some edible art! They can learn about nutrition bite by bite.

Cereal necklace. String O-shaped cereal and dried apples (with holes through the pieces) on a piece of string or dental floss. Have fun wearing it, then snacking on it!

Cottage-cheese cone. Fill an ice-cream cone about two-thirds full with a scoop of cottage cheese or chicken or tuna salad. Have the child add toppings: finely grated carrots or zucchini, chopped cucumber, or chopped olives. Top it all with a halved cherry tomato.

Breakfast banana split. Cut a banana in half lengthwise and place it in an ice-cream bowl (a "banana split" bowl is ideal). Place two scoops of cooked, cooled oatmeal, made on the thick side, in the middle of the bowl. Drizzle lightly with fruit-only jam or apple butter. Add a dollop of yogurt to each scoop. Garnish with fresh strawberries or cherries, and top with chopped nuts or granola.

Pretty pizzas. Use pita bread or English muffins sliced in half. Spread on the tomato sauce, then make a face or design with cheese triangles, sliced olives, strips of bell peppers, sliced deli meats. Heat in the oven until the cheese starts to melt.

Pancake faces. Decorate pancakes using banana slices for the eyes (with a raisin pupil), raisins for the nose, a thin sliver of cantaloupe for the mouth, yogurt for a beard, avocado slices for eyebrows.

Fruit caterpillars. Cut up an assortment of fresh fruits (apples, strawberries, grapes, bananas, oranges). Have children skewer a mixed assortment on shish kebab sticks. Serve with vanilla yogurt for the dip.

Cup faces. Put some plain or vanilla yogurt in a plastic cup. Decorate with coconut cut into small pieces for the hair, raisins for the mouth and eyes, and a strawberry for the nose.

Pepper pots. Kids enjoy stuffing peppers. Cut the top off small red, green, or yellow bell peppers and scoop out the insides. Have your child mix together some cooked rice, beans, corn, and chopped spinach, then spoon it into the peppers and sprinkle with grated cheese and seasoned bread crumbs. Bake peppers in the oven for 15 minutes at 350 degrees.

Sandwich characters. Cut out sandwiches with cookie cutters. Then decorate them with vegetables, such as olive pieces for eyes, carrot curls for a smile, and a cherry tomato nose.

Cute cookies. Make whole wheat oatmeal cookies with half the amount of honey instead of sugar and have your child decorate them with sprinkles or raisins.

F IS FOR FEEDBACK

NUTRITIP
Children generally seek to please their parents. Dole out praise for making wise food choices and experimenting with new taste sensations.

Positive reinforcement is a very effective technique for modifying behavior. Acknowledging good eating behavior with positive feedback will produce lasting positive effects. Praise your child for making good food choices and trying new foods, and resist the temptation to nag or scold about poor choices. Avoid praising your child for cleaning his plate or for how much he eats, since linking approval with overeating can lead to obesity. You can also use a reward system with a sticker chart. If your child eats at least five vegetables and fruits each day, put a sticker on a chart on the refrigerator.

Here are some ways you can acknowledge good eating behavior:

- "I like the way you chose that piece of fruit."
- "I'm so proud that you're learning to make good food choices to help you grow strong and be smart!"

- "Wow! I see all the food groups on your plate!"
- "Yummy! Those vegetables and fruits are my favorites, too! And they are all foods that will help you grow!"
- "You're such a super helper in the kitchen. We'll be able to eat dinner much sooner since you helped."

G IS FOR "GROW FOODS"

NUTRITIP
Let the Food Guide Wheel give your kids a visual description of what they should be eating so they can grow! Teach them about "grow" and "non-grow" foods.

No longer are there just the four food groups you learned about in health class long ago. Now there is a Food Guide Pyramid with five food groups, designed to illustrate the ideal composition of a daily diet, with a new emphasis on foods from plant sources. The Food Guide Pyramid or the Food Guide Wheel makes it easier to teach children about which foods are best for the family. (See the "Food Guide Wheel," page 114.)

- Help your children make a "Grow Foods" chart for your kitchen. Draw pictures or cut them out of magazines and glue them under "Grow" and "Non-Grow" categories on a piece of poster board.

- Use another piece of poster board to make your own Food Guide Pyramid. Fill it with pictures of "grow foods" in each category.

- When dining out and ordering from the menu, ask your kids to pick out "grow" versus "non-grow" foods. Talk about the "grow" and "non-grow" foods you eat at home. Name a "non-grow" food and ask your child to name a "grow" alternative.

- Make up a song about "grow" and "non-grow" foods. (For another "G" activity, see "Grazing," page 305.)

H IS FOR HAPPY BREAKFAST

> ### NUTRITIP
> A nutritious breakfast has been proven to improve behavior and learning in schoolchildren. Happy breakfast!

Missing breakfast leads to a sad state of affairs. In the morning, the blood sugar is low after a night-long fast. This translates into sluggishness, fatigue, and a low energy state. The body therefore tries to conserve energy — including brain energy! Research shows that children who skip breakfast do not do as well on tests and don't perform other tasks as well as those who eat breakfast. Problem-solving capabilities are affected also, and a child who doesn't eat breakfast may become cranky and out of control by mid-morning.

Here are some basic guidelines to set your children up for a happier day, one that starts with breakfast:

- Get up early enough to have a relaxed atmosphere at breakfast.

- Be prepared to sell your children on the benefits of breakfast: "It will help you grow, learn, and feel better all morning long."

- Choose breakfasts that provide sustained energy as well as quick energy. The best breakfasts contain protein plus complex carbohydrates. Include a food high in protein (e.g., eggs, cottage cheese), bread or cereal, a fruit or vegetable, a small amount of fat, and milk or yogurt. (For nutritious breakfast suggestions, see page 310.)

- If there isn't enough time for a leisurely breakfast, prepare a fast one-dish breakfast that is easy to eat on the run, such as a smoothie made with low-fat yogurt or milk and fresh fruit (see "School-Ade," page 309). Or mix cottage cheese and fruit (e.g., mandarin oranges from a can) and use it as a spread on mini bagels.

- Start a Happy Breakfast Club. Provide an incentive for eating breakfast. After a week or a month, reward breakfast eaters with a pass to a "breakfast club" on the weekend. Take the child to a local restaurant that specializes in buffet breakfasts and pick out "grow foods" from the wide selection. Some restaurants have clubs you can join where you can earn a free meal after you eat there a number of times.

(For more breakfast information, see Chapter 31, "Feeding the Brain.")

I IS FOR INTRODUCING NEW FOODS

> ### NUTRITIP
> "Try it, you might like it!" Have children (and parents!) take turns choosing a new food to introduce to the family.

Don't fall into a food rut. Try new foods with your family and make it fun. Here are some ideas for introducing new foods:

- Offer the new food at the beginning of the meal. Serve it alongside at least one known favorite. (See the camouflage trick, page 280.)

- Offer memberships in the "One-Bite Club." When children try "just one bite," they get to celebrate by going out to a family restaurant — one that has a nutritious salad bar, of course.

• Make sure everyone gets the same new food to sample! Remember that children copy their parents' example. Put on your happiest face but don't overdo it. Your child may see through your theatrics.

• No grunts, grimaces, or negative comments allowed. More precise descriptions are okay, such as, "sour," "chewy," or the always safe "very interesting."

• Have children be on the lookout for new vegetables or fruit at the grocery store.

• Give a funny name to foods your child is reluctant to try — be creative, such as broccoli "trees" and tofu "blocks."

• Serve food warm, not hot. It's hard to taste food after you burn your tongue.

• Try one new food each week, incorporating different types of foods. By the end of each month, your family could have a new favorite menu!

• If a child doesn't want to try a certain food today, revisit it next week or next month. When you do re-introduce it, try preparing it differently, or folding it into a favorite casserole, pasta dish, or soup. And remind your children that as they grow, their taste buds change.

J IS FOR JUMP, JOG, OR JIGGLE!

> ### NUTRITIP
> Encourage an active lifestyle for your children and join them as they jump and jiggle! Choose activities that foster family togetherness and family fitness.

Get your children moving by giving them plenty of opportunities not just to play sports but to stay fit. Children of active parents are more active themselves, so look for ways that you all can exercise together.

• Jump rope, dance, swim, bike, hike, or otherwise get moving. Balance a good, healthy diet with adequate exercise. Obesity in children is often caused by a sedentary lifestyle. Often it is directly related to the amount of time spent watching television or playing video games.

• Teach your children how to make food choices based on their activity level. Provide juice after soccer practice and outlaw high-fat snacks during TV time.

• If the weather is not conducive to outdoor play, put on some music and dance around the house, or get out rhythm instruments and shake 'em!

• Look for exercise videos to share with your children. One exercise video is called *Workout with Daddy & Me* for ages three and up (produced by Schoolhouse Videos). It's fun and can be done as a family exercise program. Our seven- and ten-year-olds often joins in.

K IS FOR KALEIDOSCOPE OF COLORS

> ### NUTRITIP
> Color it nutritious! Teach your children that a colorful plate means lots of "grow foods."

What a beautiful array of colors fruits and vegetables have! You can use this eyeful of color to your advantage by teaching your child to choose naturally colorful foods. The brightest colors are found in produce that is in season, fresh, and eaten raw or lightly steamed.

WHAT DO THE COLORS ON YOUR PLATE MEAN?

Color	Foods	Nutrients	Why It's Good for You
Yellow	pumpkin, sweet potatoes, cantaloupe, apricots, carrots	vitamin A folic acid fiber beta carotene	helps kids grow; helps kids see better (improves weak eyesight); good for their skin (promotes healthier skin)
Green	broccoli, leafy green vegetables (e.g., kale, bok choy, collard greens)	vitamin A folic acid fiber	helps kids grow; helps kids see better (improves weak eyesight)
Red	strawberries, watermelon, tomatoes	vitamin C fiber lycopene	keeps kids healthy; helps make boo-boos heal faster
Orange	oranges, grapefruit, cantaloupe	vitamin C fiber	keeps kids healthy; helps make boo-boos heal faster

Activities

- Play a color-matching game: What's in the reds? Why is it good for you?

- When you're in the supermarket's produce section, send your children out on a color-finding mission. Assign one child orange and green, and another child gets the job of choosing two yellows! This can also be an excellent way of introducing new foods and getting variety into the family diet.

- When you serve fruits and vegetables, ask your children what vitamins and minerals they are high in and why these are good for them.

- Have children cut out pictures of fruits and vegetables. Then have them paste them on a sheet of paper in groups according to their colors.

- Have children draw pictures of food on paper plates. Are all the food groups represented? Use colorful markers.

- Ask your children what color foods they ate today. Talk about each food and its color. "Did you eat your yummy yellows and great greens today?"

- Create a "rainbow lunch," a tray of colorful foods cut into bize-sized servings.

L IS FOR LEARNING ACTIVITIES

> ### NUTRITIP
> Make learning nutrition fun and games! All you have to say is, "Let's play a game," and the kids will come running!

Experienced teachers know that games are a great way to learn, much more effective than lectures and quizzes. Here are some games to try at home:

• Have children cut out pictures of foods from magazines or newspapers. Make flash cards by gluing the pictures onto index cards and then gluing the cards to Popsicle sticks (so they are easier for children to grasp). Have the children take turns holding up a card. Younger children can tell to which food group the food belongs on the Food Guide Pyramid. Older children can tell which nutrients are found in the food.

• Using the food flash cards try food group versions of "Go Fish" or "Old Maid." Or cut the cards in two pieces to play matching or memory games.

• Try this with preschoolers: Collect or draw pictures of food. Give one picture to each child. Have the children stand in different parts of the room. Call out the foods the children are holding, one by one. The child who has that food holds it up, and the children run to that child and pretend to eat that food or act out the type of animals that eat that food.

• Try the shiny penny experiment. The phosphoric acid in soft drinks is strong enough to remove the corrosion from a coin. Leave a "dirty" penny in a glass of soda overnight to show your kids what soda can do to their tummies and teeth. Do they really want that stuff in their bodies?

M IS FOR MEDIA

> ### NUTRITIP
> The mass media present both good and bad information about nutrition. Teach your children to recognize the difference.

Television, magazines, and the Internet are powerful influences on children. Discuss with your child how to tell the difference between truthful information and manipulative advertising. When you see sound nutritional information on TV, share it with your child and use it as a springboard for teaching. If a delicious citrus salad flashes on television, you can say, "Wow, those oranges look delicious! The ad says they have vitamin C! Do you know what vitamin C is good for?" If a news program describes a new study on diet and health, talk about it with your child. Point out how ridiculous many commercials are. "Did you see that thin little boy? The ad says he grew up to have a lot of muscles just because he drank that protein drink. That company really wants you to believe that kids your age will get muscles like that from their product. Do you think some kids will believe this ad?"

Be an ad buster. While watching at least one hour of children's programming on a TV network such as Nickelodeon or the Cartoon Network that has food commercials targeted at children, tally up all the different foods advertised. Write down these foods and analyze their nutritional value. Share your findings with your children.

N IS FOR NUTRITION LABELS

> ## NUTRITIP
> What's in your food? Knowing how to read a nutrition label is a valuable skill for children.

Older children can learn to read and interpret nutrition labels. Comparing labels on different products is a particularly good exercise for kids. (Serving size and percentage of daily values are based on figures for adults, so this information may not be correct for children.) Try comparing two different boxes of cereal, or compare junk-food labels with more nutritious alternatives (see "Anatomy of a Junk Label," page 125, and "A Tale of Two Cereals," page 141). Point out how much fat is in the junk food and how much fiber is in the cereal. Show your child how to be a sugar detective by checking the ingredients list. Look for foods in your pantry or refrigerator that are high in iron or vitamin C, based on information on the label. (For more on label-reading, see Chapter 12, "Learning About Labels.") (Another "N" activity is the nibble tray; see page 274.)

O IS FOR OPPORTUNITIES IN THE KITCHEN

> ## NUTRITIP
> Give your child opportunities to learn about food by helping out in the kitchen. Kids will be more likely to eat what they have helped to cook.

How could getting your child to help out in the kitchen have anything to do with teaching nutrition? One study published in the *Journal of Nutrition Education* analyzed mothers' reports of their three-year-olds' involvement in food-related activities and found that children who were more involved in these activities scored significantly higher on nutrition awareness tests. Here are some age-appropriate skills your child can practice in the kitchen.

Ages 3–5:

- Help set the table.
- Tear lettuce into bite-sized pieces for salad.
- Pour ingredients into a bowl and help mix.
- Help choose a favorite food for the menu.
- Toss a salad.
- Mix frozen fruit juice concentrate with water.
- Snap fresh beans.
- Wash fruit, such as grapes and apples.
- Slice bananas, soft cheese, or a hard-boiled egg with a plastic knife.
- Squeeze a lemon or orange.
- Help with rinsing and washing unbreakable dishes.
- Peel a hard-boiled egg.
- Knead bread dough.
- Assemble pizzas.

Ages 6 and up:
In addition to the activities mentioned above, have your child try these:

- Mash potatoes.
- Measure ingredients.
- Peel vegetables.
- Read simple recipes and follow the directions.
- Open cans.
- Use the microwave oven (with supervision).
- Put away groceries.
- Make a shopping list.

P IS FOR PRESENTATION

> **NUTRITIP**
> How do you get your child to appreciate the nutritious food you serve? It's all in the *presentation.*

"That yooks yike I don't yike it!" How food looks matters to kids. Eyes and appetites are directly linked. Here are some ideas for putting pizzazz in the presentation of the nutritious foods you serve:

- Serve food in different containers. Be a little zany and see the look of surprise on your child's face! Put pieces of fruit or pasta salad in a muffin tin. Place dinner, such as rice, vegetables, and beans, in measuring cups on a plate. Serve crackers and cheese cubes on a deviled egg platter. Put veggies in a small frying pan with a dip.

- Garnish foods — and let the kids help you! They can put slices of oranges or sprigs of parsley on plates. Kids can help wash lettuce leaves and arrange them on a plate and then add cherry tomatoes, olives, raisins, or grapes as their own creative touch. Or have them make designs on the plates out of colorful pureed vegetables squeezed out of a plastic bottle.

- Personalize it! Cut slices of cheese in the shapes of your child's initials and melt the cheese on bread. (Get it out of the oven before the shape disappears!) Or decorate a piece of toast topped with the child's initials outlined in raisins or banana slices.

- Have your child help you choose tableware, perhaps adding colorful napkins or place mats.

- Experiment with different forms of the same food. For instance, if your child doesn't go for diced carrots, try carrot "coins" or shredded carrots. Instead of spaghetti, try alphabet noodles, bow-tie pasta, or shells.

- Cut foods into shapes. There are many gadgets at houseware stores that can transform ordinary veggies into zigzags, flowers, and other appetizing shapes.

Q IS FOR QUEEN (OR KING) FOR A DAY!

> **NUTRITIP**
> Let's celebrate! On special days, treat your child like royalty, while helping her make healthy meal choices.

Help your child choose a special menu for her birthday, half-birthday, or other special day. Look for excuses to celebrate and treat family members like royalty at mealtime. For example, if your child was born on March 11, you could designate the eleventh day of every month as her day to choose the menu.

Decorate the dining room for these special meals. Tie a balloon to the back of the honoree's chair. Or use a special place setting. There are paper plates available that say "It's your special day!" or "You are special today!"

R IS FOR RESOLUTION

> **NUTRITIP**
> Make a resolution with your children to improve a family eating habit. Then get them involved in carrying it out!

Is there something you want to do to improve your family's eating pattern? Here are some examples of simple food resolutions that will benefit your family's nutrition immensely:

- We will eat more fruits and vegetables and less chips and candy.
- We will order corn on the cob or salad with our burritos or burgers instead of french fries when we eat out.
- We will sit down and plan our weekly menus together, using the Food Guide Wheel.
- We will take turns picking out a new ethnic food to try each week.

Choose a resolution together as a family. Try it for a month, then revisit it. Was your plan successful? What can be done to make it work better?

S IS FOR SNACKS

NUTRITIP
Teach children to graze on good food.

Explain to your children the difference between feel-good and junk-food snacks: "Your body works better if you eat the right foods for snacks. Feel-good snack foods are those that get into your body slowly and aren't used up fast. They leave you feeling better. Feel-good foods for snacks are fruit, yogurt, bread, cereal, homemade cookies, and veggies. Junk-food snacks, such as doughnuts, sodas, cupcakes, candy, and cereals with too much sugar, get into your body quickly and get used up quickly — and you don't feel good after they get used up. This feeling comes from what is called 'low blood sugar.' Now, what snacks would you like to take to school and what snack foods shall we keep in the pantry and refrigerator for when you get hungry or get a snack attack?"

"S" also stands for "sugar." Teach your children the concept of "steady blood sugar" — that food is fuel for energy. The sugar story could go like

this: "Your body, especially your brain, needs a steady supply of food for fuel. When it runs out of fuel, you feel hungry, weak, or just not good. And if you put the wrong fuel in your body or don't put enough of it in at the right times, you don't feel good. Because your body uses up foods for energy very quickly, you have to refill your body often. Otherwise, it won't feel or work right, sort of like a car running out of gas. You know when your body is running low on fuel. You feel hungry, tired, weak, maybe even a bit fuzzy-headed. That's why it's important to snack or nibble on nutritious foods between meals. In fact, many animals nibble all day long instead of eating breakfast, lunch, and dinner like we do. This is called 'grazing.' Some people feel better and have more energy if they graze on five or six mini meals each day instead of eating three big meals."

T IS FOR TREATS

NUTRITIP
Treats don't always have to be sweets.

Today's children are bombarded with candy treats, sugary snacks, and foods that offer fun but no nutritional value. Your grandmother probably remembers the day when an orange was a special treat.

Teach your child to appreciate nutritious treats: fresh strawberries in season, the first apples of fall, fresh-picked corn on the cob, and home-baked bread. Offer your child non-food treats, too: special times with parents, books or art supplies, a walk around the block on a beautiful day. Talk about why these treats are better than sweets.

Another "T" activity is a tally sheet. Use this sheet with your child to track eating habits in a visual way. Post a copy of the Food Guide Wheel on your refrigerator at your child's eye level. Beside it post a sheet listing the healthy food groups. Fill it in with stickers or coloring as the day goes on. At the end of the day, see if you've met or exceeded your Food Guide Wheel goals.

U IS FOR UNDERWHELM

> ### NUTRITIP
> Set your child up to finish the food on his plate by starting him out with small portions. A huge plateful of food can overwhelm and take his appetite away.

Tiny people have tiny tummies. Children don't eat as much as adults. Give children a positive sense of accomplishment by giving them servings they can finish. Then they have the opportunity to say, "More, please!" You don't want your child to give up on a meal before he even starts eating, simply because the meal put in from of him seems forbidding and impossible to finish. Start small, with "underwhelming" portions. The guideline of 1 tablespoon (per food group) per year of age may be helpful.

V IS FOR VARIETY

> ### NUTRITIP
> Variety truly is the spice of life.

There are sound reasons for offering children a variety of foods, even if they seem content with a limited menu of old favorites. Even children get bored with food if they see the same ones day after day. It's hard to enjoy a meal when you're bored. People also have less chance of being affected by pollutants or allergies if they eat a variety of foods. Offer two choices of both fruits and vegetables at mealtimes. With enough variety on the table, everyone in the family will find something he or she likes to eat. Also, children like to binge eat. They like a certain vegetable for a few days, then may not touch it for a while. Instead of a balanced meal, shoot for a balanced week.

W IS FOR WATER

> ### NUTRITIP
> Teach your children to acquire a taste for water, the most vital drink of all!

Did you "water" your growing child today? Water is essential to good nutrition! Since our bodies are more than 50 percent water, we need to continually replenish our fluids. Hidden sources of water include milk or fruit juice, soups and stews, fruits, and vegetables. Have cold water readily available for your child throughout the day. Keeping it in a pitcher in the refrigerator makes it seem more special, as does an attractive cup or glass and maybe some ice cubes or a twist of lemon peel. Don't forget to offer water often during the day, especially in warmer temperatures. If a child is well hydrated, he or she is more likely to have a good appetite.

(For more tips on watering your growing child, see Chapter 8, "Becoming Water Wise.")

X IS FOR XYLITOL

> ### NUTRITIP
> Nature's desserts are sweet to eat, thanks to a natural sugar called "xylitol."

Do you like strawberries and raspberries? They contain xylitol, a type of sugar. Teach your children to enjoy nature's desserts — fruit. Since fruit has the extra advantage of being high in vitamin C and fiber, it makes sense to depend on it to satisfy the sweet tooth of your children.

Here are some ideas for healthy desserts made with fruits:

- fresh fruit kebabs
- fresh strawberries served in an ice-cream cone topped with whipped cream
- slices of fruit with yogurt dip
- baked apple or pear
- milkshake or smoothie made with yogurt and fresh fruit
- banana bread
- applesauce topped with graham cracker crumbs

Y IS FOR YOGURT

NUTRITIP
There are many high-calcium foods besides milk. Chief among them is yogurt.

Teaching your child about building strong bones and teeth goes beyond mentioning milk. There are some children who don't particularly care for milk or have milk allergies. Many of them will like or tolerate yogurt. Eight ounces of yogurt contains even more calcium than 8 ounces of milk. And yogurt can be the start of truly creative eating. Let your children add pieces of fruit,

chopped nuts, raisins, wheat germ, and other goodies to yogurt. Or, use it as a dip for vegetables or in salad dressings. (See Chapter 20, "Yummy Yogurt.")

Z IS FOR ZEST FOR GOOD NUTRITION

NUTRITIP
Let your zest for nutrition inspire your children that good eating habits help them grow, feel great, and do their best!

You want your child to not only know about good nutrition but truly relish eating. With you as a guide, your child can learn to appreciate the foods that make him feel good. He'll be eager to eat and enjoy nutritious food. Remember these three important points:

1. *You* are your children's role model for good nutrition. In fact, you are their first nutrition teacher!
2. *You* choose the variety of foods to offer them.
3. *You* can make it fun.

May you have many happy, healthy meals together, as your children learn that eating right helps them every day to feel great, do their best, and grow!

31

Feeding the Brain

NEW STUDIES ARE CONFIRMING what parents have long observed: There is a relationship between what children eat and how they think, act, and learn. Like every other system in the body, the brain needs good food. It uses 20 to 25 percent of the total energy a person consumes, and the better you feed the brain, the better it works. While most of this chapter is devoted to the nutritional principles that help children's brains learn and behave, these same principles affect how adults think, learn, and feel, too. Everyone in the family benefits from good food for the brain.

BETTER EATING BUILDS BETTER BRAINS

There is a pecking order among the organs of the body. The most vital organs get first pick of the available nutrients in the bloodstream. Since a malfunctioning brain can take the rest of the body down with it, the brain gets VIP status when the body distributes nutrients. Here's how:

The brain is composed of trillions of nerve cells called "neurons." Thought, memory, actions, and many brain functions you're not even aware of depend on speed-of-light interactions between one cell and another. From each nerve cell, tiny feelers called "axons" and "dendrites" reach out to connect with similar branches on other cells. The system looks kind of like a map of the interstate highway system, with many roadways connecting different cities. To facilitate the transmission of signals across the gap from one cell to the other, chemicals called "neurotransmitters" act like biological bridges.

Nutrition affects the brain in three ways:

1. *The cell* itself needs proper nutrition to carry on its functions, just like any other cell in the body.
2. *The myelin sheath* covers the axon of the cell, like insulation covering electrical wires. It speeds the transmission of electrical signals along the axons, the "wires" of the

---

NUTRITIP
Buzz Foods

Some foods, such as those containing caffeine, give the brain a buzz. This may be a welcome lift when the brain needs to be turned on, such as when you want to study or stay awake. Other times caffeine can be a detriment, such as when you want to turn off the brain and go to sleep or when you need to stay relaxed under pressure.

MOOD FOODS

Both research and experience are proving without a doubt that there is a connection between how we eat and how we feel. The biochemical basis of this food-mood relationship lies in the neurotransmitters, those chemical messengers that relay thought and actions along the trillions of neural pathways in the brain. It seems logical that since food affects neurotransmitter action, and changes in neurotransmitters are responsible for changes in moods, food does affect mood. It also seems that food affects some people's moods more than others'. Some children — we call them "vulnerable kids" — are exquisitely sensitive to junk foods in their diets, while others seem to breeze through fast-food joints without any mood change. While it's easy to spot these vulnerable kids, I wonder how much behavior we attribute to "just being a kid" is really the result of poor nutrition. While the nature of the food-mood connection varies from person to person, here are the usual effects of various foods.

Carbs that calm. Complex carbohydrates and foods that have a low glycemic index (legumes, unrefined grains, and fruits) are likely to have a relaxing effect because they cause fewer blood-sugar disturbances, with less release of stress hormones. (For more on the glycemic index, see pages 35 and 38.)

Carbs that rev. Sugars such as those in frostings and soft drinks tend to cause fluctuations in moods that run parallel with fluctuations in blood sugar. First, there's a high, then a low, and eventually the person becomes irritable as the mood fluctuations parallel the ups and downs of blood sugar. Junk sugars cause fewer mood fluctuations when eaten along with a fat or fiber that slows down their absorption into the bloodstream.

Happy foods. Some feel that chocolate is calming because it triggers the release of endorphins. Other happy foods, such as milk, chicken, bananas, and leafy green vegetables may produce pleasant feelings because they stimulate the release of the neurotransmitter dopamine. Tryptophan-containing foods (see "Foods for Sleep," page 364) also have a relaxing effect, so they could be called "happy foods."

Sad foods. Some people feel sad after a high-fat or high-sugar meal. Each person has unique food-mood connections, but if you pay attention, after a while you will begin to eat more of the foods that make you happy and skip the foods that bring you down.

Parents need to become the food-mood detectives for their child. Follow these steps to figure out your child's unique fingerprints for food-mood connection:

1. Make a chart on which to record what your child eats and when. Fill in one of these forms every day for a week.
2. Record times when behavior problems, bad moods, or irritability occur.
3. After a week, examine your charts and look for connections. Then decide what improvements you can make in your child's diet to improve his moods.
4. Continue keeping food-mood records to help you decide whether dietary changes have improved the behaviors.

Mood foods vary from person to person. Try to figure out your personal food-mood connection — which foods perk you up and which ones let you down. Being able to determine how foods affect your moods will help you make wise food choices.

brain. Deficiencies of the nutrients that compose myelin, such as essential fatty acids, delay nerve-impulse transmission.

3. *The neurotransmitters,* such as serotonin, dopamine, and norepinephrine, carry messages from one cell to another and affect mood as well as thoughts and actions. Some of the nutrients in the food we eat become part of the neurotransmitters that help us think. Neurotransmitters are probably the biological explanation for the food-mood connection.

Each one of these three parts needs specific nutrients to enable the whole circuit to function properly. If any of these areas are deficient in nutrients, the circuit, like a defective electrical wire, misfires. What follows is a discussion of how different kinds of foods affect the brain.

NUTRITIP
Sweet Pleasures

Sweets lovers take note! Chocolate may be more nutritious than imagined. Depending on the type, chocolate can be a good source of iron, zinc, calcium, potassium, magnesium, and flavonoids. By a fortunate biochemical quirk, cocoa butter — the fat that gives chocolate that appealing melt-in-your-mouth feel — is metabolized like a heart-healthy monounsaturated fat, even though chemically it's a saturated fat. Chocolate as a mood elevator even merits a bit of scientific support. Possibly the caffeine or phenylethylamine compounds stimulate serotonin and endorphins, both calming and satisfying the chocolate craver. Enjoy!

FOODS FOR THOUGHT

Some foods help the brain work better, and some foods drag down brain performance. Be smart and feed your children foods that will make them smart (and eat these foods yourself, too).

Brain Builders

asparagus	cantaloupe	milk	salmon
avocados	cheese	oatmeal	soybeans
bananas	chicken	oranges	spinach
beef, lean	collard greens	peanut butter	tuna
brewer's yeast	eggs	peas	turkey
broccoli	flaxseed oil	potatoes	wheat germ
brown rice	legumes	romaine lettuce	yogurt
brussels sprouts			

Brain Drainers

alcohol	colas	high-sugar "drinks"	nicotine
artificial food	corn syrup	hydrogenated fats	overeating
colorings	frostings	junk sugars	white bread
artificial sweeteners			

A.D.D. — A NUTRITIONAL DEFICIENCY?

Intuitive parents have long suspected that in some children undesirable behavior and poor school performance are linked to poor nutrition. New scientific studies of children with Attention Deficit Disorder (A.D.D.) are beginning to confirm these suspicions.

One theory about A.D.D. is that it is caused by a neurotransmitter imbalance. Children with A.D.D. use hyperactivity and undesirable behavior to stimulate production of neurotransmitters, but then they get overstressed and deplete themselves of neurotransmitters and are soon out of control. It seems logical, then, that a child with a tendency toward A.D.D. needs a diet rich in nutrients that build neurotransmitters, given the difficulties he may have regulating their production. Research supports this idea, specifically:

• A 1996 study of ninety-six boys found that those with lower blood levels of omega-3 fatty acids were significantly more likely to have learning and behavior problems than those whose levels were normal.

• Another study showed that children with Attention Deficit Hyperactivity Disorder (A.D.H.D.) tended to have low blood levels of docosahexaenoic acid (DHA) and arachidonic acid (AA), two key brain fats. Perhaps this correlates with studies that show that children who have been breastfed are less likely to have A.D.H.D., and the longer the period of breastfeeding, the less the likelihood of having A.D.H.D. The reason may be that breast milk is high in important fatty acids, such as gammalinolenic acid (GLA), alphalinolenic acid (ALA), DHA, AA, and others, unlike formulas, which at this writing contained little of these fatty acids. Studies at Purdue University in Indiana found that many boys with A.D.H.D. had low levels of the omega fatty acids DHA, GLA, and AA in their blood and tended to have higher levels of linolenic acid (LA) precursors in their blood than boys without A.D.H.D., suggesting that these children were unable to make the fatty acids their brains need from the fats in their diet. Those boys with A.D.H.D. who had the lowest levels of DHA, GLA, and AA exhibited the most anxiety, impulsivity, hyperactivity, and conduct disorders. The researchers suggested three possible explanations for their findings: The children's diets were deficient in essential fatty acids; the children had a metabolic problem that prevented the body from converting dietary nutrients to essential fatty acids for the brain; or various lifestyle and dietary factors reduced the level of essential fatty acids available to the brain.

• While a deficiency of omega-3 fats can contribute to poor behavior and learning, the ratio of omega-6 to omega-3 fatty acids in the diet is also important. A study of fifteen children with motor-coordination problems showed that motor skills improved after the children were given a diet rich in omega-3 and omega-6 fatty acids. Brain researchers believe that the ideal ratio in the diet is 1 to 1, but a study found that children with A.D.H.D. had a higher omega-6 to omega-3 ratio in their diet. When the omega-6 to omega-3 ratio gets too high, the important omega-3 fats may be less available to the brain.

A.D.D. — A NUTRITIONAL DEFICIENCY? (CONTINUED)

- Some children with A.D.H.D. have outward symptoms of essential-fatty-acid deficiency, such as excessive thirst, frequent urination, dry hair, and dry skin. These symptoms appear because the vital organs, such as the brain, seem to have a claim on the essential fatty acids in the diet and rob these vital nutrients from less important organs, such as the skin.

- The Hyperactive Children's Support Group in England, after researching the connection between A.D.D. and essential-fatty-acid deficiency, concluded that since some children may have a problem with the normal metabolism of essential fatty acids, they should supplement their diets with essential fatty acids. The group even suggested that males may require two to three times more essential fatty acids than females, since hyperactive male children seem to outnumber females by three to one.

- In a study of DHA and behavior, a group of college students were given a daily supplement of DHA beginning in August and continuing until final exams. Students who took DHA supplements displayed far less external aggression than those not taking supplements.

- Sugars can also affect the learning and behavior of children. Glucose-tolerance tests of 261 hyperactive children showed that 74 percent had abnormal glucose-tolerance tests, indicating that some children with A.D.H.D. are more prone to blood-sugar swings and the poor behavior and school performance that may accompany them. In one study, seventeen children with A.D.D. were shown to have a lower rise in plasma epinephrine and norepinephrine in response to glucose infusion, an indication that these children may have more difficulty with adrenal-hormone response to blood-sugar changes.

- Some research suggests that vitamin and mineral supplements may help children with A.D.H.D. Studies have shown that zinc deficiency in some children with A.D.H.D., along with their lower serum levels of free fatty acids, may contribute to their A.D.H.D. Studies have shown that schoolchildren receiving a daily multivitamin containing the recommended dietary allowance of essential vitamins and minerals showed better school performance. However, studies using megavitamin therapy (doses of vitamins well above the RDA) on children with A.D.D. showed no effects; researchers concluded that this type of treatment should be discouraged because of potential toxic effects from excess amounts of some vitamins.

- Other studies show that children placed on vitamin and mineral supplements tend to exhibit less violent, antisocial behavior, and show higher gains in academic performance than children on placebos. One study found that children who took 100 percent of the RDA did better on IQ tests than those receiving 200 percent or 50 percent of the RDA. The conclusion was that taking more or less than the RDA may not be helpful.

- Finally, nutritionists who reviewed studies linking diet, behavior, and school performance concluded that students who generally ate a nutritious diet showed improved conduct and academic performance. All the whys and wherefores may not have been discovered yet, but common sense prevails.

BEST BRAIN FOODS

While most nutrients provide food for thought, some foods are more brain friendly than others. How you think, act, and learn is affected not only by the types of food you eat but also by how the food is prepared, how and when you eat it, and what foods you eat together.

Sugars: Caring About Your Carbs

The brain is a sugar hog, a carbo-craver, utilizing 20 percent of the body's carbohydrate supply. Yet it's a smart hog, being selective about the types of sugars it craves and how it processes them. It prefers a nice steady supply. When the brain receives a steady supply of sugar for fuel, it chugs along smoothly at a steady pace. But when levels of sugar in the blood fluctuate, the brain doesn't get its steady fuel supply, and behavior and learning become more erratic. Blood-sugar levels depend on the kinds of food that are coming into the body. Some carbohydrates calm behavior, others excite it.

Sugar Blues

Most scientists discount the relationship between sugar and behavior, especially when it comes to the question of whether sugar plays a role in Attention Deficit Hyperactivity Disorder (A.D.H.D.). In a 1995 paper published in the *Journal of the American Medical Association*, researchers analyzed the results of sixteen different studies in which children were given foods containing lots of sugar, and their behavior was compared with a control group. The analysis concluded that sugar had no impact on behavior. Try explaining this to a mother whose child goes wild after eating a Twinkie. Researchers tend to discount parents' observations, believing that they have been conditioned by media reports and other

A.D.H.D. FOODS

The behavior and learning of children who are labeled with A.D.H.D. (Attention Deficit Hyperactivity Disorder) tend to be influenced more than other children by foods. Clues that a dietary deficiency may be contributing to your child's behavior or learning problems include excessive thirst, frequent urination, dry hair and skin, eczema, and allergies. But most important are the observations you record in your food-mood connection diary. The acronym ADHD (Add to your Daily Healthy Diet) can help you remember to include foods that improve behavior and learning, such as fish, flax seeds or flax oil, vegetables, and whole grains.

parents to expect their children's behavior to deteriorate after sugary snacks.

If a mother comes into my office and tells me that every time her child has a certain soft drink or eats a candy full of red dye he becomes a wild man for the next hour, I believe her. A research study of one hundred children who have A.D.D. might not show that the substance she complained about was a statistically significant factor, but that is simply a statistical finding. Her child may be the one in a hundred who gets squirrelly after eating red jelly beans. One study that achieved front-page prominence in a national newspaper concluded that sugar had no effect on behavior, but the study included only fifty children — twenty-five in the study group, and twenty-five in the control group.

So we're back to the science of common sense — and basic physiology. Different sugars affect the brain in different ways, so it is only logical to conclude that certain sugars can adversely affect the thinking and actions of some children. The sugars at fault include glucose, dextrose, and sucrose, and the highly refined, highly processed "junk sugars" found in candy, icings, syrups, packaged baked goods, and table sugar. These sugars enter the bloodstream quickly and reach high levels in a short time. This triggers the release of large amounts of insulin, the hormone needed to escort the sugars into the body's cells. These sugars are used rapidly, and when they're all used up, the blood-sugar level plunges to a sugar low, called "hypoglycemia." The low blood sugar triggers the release of adrenal hormones (called a "sugar high") that squeezes stored sugar from the liver, sending blood-sugar levels back up. This blood-sugar roller coaster affects moods and concentration in some children and adults, leading to "sugar highs" and "sugar blues." The ups and downs of blood sugar and adrenal hormones can also stimulate neurotransmitter imbalance, causing the child to feel fidgety, irritable, inattentive, and even sleepy.

The best sugars for the brain are complex carbohydrates, or what grandmother termed "starches" (see page 31 for a list of the top nine complex carbohydrates). Starches and fruit sugars (fructose) do not cause the roller-coaster mood swings that the junk sugars do. The molecules in complex carbs are long, so it takes longer for the

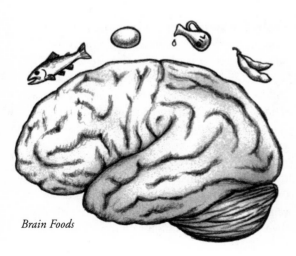

Brain Foods

intestines to break them down into the simple sugars the body can use. Thus, they provide a time-release source of steady energy rather than a sudden surge followed by a sudden drop.

Glycemic Index — The Food GI

The rate at which sugar from a particular food enters brain cells and other cells of the body is called the "glycemic index" (GI) of a particular food. Foods with a high glycemic index stimulate the pancreas to secrete a lot of insulin, which causes the sugar to quickly empty from the blood into the cells; this produces the ups and downs of blood sugar and the roller-coaster behavior that goes with them. Foods with a low glycemic index do not push the pancreas to secrete so much insulin, so the blood sugar tends to be steadier. Feeding your child carbohydrate foods with a low glycemic index is one way of helping him control his behavior and performance in school or at play. Foods with the best brain sugars include the following:

Fruits. Grapefruit, apples, cherries, oranges, and grapes have a low glycemic index. Fruits have a lower GI than fruit juices, because the fiber in the fruit slows the absorption of the fruit sugar. A whole apple will be more brain friendly than apple juice; a whole orange better than orange juice. Freshly made juice containing a lot of pulp is more brain friendly than filtered juice.

Cereals and grains. Oatmeal and bran have the lowest GI among grains. Other foods with a favorable GI are spaghetti and brown rice. Corn flakes and sugar-coated cereals have higher GI's.

Vegetables and legumes. Legumes, such as soybeans, kidney beans, chickpeas, and lentils, have the lowest glycemic index of any food group. Potatoes and carrots have a much higher GI.

Dairy products. Milk and yogurt have low glycemic indexes, slightly higher than most

LETHARGIC AFTER LUNCH

Ever wonder why schoolchildren's learning and behavior deteriorate after lunch? It's because some foods perk up the brain, while others put it to sleep. Here are some lunch tips that can improve your child's attention, behavior, and learning in the afternoon.

Have the right balance of proteins and carbohydrates. Whether your child learns well after lunch or dozes through afternoon classes can be influenced by the proteins in the lunch and the carbohydrate company these proteins keep. Protein foods that contain the amino acid tryptophan tend to sedate the brain, and protein foods containing the amino acid tyrosine wake up the brain. (See page 305 for an explanation of how these amino acids affect different neurotransmitters.) Rich dietary sources of tryptophan are eggs, bananas, dairy, sunflower seeds, and poultry. Eating a lot of carbohydrates along with tryptophan-containing foods increases their sedative effect. The carbohydrates trigger the release of insulin, which sends the amino acids that compete with tryptophan into muscle tissue. This allows more tryptophan to get into the brain. Serotonin production goes up, and sluggishness follows. Fewer carbohydrates and calories with more protein, on the other hand, makes the eater more alert after lunch. The amino acid that perks up the brain is tyrosine, found in seafood, tofu, legumes, and tuna. So, a salad of legumes with tuna, or tofu is an ideal lunch if you want your child to work and learn in the afternoon rather than drift off.

Even the order in which you eat the food in your lunch can affect afternoon performance. Whether the brain revs up or slows down depends on whether tyrosine or tryptophan gets into the neurotransmitters first. Eat the protein first and allow the amino acid tyrosine to wake up the brain. Then eat the carbohydrates, and the tryptophan ushered into the brain by the insulin will have less effect. So, if you want to wake up the brain, eat a high-protein lunch, and eat the protein before the carbohydrates; if you want the brain to relax, eat a high-carbohydrate lunch, and eat the carbohydrates before the protein.

Encourage children to eat a light lunch. A healthy lunch for school-age children contains between 600 and 800 calories, with a balance of complex carbohydrates and proteins and a minimum of fats. A high-calorie, high-carbohydrate meal, such as pasta with a fat-laden sauce, is likely to diminish your child's academic performance after lunch. A high-fat meal diminishes mental alertness by diverting blood from the brain to the stomach to help with digestion. An example of a healthy lunch would be a tuna sandwich on whole wheat bread with lettuce, tomato, and a low-fat mayonnaise made with canola oil, a side salad, a piece of fruit, and a glass of milk. Encourage your child to skip dessert after lunch and to save his daily dessert treat for after dinner.

Lobby for healthy school lunches. In many schools, the hot lunch program is a nutritional failure. Based on the lunches that are served, many schools deserve the behavior they get from children after lunch. Fast-food favorites are now taking over the counter space in school cafeterias, teaching children that the four food groups are burgers, fries, pizza, and chicken nuggets. Get involved in your PTA and make the topic of healthy school lunches a high priority. Also, monitor what is sold in the vending machines, and lobby for juices rather than heavily sugared, high-caffeine sodas.

legumes but lower than most fruits. Of course, plain yogurt has a lower glycemic index than yogurt with fruit preserves or added sugar.

The company a food keeps and how it is prepared also affect the glycemic index, that is, how fast and steadily the sugar enters the brain.

- A food with a high glycemic index, such as juice, candy, or a sweet treat, is better consumed with or right after a meal. The company of other foods slows the entry of sugar into the bloodstream and therefore the brain. Indulging in highly sugared snacks between meals is likely to hinder learning and behavior.

- Fat can slow the absorption of sugars, which is why the sugar in ice cream has a lower glycemic index than the sugar in nonfat yogurt.

- Because salads contain mostly foods with a low glycemic index, they are an excellent school lunch, contributing to maximum mental performance. Especially good are salads containing cruciferous vegetables and beans, chickpeas, and other legumes.

- Eating foods with a low glycemic index along with highly sugared foods lessens the effects of the fast-acting sugars on the blood sugar.

For more on the glycemic index, see pages 35 and 38.

Proteins: Feeding Your Neurotransmitters

Proteins in the diet affect brain performance because they provide the amino acids from which

---

GRAZING

We have noticed that children's behavior often deteriorates in the late morning and late afternoon, or three to four hours after a meal, whether the child has A.D.H.D. or not. Children simply run out of fuel. When blood-sugar levels go down, stress hormones kick in to raise it up again, and this can cause behavioral problems and diminished concentration. To smooth out the blood-sugar mood swings, try the fine art of grazing. Let your child nibble, or graze, on nutritious foods throughout the day. Make them easily accessible in a lunch pack at school. (Smart teachers allow even upper-grade children to have a mid-morning snack.) Carry snacks with you when you are away from home. While at home, keep a supply of healthy snacks readily available in the pantry or refrigerator.

Here's a trick from the Sears family kitchen for the preschool child. Prepare a nibble tray. Use an ice cube tray, a muffin tin, or a compartmentalized plastic dish and fill each section with bite-sized portions of colorful and nutritious foods. Give the foods fun names, such as avocado boats (a quarter of an avocado sectioned lengthwise), banana or cooked carrot wheels, broccoli trees, cheese blocks, little O's (O-shaped cereal), canoe eggs (hard-boiled eggs cut lengthwise in wedges), moons (peeled apple slices, thinly spread with peanut butter), or shells and worms (different shapes of pasta).

Don't forget that children love to dip. Reserve one or two compartments in the tray for your child's favorite dips, such as yogurt or guacamole (made without the spices). Encourage the child to sit and nibble from the tray frequently throughout the day, especially late in the morning and in the mid to late afternoon, when the fuel from the previous meal begins to wear off. Shorten the spaces between feedings and you are less likely to have spacey children.

PURE MOMS

Over my twenty-five years in pediatrics practice, I have noticed a striking connection between how children are fed and how healthy they are. Mothers who consistently do not allow any unhealthy food to pollute the minds and bodies of their children seem to have healthier children. I have noticed that these children have fewer office visits and colds, and when they do come for periodic checkups they seem more settled and better behaved. These "pure children" seem to get tagged with fewer labels, such as "A.D.D." or "learning disabled." Even when these children do warrant such tags, they seem to cope better with behavioral and learning differences and these seem less severe. These moms have made a believer out of me. I truly believe that there is a connection between how kids are fed and how they act and learn.

neurotransmitters are made. Think of neurotransmitters as biochemical messengers that carry signals from one brain cell to another. The better you feed these messengers, the more efficiently they deliver the goods. Some neurotransmitters are neuron turn-ons that perk up the brain. Others have a calming or sedative effect.

The two important amino acids, tryptophan and tyrosine, are *precursors* of neurotransmitters, the substances from which neurotransmitters are made. Tryptophan is an essential amino acid, meaning, the body does not make tryptophan; it must be gotten from the diet. Tyrosine, on the other hand, is not an essential amino acid, because the body can make it if there is not enough in the diet. So, dietary deficiency is more likely to affect tryptophan than tyrosine. These two amino acids influence the four top neurotransmitters,

called "serotonin," which is made from the amino acid tryptophan, and "dopamine," "epinephrine," and "norepinephrine," which are made from the amino acid tyrosine. Serotonin is the neurotransmitter that relaxes the brain; the other three, collectively known as "catecholamines," are neurotransmitters that rev up the brain. Popular anti-depressant drugs called "SRI's" (serotonin re-uptake inhibitors), such as Prozac, work by increasing the amounts of serotonin in the brain. Since carbohydrates favor serotonin production, perhaps carbo-cravers self-medicate to increase their own serotonin (see "The Chemistry of Cravings," page 44).

Two factors influence whether the brain perks up or slows down following a meal: the ratio of protein to carbohydrate, and the ratio of the amino acids tryptophan and tyrosine. High protein–low carbohydrate–high tyrosine foods that are likely to jumpstart the brain include seafood, soy products, meat, eggs, and dairy. High carbohydrate–low protein–high tryptophan foods that are likely to relax the brain include chocolate, pastries and desserts, bean burritos, nuts and seeds (e.g., almonds, filberts, sunflower seeds, and sesame seeds), and legumes. (For a discussion of how different amino acids in foods perk up or slow down the brain, see "Foods for Sleep," page 364.)

The Carb-Protein Partnership

Brain performance following a meal is also affected by the carbohydrates consumed with the protein. Carbohydrates stimulate the release of insulin, which helps more tryptophan to enter the brain, where it makes more serotonin. The more simple sugars in the meal, the more serotonin is produced, and the more the brain is sedated. Complex carbohydrates — slower insulin-release sugars — on the other hand, will cause less drastic serotonin production. A high-calorie meal will contribute even more to serotonin production, leading to "serotonin slump" (see "Lethargic After

Lunch," page 304). Eating too much at any meal, regardless of the carbohydrate or protein content, seems to diminish mental performance. So, to perk up the brain, eat a meal that is:

- high in tyrosine-containing proteins;
- moderate in the amount of sugars, containing mainly complex carbohydrates;
- relatively low in calories.

To relax, or even sedate, the brain, eat a meal that is:

- high in tryptophan-containing proteins;
- high in carbohydrates;
- high in calories.

You can plan your meals according to how you use your brain during the day. A low-calorie, high-protein meal that also contains complex carbohydrates makes you more alert and is perfect for breakfast and lunch. A higher-calorie, higher-carbohydrate, lower-protein meal can help you relax and fall asleep in the evening. Skip the dessert at lunchtime if you have a lot of work or learning to do in the afternoon. If you want to be alert after the evening meal, skip dessert or save it for a bedtime snack, unless, of course, you are trying to trim your weight. Remember the saying "What you eat after eight puts on weight."

The balance of calories, carbohydrates, and protein in a meal affects different people in different ways. This is not an exact science. You need to figure out what combinations work best for you, giving you energy and alertness when you need it. Keeping a diary of what you eat and how you feel can help you make corrections. For parents, careful observation of your school-age child is important when you're trying to figure out which foods enhance behavior and school performance and which foods make it worse. This is a challenging game, but one that every home nutritionist can play.

Fats: Feeding Your Brain

Fats, too, can influence brain development and performance, especially at either end of life — growing infants and elderly people. In fact, these are the two windows of time in which the brain is especially sensitive to nutrition: the first two years of life and the last couple of decades of life for a senior citizen. Both growing and aging brains need nutritious fats.

*Fats for Growing Brains**

The most rapid brain growth after birth occurs during the first year of life, with the infant's brain tripling in size by the first birthday. During this stage of rapid central-nervous-system growth, the brain uses 60 percent of the total energy consumed by the infant, and the brain itself is 60 percent fat. Fats are major components of the brain cell membrane and the myelin sheath around each nerve. So, it makes sense that getting enough fat and the right kinds of fat can greatly affect brain development and performance. In fact, during the first year, around 50 percent of an infant's daily calories come from fat. Mother Nature knows how important fat is for babies; she provides around 50 percent of the calories in mother's milk as fat.

It's not only the amount of fat that's important for growing brains, it's the type of fat. Different species provide different types of fat in their milk, fine-tuned to the needs of that particular animal. For example, mother cows provide milk that is high in saturated fats and low in brain-building fats, such as docosahexaenoic acid (DHA). This helps their calves grow rapidly, though it does not do much for their brains. In adult cows, the brain

---

* *An informative book on the best fats for growing brains is* Smart Fats: How Dietary Fats and Oils Affect Mental, Physical, and Emotional Intelligence, *by Michael A. Schmidt (Frog, 1997).*

NOURISHING TEEN BRAINS

Even though the brain has completed most of its growth by adolescence, it continues to make vital connections during the teen years. This is another window of opportunity for brain growth, when a healthy diet is important. However, adolescence is a time when there tends to be a lack of essential fatty acids in the diet for several reasons: Adolescents tend to eat a lot of saturated-fatty foods and foods that contain hydrogenated fats. Also, due to pressure to please their peers and compete in athletics, teens often restrict their fat intake in order to keep fit and trim. When they cut out fat in general, they also cut out healthy fats. Teen brains need more fish and fewer fries.

is small compared with the body. Cows don't have to do a lot of thinking to survive. In human infants, the brain grows faster than the body. Highly developed brains are important to human beings, so human milk is low in body-building saturated fats and rich in brain-building fats, such as the fatty acid DHA, an omega-3 fatty acid.

DHA is the primary structural component of brain tissue, so it stands to reason that a deficiency of DHA in the diet could translate into a deficiency in brain function. In fact, research is increasingly recognizing the possibility that DHA has a crucial influence on neurotransmitters in the brain, helping brain cells better communicate with each other. Asian cultures have long appreciated the brain-building effects of DHA. In Japan, DHA is considered such an important "health food" that it is used as a nutritional supplement to enrich some foods, and students frequently take DHA pills before examinations.

Just how important is DHA for brain development? Consider these research findings:

- Infants who have low amounts of DHA in their diet have reduced brain development and diminished visual acuity.

- The increased intelligence and academic performance of breastfed compared with formula-fed infants has been attributed in part to the increased DHA content of human milk.

- Cultures whose diet is high in omega-3 fatty acids (e.g., Eskimos, who eat a lot of fish that contain DHA) have a lower incidence of degenerative diseases of the central nervous system, such as multiple sclerosis.

- Experimental animals whose diets are low in DHA have been found to have smaller brains and delayed central-nervous-system development.

- Some children with poor school performance because of A.D.D. have been shown to have insufficient essential fatty acids in their diet (see "A.D.D. — A Nutritional Deficiency?," page 300).

NUTRITIP
Fat Food for Growing Brains

While a baby is in the womb, the brain grows more rapidly than at any other stage of infant or child development. And during the first year after birth, the brain continues to grow rapidly, tripling in size by an infant's first birthday. It makes sense for a pregnant and lactating mother to supplement her diet with brain-building nutrients, primarily the omega-3 fatty acids found in fish and flax oil (1 tbsp. of flax oil daily, 4 ounces of tuna or salmon three times a week). In fact, some nutritionists recommend that pregnant and lactating women take 200 milligrams of DHA supplements a day.

SCHOOL-ADE

Here is a Sears family recipe for a smoothie we give our children and ourselves for a quick and nutritious breakfast as they are hurrying off to school and I am rushing off to work.*

3 cups milk or soy or rice beverage
1½ cups plain nonfat yogurt
4 servings SCHOOL-ADE™† or similar
   multinutrient supplement
1 frozen banana, cut up
1 cup frozen blueberries
½ cup each of your favorite fruit, frozen (e.g., organic
   strawberries, papaya, mango)
2 tbsp. flax oil or ½ cup flaxseed meal‡
4 ounces tofu
1 serving soy isolate powder (optional)
2 tbsp. peanut butter (optional)

Combine all the ingredients and blend until smooth. Serve immediately after blending while the mixture still has a bubbly milkshake-like consistency.

This family-size recipe makes four 16-ounce servings (approximately 550 calories per serving). Adjust the recipe to the desired taste and volume. Besides being tasty, it's nutritionally balanced, with each serving containing approximately 25 to 30 grams of protein, 55 to 60 grams of carbohydrates, 8 to 16 grams of fat (mostly healthy omega 3's), and 5 to 10 grams of fiber. Enjoy!

School-Ade Quick

2 cups milk or soy or rice beverage, or 1 cup milk
   and 1 cup yogurt
1 serving SCHOOL-ADE™†
2 tsp. flax oil
1 small frozen banana, cut up
½ cup each of your favorite fruit, frozen (e.g.,
   blueberries, strawberries, papaya)

2 ice cubes if fruit is not frozen or if you want a
lighter taste

Makes one 20-ounce serving (approximately 550 calories).

---

* We formulated this recipe based on the principle of "synergy." These nutrients consumed together enhance each other's benefits, so the whole nutritional effect is greater than the sum of its parts. I have prescribed this recipe for several hundred schoolchildren and their parents, and we drink it ourselves four to five mornings a week. It's a powerful performance booster for working parents and school-children.

† A multinutrient breakfast supplement enriched with omega 3's (DHA). For more information about this supplement, see www.schoolade.com.

‡ Because fiber steadies the absorption of carbohydrates and therefore contributes to a steadier blood sugar, we suggest using rich sources of fiber, such as flaxseed meal (i.e., ground flax seeds, containing both the oil and fiber), although flax oil has a more palatable consistency than flaxseed meal. For additional fiber if you don't mind an even grainier texture, add 1 tbsp. or more of oat bran.

BREAKFASTS FOR GROWING BRAINS

"Breakfast" means just that: *break* the overnight *fast*. Eating breakfast allows you to restock the energy stores that have been depleted overnight and begin the day with a tank full of the right fuel. Sending yourself to work or your child to school without breakfast is like trying to use a cordless power tool without ever recharging the battery. If you don't refuel your child's body in the morning after an overnight fast, she has to draw fuel from her own energy stores until lunchtime. The stress hormones necessary to mobilize these energy reserves may leave her feeling irritable, tired, and unable to learn or behave well. If you want your child to rise and shine rather than limp along sluggishly at school all morning, make sure her day gets off to a nutritious start.

Breakfast Basics

Throughout the brain, biochemical messengers called "neurotransmitters" help the brain make the right connections. Food influences how these neurotransmitters operate. The more balanced the breakfast, the more balanced the brain function. There are two types of proteins that affect neurotransmitters: (1) neurostimulants, such as proteins containing tyrosine, which affect the alertness transmitters dopamine and norepinephrine, and (2) calming proteins that contain tryptophan, which relaxes the brain. A breakfast with the right balance of both stimulating and calming foods starts the child off

with a brain that is primed to learn and with emotions prepared to behave. Eating complex carbohydrates along with proteins helps to usher the amino acids from these proteins into the brain, so that the neurotransmitters can work better. Complex carbohydrates and proteins act like biochemical partners for enhancing learning and behavior. This biochemical principle is called "synergy," meaning that the combination of two nutrients works better than each one singly, sort of like 1 + 1 = 3.

Breakfast Research

If your hectic household has a morning rush hour like the one in our home, you may feel that you don't have time for a healthy breakfast. But consider what studies have shown:

- Breakfast eaters are likely to achieve higher grades, pay closer attention, participate more in class discussions, and manage more complex academic problems than breakfast skippers.
- Breakfast skippers are more likely to be inattentive, sluggish, and make lower grades.
- Breakfast skippers are more likely to show erratic eating patterns throughout the day, eat less nutritious foods, and give in to junk-food cravings. They may crave a mid-morning sugar fix because they can't make it all the way to lunchtime on an empty fuel tank.
- Some children are more vulnerable to the effects of missing breakfast than others. The effects on

BREAKFAST FOR GROWING BRAINS (CONTINUED)

behavior and learning as a result of missing breakfast or eating a breakfast that is not very nutritious vary from child to child.

- Whether or not children eat breakfast affects their learning, but so does what they eat. Children who eat a breakfast containing both complex carbohydrates and proteins in equivalent amounts of calories tend to show better learning and performance than children who eat primarily a high-protein or a high-carbohydrate breakfast. Breakfasts high in complex carbohydrates with little protein seem to sedate children rather than stimulate their brain to learn.
- Children eating high-calcium foods for breakfast (e.g., dairy products) show enhanced behavior and learning.
- Morning stress increases the levels of stress hormones in the bloodstream. This can affect behavior and learning in two ways. First, stress hormones themselves can bother the brain. Second, stress hormones such as cortisol increase carbohydrate craving throughout the day. The food choices that result may affect behavior and learning in children who are sensitive to the ups and downs of blood-sugar levels. Try to send your child off to school with a calm attitude as well as a good breakfast.
- Breakfast sets the pattern for nutritious eating throughout the rest of the day. When children miss breakfast to save time or to cut calories, they set themselves up for erratic bingeing and possibly overeating the rest of the day.

Best Breakfasts

An ideal, nutritious breakfast contains a balance of complex carbohydrates and protein. Think grains, plus dairy, plus fruits. Here are some examples of balanced breakfasts:

- granola cereal, yogurt, a sliced apple
- scrambled eggs, toast, orange juice
- veggie omelet, bran muffin, fruit with yogurt
- whole-grain pancakes or waffles topped with berries and/or yogurt, milk
- whole wheat zucchini pancakes topped with fruit, milk
- french toast topped with fruit, orange juice or milk
- low-fat cheese melted on toast, a piece of fruit
- low-fat cream cheese on a whole-grain bagel, orange juice
- peanut butter and banana slices on an English muffin, milk
- For a breakfast-on-the-run smoothie, see "School-Ade," page 309.

Of course, it's what you eat, not what you say, that impresses a child most. By treating yourself to a healthy breakfast, you model to your children that eating a healthy breakfast gives the whole family a smart nutritional start.

Smart fats. Besides being found in human milk, DHA appears in high levels in cold-water fish (sardines, salmon, albacore tuna). In addition, vegetable oils, primarily flaxseed, soy, and canola, are also rich sources of omega-3 fatty acids, with flaxseed oil being the best. The two F's, fish and flax, are the top brain-building foods for growing children and adults.

Dumb fats. Avoid factory fats, which are biochemically altered fats and recognizable by the words "hydrogenated" or "partially hydrogenated" in the fine print on the package label. The hydrogenation process produces trans fatty acids, which may affect brain function and health in two ways. First, the trans fats enter the cells of the central nervous system, where they may compete with the action of natural fats, so that the nerves in the brain don't function as well as they were designed to. Also, hydrogenation turns unsaturated fats into saturated fats, in which the fat molecules are packed together tightly, like lard. Brain researchers worry that the same type of packing could occur in blood vessels, compromising the blood flow to the brain. Avoiding hydrogenated fats is especially important for the growing brains of children, since children who fill up on these undesirable fats are likely to eat less of the omega-3 fatty acids that are good for the brain. (For more about the effects of hydrogenated fats on health and well-being, see pages 6 to 10.)

VITAMINS, MINERALS, AND FIBER

Vitamin Supplements

Studies indicate that schoolchildren whose diets are supplemented with vitamins and minerals to ensure that they receive the standard recommended dietary allowances show improved learning and score higher on intelligence tests. Here are some of the vitamins that have been shown to affect behavior and learning:

NUTRITIP
Feeding Senior Brains

Once upon a time it was believed that the brain didn't keep growing as people got older. New research, however, has shown that the brain cells continue to branch out and make connections throughout a person's life. Eating the right diet can help the brain make the right connections — at all ages.

- *Vitamin C* is required by the brain to make neurotransmitters. In fact, the brain has a special vitamin C "pump" that draws extra vitamin C out of the blood and concentrates it in the brain.
- *Vitamin B-12* is vital to maintaining healthy myelin, the sheath that covers and insulates nerve tissue.

NUTRITIP
Brainy Breakfasts

A nutriperk in yogurt could theoretically improve school performance by perking up the brain. Yogurt is relatively high in the amino acid tyrosine (a neurostimulant) and low in the amino acid tryptophan (a neurosedative). Add yogurt to other brain foods, such as flax oil (for brain-building fatty acids) and soy foods (for protein and blood-sugar stabilization), and you have three synergistic foods that form the basic ingredients for our "School-Ade" recipe (see page 309). I have personally felt the effects of this nutriperk by drinking a smoothie with these three basic ingredients each morning before I go to work.

- *Vitamin B-6* deficiency causes hyperirritability and fatigue.
- *Folic acid* deficiency seems to affect neurotransmitter function, resulting in symptoms associated with depression.

Minerals

Iron. The symptoms of iron deficiency include irritability and diminished mental alertness. Studies show that when the iron level of students increases, they concentrate better and learn better. Iron is necessary for healthy brain tissue and for adequate neurotransmitter function. (For information on a blood test to accurately check nutritional iron status, see page 61.)

Calcium. Calcium is important not only to growing bones but also to growing brains. Children with calcium deficiency may show impaired behavior and learning. In his book *Feeding the Brain: How Foods Affect Children* (Plenum,

1989), Dr. C. Keith Conners reports that children who were more hyperactive had significantly lower calcium intakes than less hyperactive children. Other studies have shown that schoolchildren who are in the habit of skipping breakfast exhibit calmer behavior when given milk in the morning. (See "Breakfasts for Growing Brains," page 310.)

Fiber

An apple a day may keep the A.D.D. doctor away. While fiber is not directly involved in brain function, it does influence how other nutrients affect the brain. Soluble fiber, such as fruit pectin, helps lower the glycemic index of foods, thereby having a stabilizing effect on blood sugar. As we discussed above, the more stable the blood sugar, the better the brain functions. A bowl of bran for breakfast and an apple as a mid-morning snack keep your brain working at top form until lunchtime.

32

Tracking Down Food Allergies

APPROXIMATELY 3 TO 7 percent of children and adults have some degree of food allergies. Food allergies have been called the great masqueraders because they are a hidden cause of so many problems, ranging from mere annoyances to downright disease. Food allergies tend to be underdiagnosed by physicians and overdiagnosed by everyone else. The truth about their prevalence is somewhere in between. In one study of children whose parents were convinced that their child had food allergies, only 39 percent of the allergies could be confirmed scientifically. Perhaps with no other medical problem is partnership between physician and patient more vital. The patient's role is to be a keen observer and accurate reporter. The physician's role is to take the information gathered by the patient (or parent) and work out a step-by-step plan for tracking down hidden food allergies and figuring out what to do about them. Here are some facts you should know about food allergies and what to do about them.

ALLERGY TERMS YOU SHOULD KNOW

Allergy. The term "allergy" comes from two Greek words, *allos* ("other") and *ergon* ("work"). If you are allergic to something, you have a reaction other than what you would expect. You don't expect to get hives when you eat a red tomato. That kind of reaction is an allergy. An allergy may manifest itself in various target organs, meaning sites where allergy signs occur. These are typically one or more of four places: the skin, the intestines, the respiratory passages, and the brain (i.e., behavior changes).

Intolerance. The term "food intolerance" means that a food upsets your intestines but does not bother any other target organ. Food intolerances are usually due to an enzyme deficiency, such as lactase, which causes lactose intolerance. Or the intestines may be oversensitive to certain foods, resulting in abdominal discomfort, diarrhea, and bloating. Food allergy is usually a reaction to the protein content of a food, but it is possible to be

---

NUTRITIP
Beware of Combination Allergies.

Allergens may appear in the most unlikely places, so get used to reading the ingredients list. A candy bar, for example, may contain corn, dairy products, gluten, soy, colorings, and additives — all of which are potential food allergens.

FOOD SUSPECTS

Most Allergenic Foods

berries	coconut	nuts	soy
buckwheat	corn	peanut butter	tomatoes
chocolate	dairy products	peas	wheat
cinnamon	egg whites	pork	yeast
citrus fruits	mustard	shellfish	

Least Allergenic Foods

apples	cauliflower	mangoes	rye
apricots	chicken	oats	safflower oil
asparagus	cranberries	papayas	salmon
avocados	dates	peaches	squash
barley	grapes	pears	sunflower oil
beets	honey	poi	sweet potatoes
broccoli	lamb	raisins	turkey
carrots	lettuce	rice	veal

Read Labels

Potentially allergenic foods may be listed under another name in packaged foods. Here are the most common:

- wheat flour: durum, semolina, farina
- egg white: albumen
- dairy products: whey, casein, sodium caseinate

   Careful label reading will help you discover what you are eating:

- Cocoa mixes, creamed foods, gravies, and some sauces contain milk.

- Margarine usually contains whey.
- Noodles and pasta contain wheat and sometimes eggs.
- Canned soups may contain wheat and dairy fillers.
- Most breads contain wheat and dairy products.
- Hot dogs, cold cuts, and "nondairy" desserts contain sodium caseinate.
- For persons who keep kosher, the word "pareve" or "parve" on a label means the food contains no milk or meat; however, recent studies on persons who suffered severe allergic reactions to "pareve"-labeled foods revealed milk residues.

AN OUNCE OF ALLERGY PREVENTION

If one parent has food allergies, the risk of the children having food allergies may double; the risks are even higher if both parents are allergic. On the other hand, a child may have a completely different food allergy from that of the parent. If you and your spouse are passing along genes that will place your child at high risk for developing food allergies, the following wise allergy-prevention measures can lower your child's chances of sneezing, wheezing, and itching by around 50 percent.

Prevent allergies prenatally. Some studies suggest that mothers who are allergic to certain foods, especially dairy products, can lessen the chances of their infants' being allergic to that food by limiting the child's exposure prenatally. Avoid bingeing on common allergens during pregnancy and while breastfeeding.

Breastfeed your baby as long as possible. The longer you breastfeed, the less chance your child has of developing allergic diseases such as eczema and asthma. Breast milk is rich in an immunoglobulin called secretory IgA, which acts as a protective paint, coating the intestines and keeping food allergens out of the bloodstream. Breast milk keeps the intestinal lining healthy and better able to break down proteins into individual amino acids. The amino acids themselves are not likely to cause allergies when they get into the bloodstream. Intestines that are damaged due to infection or inflamed by foreign milk or formula may allow whole protein molecules to seep through, setting up an allergic reaction in the bloodstream. To further decrease the risk of your child's developing food allergies, the wise breastfeeding mother will keep the most allergenic foods out of her diet until her baby is at least one year of age.

Delay the introduction of solid foods. Mature intestines are better able to screen out potential allergens and keep them from entering the bloodstream. If you feed your infant solid foods (especially those containing protein, such as wheat, soy, and dairy) before the intestinal lining is mature, food allergens can seep into the bloodstream, causing baby to build up antibodies to those allergens and later become allergic to those foods. When you do start solids, introduce the least allergenic (i.e., lowest in protein) foods first, such as fruits, vegetables, and rice. Wait until at least eighteen months before introducing potentially allergenic foods, such as egg whites, tomatoes, shellfish, and peanut butter. Make citrus fruits the last fruits you introduce. Also, if you're formula feeding, discuss with your doctor the use of a hypoallergenic formula, such as Alimentum or Nutramigen, instead of soy formulas. Also, delay introducing cow's-milk products until at least one year of age. By twelve months of age, your child's intestines are mature enough to screen out most of the food allergens.

Variety, variety, variety. The less children eat of one particular food, the less likely they will become allergic to it, since most food allergies are dose related. Encourage your children to eat a variety of foods. Continuing to bombard the body with the same food risks turning on the food-antibodies response. Rotation diets make good sense for every eater, and especially for the allergic person.

Be a pure parent. During the early years, make your child's diet as fresh and as additive-free as possible. The fewer cans, boxes, and packages you open, the less likely your child is to be exposed to allergens. Be especially vigilant about keeping food colorings out of your child's tummy, namely, yellow dye #5 and red and blue dyes. (See the related discussion of "leaky gut syndrome," page 374.)

intolerant of any part of the food, including sugar or any additives.

Food hypersensitivity. This term essentially means the same as "allergy." It's possible to lump all three of the terms ("allergy," "intolerance," and "hypersensitivity") together and simply call them "food sensitivities." Practically speaking, people don't really care about definitions; they just know that certain foods bother them (or their child) more than other foods.

Here's what goes on in your body when you're hypersensitive to a food. The suspect protein is known as an "allergen." When an allergen gets into your body, it comes into contact with the target organs, usually the skin or the lining of the breathing passages or intestines. As happens whenever something gets into your body that it doesn't like, your body mobilizes defense troops called "antibodies." When the fight breaks out be-tween these allergens and antibodies, microscopic explosions occur that release chemicals such as histamines (hence, allergy medicines are called "antihistamines") that disturb the integrity of tis-sues. Your blood vessels then dilate and produce a rash, or fluid leaks out through the injured blood vessels, causing a runny nose or puffy and watery eyes, or the muscles in the breathing passages go into spasms of wheezing. Even the brain can be bothered by an allergic reaction. A new field of re-search interest, called "brain allergy," describes the behavioral reactions of the brain when it's both-ered by certain foods.

COMMON SIGNS OF FOOD SENSITIVITIES

While individual signs and symptoms of food al-lergy are as unique as fingerprints, usually at least one of the four common target organs is involved:

COMMON SIGNS OF FOOD ALLERGY

While any food could cause just about any reaction, the following are the most common signs and symptoms of food allergy.

Skin	Respiratory Passages	Intestines	Behavior
hives	sneezing	burnlike rash around	fatigue
red, sandpaper-like	runny nose	anus	migraine headaches
facial rash	stuffy nose	abdominal discomfort	hyperactivity
dry, scaly, itchy skin	wheezing	mucusy diarrhea	crying
(mostly on face)	watery eyes	constipation	irritability
swelling in hands and	rattling chest	intestinal bleeding	night waking
feet	persistent cough	poor weight gain	anxiety
puffy eyelids	congestion	bloating, gassiness	crankiness
dark circles under eyes	bronchitis	excessive spitting up	sore muscles and joints
lip swelling	recurring ear infections	vomiting	
tongue soreness and			
cracks			

the respiratory passages, skin, intestines, or brain. While it's relatively easy to spot a rash, a wheeze, a bout of diarrhea, or abdominal cramps and attribute the problem to food allergy, brain changes are more difficult. In our experience, some children can experience behavioral changes due to food sensitivity without showing any other signs or symptoms. Most food allergies, though, attack more than one target organ. Don't be too quick to pin the rap for your child's school failure on food allergy, at least not without symptoms beyond the academic ones. Here are some facts you should know about the subtleties of food allergy:

- Food allergy symptoms vary in severity. While one mother may have to rush a wheezing child to the nearest emergency room within minutes of his eating a peanut butter sandwich, another child may develop only a nuisance-like rash around the mouth.

- It may take a few minutes, a few hours, or a few days for a food to cause a reaction. Monday's chocolate bar may be the cause of Tuesday's rash. Food allergies are often known as the "eat now, pay later" phenomenon.

- Food sensitivities are often dose related. A teaspoon of peanut butter may be no problem, but a couple of tablespoons can trigger wheezing. Some people will do just fine with one glass of milk but may get bloated after drinking three glasses. Eating shellfish every day could make you break out in an all-over body rash, while having a few shrimp every four days may be no problem.

- Even though it's possible to be allergic to just about any food, over 90 percent of food allergies, especially in young children, are caused by nine foods: dairy products, soy, shellfish, wheat, tree nuts, peanuts, egg whites, citrus fruits, and food additives.

- If you're allergic to one food in a food group, you may or may not be allergic to other foods or all the foods in that group. If you're allergic to peanuts (which is a legume, not a nut), you may be able to eat almonds, but not other foods in the legume family.

- Don't be surprised if you actually crave the food you're allergic to. When you go on an elimination diet, your body may go through withdrawal symptoms, triggering cravings for the very food that is not good for it. Sometimes the wisdom of the body breaks down. This food-craving paradox is especially true in children who are hypersensitive to sugar. When the blood sugar rises and then falls, children crave the food that will send their blood sugar skyrocketing.

- Food allergies do not interfere with a child's growth. Few foods are absolutely essential for growth. A child who is allergic to one food can certainly get the same nutrition in many other foods.

- Allergy symptoms change with age. The good news is that most children outgrow their food allergies by three years of age. The tomato-allergic toddler may become the preschooler who can safely indulge in ketchup. In particular, children tend to outgrow their sensitivity to milk and soy products; other food allergies, such as nuts and shellfish, tend to persist.

- The incidence of food allergies may be on the rise because more people are eating processed foods containing preservatives and additives. It's no wonder that the body rebels against all the foreign substances added to food in factories.

TRACKING DOWN HIDDEN FOOD SENSITIVITIES

Here's a three-step method for uncovering the food that could be bothering you or your child.

TESTING FOR FOOD ALLERGIES

At present there are no medical tests for food allergies that are more accurate than the detective work of a parent who is a keen observer and accurate recorder. In most cases, a carefully done elimination diet will uncover what the allergy is to. Your doctor or allergist can help by performing one or both of the following tests:

- *Skin test.* A skin test is helpful in uncovering hidden food allergies, but it has a high incidence of false positives, meaning, the skin test is likely to show that you or your child is allergic to a food when really you are not. A negative skin test (i.e., your child does not react to a certain food allergen injected in his skin) is a reliable indication that he is unlikely to be allergic to that food.

- *Blood test.* This test, called a RAST (Radio-Allergo-Sorbent Test), measures the antibodies in the bloodstream to certain food allergens. Unlike the skin test, a RAST has a high degree of false negatives, meaning, it does not detect food allergies that your child really has. A positive test is a reliable indicator that he is likely to be allergic to that food.

If a certain food, say peanuts, shows up positive on a RAST, that means you are more likely than not to be allergic to peanuts. If a skin test and a RAST agree, you can give the results even more weight. But keep in mind that neither skin test nor blood test is as reliable as your own observations, and they are certainly more costly. Testing may be most helpful when the results of an elimination diet are confusing.

Step 1: Keep a Food Record

Over a four-day period record everything that gets eaten. If you are keeping records for yourself, be sure to include snacks or meals you eat at work or at restaurants. If you're keeping a food record of what your child eats, do it during a four-day period when your child is home all day so you know exactly what he eats. Don't make an issue of your child's food choices during this time or he may sneak (because he craves) the very foods he's sensitive to. Enlist your child's cooperation so that together you can keep an accurate record. Also, keep track of any symptoms that you feel may be caused by food allergies.

Step 2: Try an Elimination Diet

On your list, circle the foods that you most suspect, paying particular attention to the nasty nine: dairy products, soy, egg whites, wheat, peanuts, tree nuts, citrus fruits, shellfish, and food additives. If you have no hunch about what you or your child may be allergic to, seek medical help from your doctor or an allergist (see "Testing for Food Allergies," above). Start your elimination diet at a time when there are no outside influences that make the diet impossible to follow, such as during holidays, birthdays, vacations, parties at work, and so on. Once you have picked out the most plausible offenders (with or without your doctor's allergy-testing help), eliminate these foods for at least ten days (preferably two weeks) and keep track of any reactions (see sample chart, next page). Avoid multiple-ingredient foods during this time, since these may contain multiple potential allergens, making it difficult to isolate the single offender. Focus on objective signs and symptoms; changes in mood or behavior are harder to evaluate.

Suspected Foods	Associated Symptom	Results After Elimination	Notes
milk	facial rash	rash dried up	couldn't tolerate milk; yogurt and cheese ok
strawberries	diarrhea	diarrhea lessened	
peanuts	cough watery eyes waking up 3 times a night	cough lessened drier eyes waking up once only	

Step 3: Challenge Your Findings

It's humanly impossible to be absolutely positive about offending foods and what quantities of them cause reactions. Because you don't want to eliminate nutritious foods from your own or your child's diet without good reason, it's a good idea to test your findings by reintroducing suspicious foods one at a time, seeing if the concerning signs and symptoms reappear. If they do, that food goes on your no-no list, at least for a few months. Later you can find out whether or not your allergy is dose related by reintroducing the food, beginning with a small amount once every four days and then increasing both the amount you eat and how often you eat it until your most annoying signs reappear. This threshold effect is especially characteristic of dairy allergies. Some people cannot drink even one glass of milk a day but can tolerate a cup of yogurt every other day.

The Quick-Detection Method for Zeroing In On Food Allergies

Use this method if you are a well-disciplined adult. It is more difficult to use successfully on a child.

RESTRICTIVE DIETS WHILE BREASTFEEDING

Research shows mixed results about whether maternal food restrictions during breastfeeding will lessen the risk of food allergies in babies. In fact, a study presented at the 1996 meeting of the American Academy of Allergy, Asthma, and Immunology showed a surprising result: The children of breastfeeding mothers who withheld allergenic foods from their diet later showed an *increase* in food allergies.

At present, there is some scientific basis for believing that cow's-milk products in a mother's diet can cause colicky symptoms in a baby, and therefore it would be wise for a breastfeeding mother with a family history of cow's-milk allergies to withhold dairy products from her diet, at least during the first year. It would be wise for a breastfeeding mother to seek nutritional advice from a doctor or nutritionist before going on a restrictive diet; otherwise she (and perhaps her baby) could run the risk of nutritional deficiency.

1. Eliminate the possible suspect foods, beginning with the nasty nine (see page 319), for a period of at least a week or ten days. During this time eat only the least allergenic foods, such as fresh fruits (except berries and citrus fruits), avocados, rice, barley, millet, poultry, and lamb. All the foods, if possible, should be organic and free of additives, dyes, and colorings.
2. Reintroduce one food each week to see if your symptoms reappear. How much time, energy, and expense you are willing to go to in order to track down food allergies depends on how much they bother you or your child, and whether your symptoms are getting better or worse. The good news is that most food allergies in children either become less severe or entirely disappear as they grow older. Of course, if the child is miserable and making everyone else miserable, too, you may not want to wait for him to grow older to do something about them.

LIFE-THREATENING ALLERGIES

Some food allergies, especially to nuts and shellfish, can be life threatening in very sensitive people. The windpipe may go into spasms, or the cardiovascular system may go into shock (called "anaphylaxis") within minutes of your eating a particular food. If you or your child has had one serious reaction to a food — even severe hives or wheezing — discuss with your doctor or allergist the possibility of keeping an Adrenalin-filled syringe (such as a bee-sting kit) with you for emergencies. This can be a life saver if you are not within minutes of an emergency room. To prepare yourself for using the real medicine, use a practice kit to learn what to do and how to do it. If you or your child accidentally eats a food that has caused a severe reaction before, go immediately to the nearest emergency room and sit in the waiting room for a couple of hours, just as a precaution. If the reaction is not severe enough to merit emergency treatment, you can go back home. Adults and children who are very allergic should wear a medical-alert bracelet.

SWEETENER ALLERGY

Once upon a time we physicians were all taught that the body can become allergic only to proteins. But once again, the observations of many people are at odds with scientists' findings. Many wise parents report that their infant or child goes berserk after high doses of sweeteners, such as corn syrup. Even the purists among allergists are beginning to believe in the concept of "brain allergy," meaning the chemicals a person eats can have a profound effect on biochemistry — thinking, feeling, and behaving. Corn syrup is a common sweetener in processed foods, baby formulas, and sodas. The fact that corn syrup has become so prevalent in the American diet may account for an increasing number of allergies to it. As one breastfeeding mother who successfully tracked down her infant's gassiness, diarrhea, night waking, and fussy behavior to corn syrup in her diet wrote us, "I feel that there is a corn syrup conspiracy going on in our country."

RESOURCES FOR FOOD ALLERGIES

Food Allergy Network, 10400 Eaton Place, Suite 107, Fairfax VA 22030-2208 (703-691-3179 or www.foodallergy.org). Ask for their booklet *Learning to Live with Food Allergies* or their bimonthly newsletter, *The Food Allergy News.*

Tracking Down Hidden Food Allergy, by William G. Crook, M.D. (Professional Books, 1980)

Resource for testing for food allergies: Immuno Laboratories, 1620 W. Oakland Park Blvd., Fort Lauderdale FL 33311 (800-231-9197 or www.immunolabs.com)

IV

TRIMMING THE FAMILY FAT

Most of us either carry around excess fat or fear that we do, and many of us have tried countless diets through the years that haven't worked. In this section you will learn how to keep your family lean, which requires healthy living habits as well as healthy eating habits. Besides showing you how to prevent infants and children from getting and staying fat, we'll introduce you to a new and exciting family fitness program, which we call the L.E.A.N.® (Lifestyle, Exercise, Attitude, and Nutrition) program. The L.E.A.N. program not only helps you trim down but, more important, helps your mind and your body work better for you so that you can follow the wisdom of the body to genuine well-being.

33

Fat Facts Every Family Should Know

WE OWE IT TO OUR CHILDREN to keep them from being overfat. The risk of just about every disease increases in proportion to the extra fat the body has to lug around. This is especially true when it comes to the big three killers: cancer, heart disease, and stroke. The plain fact is, *lean people are healthier and live longer.* You have probably noticed that we prefer to use the terms "fat control" and "overfat" rather than "weight control" or "overweight." Fat is the real issue. Many healthy, large-boned, muscular people are overweight according to charts and scales, yet they are lean. Muscle and bone weigh more than fat; being overfat is what harms your health. We don't want you and your family to have the goal of being thin. Rather, we want you to be lean.

WHAT "LEAN" MEANS

Scales and charts do not paint a true picture of health, which is why we don't stress the concept of "weight control," especially in growing children, who naturally must get heavier. Concerning weight control (oops, fat control), here is the master verse: *"Lean" is the most important health word you will learn.*

"Lean" means having the right percentage of body fat for your individual body type. It is feeling just a pinch of fat under your chin or seeing just a bit of pudginess around your middle. Scales tell you little about your leanness, and you can lower the figure on the scale with a crash diet that causes you to lose water and muscle weight rather than fat. You may weigh less, at least for a while, but you won't be any leaner.

Being lean is not to be confused with being skinny or scrawny, which imply an unattractively low or even unhealthy percentage of body fat due to undernourishment. Nor does lean mean lanky, which describes a person's bones and muscles, a body build influenced more by genes than by diet. Being lean means being trim, a goal that can be accomplished by anyone, regardless of genetic makeup (though, admittedly, some genes make it easier to stay lean than others).

Five factors determine how easy or difficult it is for you to be and stay lean.

Genes

Kids, look at your parents, and parents, look at your parents and grandparents. If they are (or at least in their youth were) trim, you've got a slimmer chance of ever becoming overfat (see "Hered-

EATING RIGHT FOR YOUR TYPE

A person's body type reflects what's happening on the inside. The three body types — ectomorph (tall and lean), mesomorph (medium or stocky), and endomorph (short and round) — can be remembered by relating them to fruit. An ectomorph is like a banana; a mesomorph like a pear; and an endomorph like an apple. And these three types burn calories and store fat in different ways. Apples and pears envy bananas. They can eat more food, but put on less fat. They also seem to have more reliable appetite controls. They are more likely to refuse the extra piece of cake if they're full than endomorphs and mesomorphs, who are more likely to give in to an extra piece. While the ectomorph is likely to leave a few bites on the plate, mesomorphs and endomorphs clean their plates. Genetically lean persons tend to be fat burners. Other body types tend to be fat storers. The ectomorph, or genetically lean person, tends to burn more calories during digestion and metabolism than other body types, so a greater percentage of

calories from food are burned before they even have a chance of becoming body fat. An ectomorph mom in our practice described her fat-burning metabolism this way: "I eat once, my body eats twice."

There are gender differences in how people carry around excess fat. Men tend to be apples, being wider and rounder around the chest and belly, whereas women tend to be pears, wider around the hips and thighs. It's easier to lose weight from the upper body, so apples on the L.E.A.N. program (see Chapter 35) may have quicker results than pears.

You can't change the body type you are born with any more than an apple or pear can become a banana. Even tall and lanky people can become more pear- or apple-like if they don't actively stay lean as they age. No matter how religiously you follow the L.E.A.N. program, most often an apple will remain an apple and a pear will remain a pear. The good news, though, is that you can become a leaner apple or pear.

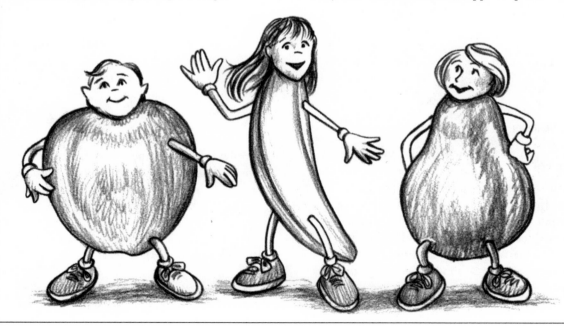

ity," below). If one or both parents or your grandparents were overfat, you can still be lean, but you'll have to work harder at it.

Body Build

Some body types stay lean more easily than others. Lean and tall (also known as "ectomorph") body types are longer and lighter than the average on the growth chart. Ectomorph babies, children, and adults are recognized (even at birth) by spindly "piano fingers" and long, slender feet. Ectomorphs seem to put more calories into height than weight. Persons with ectomorph body types are hypermetabolizers; they burn off calories more easily than other types and can better adjust their food intake to their activity level. They can eat a lot but not gain weight (which is likely to make them the envy of their calorie-watching friends). Stocky children and adults (called "mesomorphs") have average height and weight, and both height and weight are near the same percentile on the growth chart. These square-shaped bodies have a greater tendency toward being overfat than their rectangular ectomorph friends. Short and wide persons ("endomorphs") have the greatest chance of becoming and staying overfat. Few persons are pure body types; many have a combination of features.

Metabolism

Some people are born with a high metabolism. We call them "burners." They burn fat easily. Others have slower metabolisms and burn fat slowly. We call them "storers." Whether you are a fat burner or a fat storer is, like body build, an inherited tendency. On occasion I will see two children in the same family, one trim, the other overfat, yet both eat similar diets. "No fair," says Susie Overweight. "My sister gobbles up banana splits, but I'm a size sixteen, and she's a size eight."

Temperament

Active people with lots of energy burn energy, whereas couch sitters store fat. You can spot these tendencies in infancy. A lanky, wiry, very active baby, especially one with active parents, has a slim chance of becoming fat. Mellower, rounder, quieter babies tend to burn fewer calories and are at increased risk of becoming fat.

Eating Habits

Persons who eat nutrient-dense foods in proportion to their individual energy needs are more likely to stay lean. Persons who eat too many high-fat, empty calories are less likely to be lean. Any fat-control program needs to take into consideration not only the quantity, but the *quality* of the food.

The three most important facts to understand about fat control are:

1. why you get fat (Answer: You eat more calories than you burn.)
2. how you get lean (Answer: You burn more calories than you eat.)
3. how you stay lean (Answer: You program your body toward leaner eating habits and set your metabolism higher to promote fat burning. You can stay lean by eating differently, exercising more, or doing a bit of both.)

For 90 percent of children and adults, fat control is as simple as these three facts. For around 10 percent of people it's not that simple because of metabolic quirks that don't follow these rules.

HOW DO YOU GET FAT?

Some of the reasons people are overfat are under their control and some aren't. Some reasons are

THE DISEASE CONSEQUENCES OF OBESITY

Just about every organ of the body works less well when you're obese. Here are the major health problems associated with being overfat.

- *Cardiovascular disease.* With excess body fat come higher levels of blood lipids: Cholesterol, LDL (bad) cholesterol, and total triglyceride levels all increase, while HDL (good) cholesterol decreases. These lipid levels lead to bad things for your cardiovascular system. The incidence of high blood pressure also rises when you're overfat.
- *Diabetes.* Excess fat reduces the efficiency of insulin. As a result, the pancreas needs to produce more insulin and may eventually wear out, leading to diabetes.
- *Psychological and emotional problems.* Being obese definitely affects the psychosocial development of the child and adolescent. Our society places less value on fat people. Our culture rewards leanness and penalizes fatness, particularly in women. Studies have shown that obese children are more likely to develop a poor self-image and low self-esteem. They are prone to social isolation and, because they compete poorly in athletics, often choose more sedentary activities, which further increases their fat. Obesity is a problem not just of the body but also the mind. Obsession with being

fat and becoming thin presents its own problems, such as anorexia and bulimia.
- *Sleep apnea.* A study showed that 33 percent of severely obese persons had sleep apnea, a problem with breathing during sleep, that was severe enough to cause restlessness at night and interfere with the ability to work and think the following day.
- *Orthopedic problems.* Especially in growing children and adolescents, increased weight bearing on the hips and knee bones tends to cause bowed legs, to the extent that the leg bones are more likely to slip out of the hipbones (a condition called "slipped femoral epiphysis"). Arthritis is also more common in obese persons. Losing weight eases the workload for arthritic joints.
- *More infections.* One study showed that fat babies get twice as many infections as slim babies. Another study demonstrated that the ability of white blood cells to fight infection is reduced in obese persons.
- *Increase in other health problems.* The risks of gallstones, headaches, kidney problems, and colon cancer all increase when you're overfat.

Medical studies show that leaner people live longer. Get lean for life and you'll enjoy life longer.

---

obvious and some are not so apparent. Here are the facts you should know about your body's fat-storing habits.

Heredity

Do fat parents usually produce fat children? Statistics say yes. Lean parents have only a 7 percent

chance of having an obese adolescent. If one parent is obese, there is a 40 percent chance, and if both parents are obese, the probability of the child's being obese may be as high as 80 percent. Genes may actually be a more powerful determinant of obesity than diet. Studies on adopted children show that their body weight tends to be more like their biological parents' than their adopting ones'. Studies of identical twins reared in different environments with different parental eating habits showed a tendency toward similar fatness or leanness. But don't be too quick to blame your parents. Genes influence whether or not children or adults become fat, but diet and lifestyle, both of which are under your control, also play a role. It's what you do with the genes you inherit that determines whether you will wind up fat or lean.

Are fat children more likely to become fat adults? Yes and no. One study showed that nine out of ten obese infants became lean by the time they were seven. Yet, obese infants are still three times more likely to be fat at age seven than infants who have been lean from the start. Studies have also shown that 40 percent of obese seven-year-olds are likely to become obese adults, 70 percent of obese preteens are likely to become obese adults, and around 80 percent of obese adolescents are obese as adults. The fatter children are in the first few years of life and the longer they keep their excess fat, the greater the likelihood they will remain fat into adolescence and adulthood.

Diet

Does overeating lead to overfattening? Most studies show that fat children and adults do not eat more than lean ones, and some may even eat less. Believe it or not, some overeaters may actually have nutritional deficiencies. What's significant, however, is that while fat persons do not necessarily eat more food, they do eat more calories than they burn off through exercise. The fat person may also have a slower metabolism than the lean person. Also, studies show that fat persons are more likely than lean persons to eat foods higher in fat. They may get around 40 percent of their calories from fat instead of the recommended 20 to 25 percent.

A fat calorie is fatter than a protein or carb calorie. It's a myth that a calorie is a calorie is a calorie. Calories from fat are more fattening than calories from proteins or carbohydrates. Our bodies tend to store excess calories from fat as fat more readily than they do excess calories from carbohydrates or proteins. And not only does the body store fat calories more easily, it also burns them less readily. The body, plotting to protect itself from starvation, will use up carbohydrate stores for energy before dipping into the fat reserves. In addition, the body uses more energy (or calories) to metabolize carbohydrates and proteins than it uses to burn fats. Fatty foods tend to pack more calories into a smaller volume than do carbohydrate and protein foods. Because the stomach takes its cues for fullness based upon food volume rather than calories, calorie for calorie fat is less satisfying.

Sugar can make you fat, too. The hormone insulin doesn't just control sugar, it also controls fat. Insulin also helps the body store excess sugar as fat. Junk sugars and other carbohydrates with a high glycemic index (for an explanation of the GI, see page 35) are the most likely to be stored as fat. Insulin bursts following the ups and downs of blood sugar also contribute to fat storage, which is why five mini meals a day that keep your blood sugar steady are more likely to keep you lean than three big meals. Once you get overfat from sugar, a vicious cycle may begin, according to a new metabolic theory called *"insulin resistance"* (IR).

This is how IR works: When sugar enters the bloodstream, the pancreas secretes a dose of insulin high enough to usher the sugar into the muscle cells and other organs, where it's needed for energy. If a lot of sugar enters the bloodstream, the pancreas releases a lot of insulin. Some people develop a metabolic quirk in which the cells begin to resist the insulin. When this happens, glucose levels in the blood do not drop, so the body secretes even more insulin, which can cause two problems: The overworked pancreas may gradually wear out, resulting in diabetes; and the excess insulin promotes more fat storage. The theory of insulin resistance also explains why some people become fat even if they do not take in too many calories. They just eat too many carbohydrates *for them.* Not all nutrition experts believe in the concept of insulin resistance, but, because we have a daughter with this metabolic quirk, we have thoroughly researched the issue and have concluded that for some people there really is a possibility that being overfat is more the result of producing too much insulin than of overeating.

Actually, fatness produces more fatness. The more sugar you eat, the higher your blood sugar rises, so the more insulin you secrete. This causes the blood sugar to fall, which makes you hungry again, so you eat more and continue the cycle. It's interesting that a diet with adequate amounts of omega-3 fatty acids (found in fish and flaxseed oils) will improve insulin efficiency by helping the body use up carbohydrates and fats for fuel. Imagine — a fat that fights fat!

Endocrine Disorders

"Doctor, could it be her thyroid?" is a common question of parents seeking counsel for their obese adolescent. Generally, but not always, if an endocrine disorder is causing the obesity, it will also cause children to be short. Most children who are obese, especially from overnutrition, tend to be taller than average, or at least average height. A short, fat child should always undergo a complete medical evaluation.

Metabolism and Fat Type

New insights into obesity are showing that for an increasing number of persons, obesity is a metabolic as much as a behavioral problem. True, many people are overfat because of unhealthy eating behaviors, but new medical discoveries suggest that problems such as insulin resistance (see page 328) and differences in how people metabolize fat are also important contributors to obesity.

Another possible explanation comes from the difference between white fat and brown fat. White fat is the fat that pads the body near the surface. It makes up 90 percent of total body fat. Brown fat, which makes up the other 10 percent, is located deeper in the body, primarily within the upper back, around the nape of the neck, the armpits, between the shoulder blades, and deep in the chest cavity. Brown fat primarily burns calories, whereas white fat stores calories. Some overfat people either have less brown fat than most people, or else the brown fat they have is not as easily triggered into fat burning as it should be, so they tend to store fat rather than burn fat.

The Fat Cell Theory

You may have heard the theory that a person is destined to become lean or fat based on the accumulation of fat cells early in life. The fat cell theory states that during the first two years of life (considered to be one of the critical periods for fat cell development), there is normally an increase in fat cell number. Other spurts in the number of fat cells come in middle childhood, around seven years of age, and again during adolescence. After a person is finished growing and reaches adulthood, the number of fat cells remains constant. The size of these cells may change, but they will not decrease in number. Thus someone who is overnourished in childhood (or genetically programmed to grow more fat cells) will have an excess number of fat cells, making it more difficult to control his weight as an adult. While there may be some truth to this fat cell theory (one of the reasons we stress the importance of raising a lean child), new insights suggest that neither the number nor the size of the fat cells is genetically fixed or set for life. It is certainly possible for previously overfat children or adults to become lean for the rest of their lives.

Senior Fat

As you age, your body tends to gain fat. The good news is that this happens only if you let it. One of the reasons that there is more fat in an older body is that people at retirement age, especially males, may actually have 25 percent less muscle mass than they did in their twenties. Since muscle burns calories, a sixty-year-old person eating the same number of calories as he did in his twenties is going to get fat. Add to this the fact that an older person may not be as active or as able to exercise. Exercising more and eating more wisely will combat this trend. Many people by the time they are sixty years of age are more motivated to watch what they eat in order to avoid disease. Unfortunately, many people don't discover the nutrition-disease connection until they've already gotten some disease. As a tribute to the wisdom of the aging body, most persons in their fifties can simply not "stomach" the quantity of junk food that makes up the diet of most young folk. The key to having an older yet healthier body is acquiring nutritional wisdom when you are young.

34

Lean from the Start: Trimming Kids' Fat

THE EARLIER YOU START growing a lean child, the greater the chance you'll be the parent of a lean adult.

TRIMMING BABY FAT

You've heard that the first three years are formative years for intellectual and psychological development. Well, these are also important years for forming healthy eating habits. The nutritional habits acquired by the toddler become her norms. This is when she learns what eating is all about and recognizes how her body is supposed to feel. If the toddler grows up lean, with a lean set point (for an explanation of the term "fat point," see page 341), the child is more likely to stay lean. Try these seven ways to start your baby off lean.

1. Breastfeed. Many experts believe that breast-fed infants are less likely to become obese than formula-fed infants, but studies comparing the two groups have not produced clear results, partly because of problems with study design but also because many other factors also contribute to obesity. Let's approach this question instead from the commonsense point of view. It seems to us that a breastfed baby is more likely to learn healthy appetite-control habits, a major factor in determining leanness or obesity.

Breastfeeding leaves the infant in control of the feedings, how much he takes, and with a responsive mother, how often he eats. The bottlefeeding mother can take control of the feeding away from the baby. She counts ounces and watches the clock. A breastfeeding mother is more likely to watch the baby for cues. As she reinforces the baby's cues, he learns to trust his body's signals. An interesting study showed that formula-fed infants, if allowed to determine for themselves how much formula to drink, can self-regulate their total daily calories quite well. Six-week-old infants can adjust their formula intake according to their calorie needs. If the experimenter substituted a more dilute, lower-calorie formula, the infants drank more, making an adjustment for the lower energy levels. With bottlefeeding, maternal control can override the infant's automatic regulatory ability, as mother urges the baby to take "just a little bit more." Baby comes to expect that "stuffed" feeling after a meal and eventually seeks it out for herself.

A breastfed baby gets custom-calorie milk. The fat content of breast milk changes during each feeding and also at different periods of the day. At the beginning of a nursing, when a baby is most hungry, she gets a large volume of foremilk, rich

KIDS (AND ADULTS) AT RISK OF GETTING FAT

Low Fat Risks	High Fat Risks
• slim genes from parents or grandparents	• fat genes in family
• naturally slim body build	• stocky body build
• a high metabolism (fat burner)	• low metabolism (fat storer)
• active temperament and lifestyle	• sedentary temperament and lifestyle
• watches little TV	• watches a lot of TV
• lean eating habits	• fat eating habits

In counseling parents about their children's weight issues, that is, whether or not they need to worry about how much guidance a child needs, I first look at the parents themselves, second at the child, and third at the eating and lifestyle habits of the family. I look at the growth chart and the scale last. Children who are in the low-risk category don't need much fat-control counseling. Families in the high-risk category need a high level of early intervention, which can prevent obesity in adulthood. Children and adults do not inherit obesity, they simply inherit the tendency. How they learn to eat and live with this tendency determines whether they will grow up to be fat or lean.

in protein and carbohydrates but low in calories. If the baby is very hungry, she continues sucking, and the fat levels in the milk rise (the hindmilk). This tells the infant that it's time to slow down because she is getting satisfied. When you watch breastfeeding babies at the end of a feeding, you will notice how they radiate contentment, sucking needs and appetite both completely satisfied. When a breastfeeding baby is thirsty rather than hungry, or just wants to soothe herself, baby sucks in a way that makes the breast deliver only the lower-calorie foremilk for a quick pick-me-up or some "calm me down" comfort. A formula-fed baby receives the same kind of formula, regardless of whether he is hungry, thirsty, or just needs to suck for comfort. Responding to the baby or toddler's different needs for food and comfort is more complicated with bottle feedings. Allowing a toddler to walk around with a bottle just to "keep him quiet," or offering formula at every peep from an infant could condition the child to connect eating with comforting. Breastfeeding conditions the child to connect comfort with a person. Developmentally these are known as "patterns of association," whereby an infant stores in the file library of his developing brain these associations to be replayed later on.

The fat content of mother's milk changes as baby's growth decelerates. Breast milk changes from "whole milk" to "reduced-fat milk" sometime during the second half of the first year, another biological sign that leanness is nature's intent. In fact, recent research has shown that breastfed babies, after the first four to six months, are leaner than their formula-fed peers, as they gain proportionally more height than weight. Formula-fed babies tend to get solid foods earlier and gain proportionally more weight than height, suggesting an early tendency away from leanness.

2. Delay solids. The longer you wait to start your baby on solid foods, the lower the risk of your baby getting overfat, especially a baby who neither looks lean nor has lean parents. When you do begin solids, begin with the most nutrient-dense foods, those that pack the most nutrition in the fewest calories, such as vegetables rather than fruit, and whole grains over sweets.

3. Watch for low-cal cues. It's easy to interpret every cry as baby needing food, but maybe baby is thirsty, physically uncomfortable, lonesome, or just wants to be held. Especially if you are formula feeding, sometimes try to pacify your baby by holding him or playing with him rather than simply plugging a bottle into him. If you are still unable to calm baby, try a bit of water or a pacifier, since baby may just be thirsty or in need of sucking.

4. Don't fill your baby with juice. Juices are not nutrient-dense foods. Fruit juices straight out of the carton contain nearly as many calories as the same volume of milk or formula but are much less nutritious and filling. Babies can consume a much larger quantity of juice than breast milk or formula without feeling full. Excess juice can be a subtle cause of infant obesity. Instead of full-strength juice, dilute the juice at least half with water, or if you feel baby is simply thirsty, use a small amount of juice simply to flavor the water.

5. Get baby moving. Most babies when awake are in constant motion anyway, so you don't actually have to put your baby on an exercise program. But there are some mellow babies who are content with visual stimulation. They like to lie and look rather than wiggle and crawl. The plumper the baby, the less baby likes to budge, leading to the cycle of inactivity and fatness. Get down on the floor and play with your baby. Or put on some music and dance around with your toddler.

6. Respect tiny tummies. Babies' tummies are about the size of their fists, so that small, frequent feedings (the breastfeeding pattern) are more physiologically correct than larger, less frequent feedings (the bottlefeeding pattern). To appreciate this bottle–tummy size mismatch, compare a full bottle to baby's fist. You will be less likely to urge baby to "finish the bottle."

7. Respect toddler tummies. Just about every day in my pediatrics practice, some parent complains, "My toddler is such a picky eater." Over the years I've come to realize that toddlers pick and peck at food because toddlers are made that way. During the first year, babies eat a lot because they grow a lot, tripling their birth weight by one year of age. Between the first and second birthdays, the normal toddler may get only one-third heavier. Many toddlers grow proportionally more in height than in weight in the second year, burning off excess baby fat and gradually becoming more lean. If you understand this as a normal stage that most toddlers go through, you will be less obsessed about your toddler's eating patterns.

TRIMMING CHILDHOOD FAT

Obesity affects one in four children in the United States. The National Health and Nutrition Examination Survey (NHANES) done between 1988 and 1994 showed that 11 percent of American children and adolescents are overfat and an additional 14 percent are at risk of becoming obese. This represents a 30 percent increase in childhood obesity over the previous decade. Whereas nutritional deficiency is the most prevalent nutritional problem in developing countries, overnutrition, or obesity, is the number-one nutritional disease of children, adolescents, and adults in the United States. As children get older, it becomes more difficult to keep them lean. You have less control over what they eat at home and especially away from home. Peers and television compete with family as models for eating habits. But you are still the most important influence on your child's behavior. Here are sixteen ways to help your child stay lean.

1.   Monitor snacks. Children like and need to graze. As we have previously discussed, grazing on many mini meals throughout the day is less likely to make you overfat than packing in three big meals a day. Since children get a large percentage of their calories from between-meal snacks, encourage them to snack on nutrient-dense, low-fat foods rather than on foods that pack a lot of calories and little nutrition. (For examples of nutrient-dense foods, see page 352).

2.   Avoid the "clean plate syndrome." Don't feel it is your responsibility to fill your child up, since children need to develop and exercise their own internal appetite-control signals. Your job is to make nutritious food available and to serve it creatively. The rest is up to your child. The fact is, many children don't empty their plates because parents put too much food on them in the first place. Better to dole out small dollops of food and replenish the plate when the first helping is gone.

3.   Discourage boredom eating. Children often turn to the refrigerator for satisfaction when what they are really craving is something to do and someone to do it with. It may be tempting for a caregiver to offer snacks rather than devote time and energy to nurturing the whole child. Discourage your child from eating alone in front of the television set. Encourage activities that boost children's interests rather than their body fat. Get them busy with things they enjoy doing.

4.   Resist using food as a reward. Using food as a reward or as a source of pleasure outside of nutritional needs may instill unwise eating habits in children who are already at risk for becoming obese. It's okay to associate a trip to grandmother's house with chocolate chip cookies or social occasions with special meals. Food for pleasure or food for a reward deserves a PG rating — that is, parental guidance is necessary. A special outing with mom or dad or a special friend is a more effective reward than a lollipop for a job well done.

RAISING ACTIVE KIDS

Most children certainly do not need a planned exercise program since, as one photographer father told us, "There is no such thing as a still shot of my children." Most children are by nature wiggly, jiggly, always moving little bodies that burn calories and exhaust their caregivers. Yet there are some quiet-by-nature children who need a little parental guidance to get moving. Here are some family exercise tips:

- *Plan a workout for two.* If you go to the gym or have a regular exercise program yourself, include your child. Work out together at home, in the park, at the gym, or in the pool.

- *Work out while you watch.* Put exercise machines in the TV room and work out while you watch. Mini trampolines, exercise bikes, and jump ropes are great fat-burning equipment to have in parts of the house where kids hang out.

- *Take up a family sport.* This could be bike riding, hiking, jogging, games of tag in the park, soccer, or even games such as hide-and-seek. When we took up ballroom dancing, our kids caught the spirit. Occasionally, the main activity in the rec room turns from TV watching to swing dancing. Take up whatever lifestyle exercises your family enjoys to get everyone moving.

TRAFFIC-LIGHT EATING

Bring your children up to understand that different foods have different values. "Green-light" foods are "go for it" foods. They're great for you — eat all you want of these. "Yellow-light" foods are "think about it" foods. They are okay in moderation but should be reserved for treats and eaten only occasionally, not as a steady diet. "Red-light" foods are "stop, say no, bad for you" foods. At the very least avoid eating too many of them. Here are samples of each catogory:

Green-Light Foods	Yellow-Light Foods	Red-Light Foods
vegetables	pies	hot dogs (most)
legumes	cakes	nitrite-containing meats
fruits	butter	packaged foods with
whole grains	cookies, pastries	hydrogenated oils
fish	candy	marshmallows
pasta	fast foods	punches and drinks with
nuts and seeds	fruit drinks	added colorings
soy products; tofu	white bread	cotton candy
eggs	doughnuts	crushed ice drinks (mostly
meat and poultry (lean)	sodas	syrup and dyes)
dairy products (low-fat or	frozen yogurt	cereals with dyes and
nonfat)		hydrogenated oils
vegetable oils		fast foods fried in
(unhydrogenated)		hydrogenated oils
healthy treats		
(unhydrogenated)		

These activities are more likely to feed the child's self-esteem than simply more icing on the cake is. You'll also avoid sending confusing signals about food.

5. Encourage impulse control and delayed gratification. Help your child learn to say no to that second scoop of ice cream or extra piece of cake. Just say no to the candy racks at supermarket checkout counters. Promise a nutritious treat instead or, better still, special time with you when the shopping is done. If your child throws a tantrum about not getting three scoops of ice cream, or even two, talk her through it in terms she can understand: "Your tummy isn't big enough to hold that much ice cream and you'll feel yucky afterward." Children don't like to wait for anything, especially food, but try this promise: "If you still want another piece of cake later, you may have one." Later the child may be so engrossed in another activity that he forgets about that promised extra piece of cake, or he'll find he just doesn't want it.

6. Trim TV watching. Today's preschool and school-age children watch an average of twenty-five to thirty-five hours of TV a week. This contributes to obesity for two reasons: lack of fat-burning exercise and a slowed metabolic rate associated with TV watching. Here are some other

SIT STILL AND EAT YOUR CHIPS — NOT!

Children today are approximately 10 pounds heavier for the same height than they were ten years ago, and over the past ten years, the rate of obesity has doubled. These trends have been attributed to two main factors: the increasing number of hours that children spend watching TV and the fact that packaged and fast foods make up an increasingly large proportion of a child's diet. TV watching may contribute to obesity for two reasons: It's a sedentary activity to begin with, and studies have found that a person's metabolic rate may actually slow during TV watching, burning even less fat than might otherwise be expected in a body that's sitting still. A third contributor to the modern obesity trend is unsupervised eating. Children left alone will often overdose on junk food. So, while a medically legitimate cause for obesity may occur in around 10 percent of children and adults, the other 90 percent are overfat because they eat too much, exercise too little, or both. A study by the National Institutes of Health in 1994 showed that young adults in the twenty-five-to-thirty age group were on average 10 pounds heavier than the same age group in 1986. Their conclusion was that Americans are getting fatter for three reasons: a decrease in the quality of eating habits, a decrease in the nutritional quality of the food, and a decrease in exercise. Also, early habits do influence later obesity. Children who are less active have a greater tendency to become fatter adults.

concerns about the connection between obesity and TV watching:

- Studies indicate that for adolescents, fatness correlates directly with the amount of time spent watching TV.

- TV watching encourages both inactivity and the consumption of high-calorie snack foods, a double-whammy for getting overfat. While tuning in the tube, it's easy to tune out your body's signals for appetite control. Next thing you know you've downed a whole bag of chips without realizing it, and you probably won't feel like taking a long walk to burn it off either.

- Advertising definitely affects children's eating habits. The largest share of advertising during children's programming is for food products, and according to one study, 80 percent of these advertisements are for foods with low nutritional value, including highly sugared cereals and highly sugared and high-fat snack foods. And the advertising pays off. Studies show that children's requests for foods are related to the frequency with which they see those foods on TV, and children exposed to food advertisements select more sugared foods than children who have not viewed any advertisements. The conclusion of these advertising studies was that repeated exposure to advertising may foster children's preferences for high-calorie and nutrient-poor foods, contributing greatly to childhood obesity. Commercials teach children that food should be a source of fun and entertainment rather than a source of balanced nutrition. Unfortunately, many children believe that what the commercials promise is true, especially when they see their parents eating or drinking what's advertised. Teach your child to be skeptical about advertising and not to believe something just because it's on television.

7. **Model good eating habits.** As you eat, so your child eats. If your child sees you overindulge, he most likely will overindulge, too. It is much easier for your child to learn to discipline his ap-

petite when he sees you eating appropriate amounts of healthy food. Children are very quick to pick up on the ways parents use food for gratification. Studies show that children follow the example of their parents and caregivers when it comes to eating habits. Dieting mothers are more likely to have dieting daughters, and parents with compulsive eating problems are more likely to have children with the same eating patterns. Girls seem to be more influenced by parental eating habits than are boys. Parents shape their children's behavior in all aspects of life, and they are particularly influential in shaping their children's eating habits.

8. Back off on power struggles. Don't make food a control issue. You're like to lose, if not in the short run, certainly in the long run. Eating, like toileting, is a function children need to control. Eating, like sleeping, is an activity you can't force a child into. Parents have a natural tendency to coerce, beg, threaten, or bribe children to "clean your plate," "eat your veggies," or "don't expect dessert unless you finish your broccoli." To many parents, a clean plate is reassurance that they are doing their job well. The unspoken message may even be "love me, love the food I put in front of you." Studies show that parental attempts to assert control over food habits often backfire. In fact, the more parents encourage a child to eat a particular food, the more a child may dislike that food. Constant pressure to eat veggies makes children less likely to eat their vegetables. Parents can get better results by simply eating the vegetables themselves and letting their children "catch" the good eating habit. Restricting or forbidding a particular food increases the child's desire for that food and even his consumption of it. The occasional use of food as a reward for doing non-food-related jobs may increase the child's appetite for that food. Give choices: "Do you want broccoli or a salad?" "Which salad-bar restaurant do you want to go to?" Compliment the child: "Good choice!"

as she chooses corn on the cob instead of a sweet treat.

Even subtle parent prompts can shape children's eating habits in unexpected ways. The "poor, starving children in Africa" speech may get plates cleaned at dinnertime, but these members of the clean-plate club may grow up to overeat and be overfat. Studies show that parents who try to exert a high degree of control over a child's eating habits tend to produce children who are unable to control their eating on their own and who eat more high-fat foods. Girls are more likely than boys to be affected by parental dietary controls. Just as in all aspects of discipline, the key is to shape your child's eating behavior, not control it.

9. Take baby steps. Suddenly switching from a junk-food family to a bunch of "health nuts" is likely to drive children into temptation at the junk-food family next door. Like introducing solids to babies, the key is to do it *gradually*.

10. Get your child moving. The National Health and Nutrition Examination Survey (NHANES) showed some surprising changes in the American diet between 1988 and 1994. Daily calorie intake in young children and adolescents remained the same, with calorie intake increasing in proportion to their level of exercise. Older adolescents and adults, however, did show an increase in daily calorie intake; that is, they ate too much. Surprisingly, the percentage of calories from fat in the American diet continued a downward trend. The most disturbing finding was that children exercised less in 1994 than 1988, and this seems to be one of the most important factors influencing the trend toward obesity in children and adolescents. Obese children more often choose sedentary pastimes, and even when they participate in team sports, they are less active than their lean teammates.

We are left with the chicken-or-egg question, which came first, the inactivity or the obesity?

Studies suggest that these inactive children are that way from infancy. Infants with only moderate food intake but with quiet, placid personalities are more likely than more active children to become obese. An infant with a very active temperament may not become fat even with a high calorie intake. Unfortunately, with time, a vicious cycle results. The less active the child, the more chubby he becomes, which leads the child to become less interested in physical activity. His sports skills may have been meager to begin with, and as his abilities fall further behind those of his peers, the less he'll want to participate.

To help our family stay lean, we have put exercise equipment in the TV room. We have also outlawed snacking while watching TV. Our family TV is now flanked by a treadmill and an exercise bicycle. The children watch me exercise while I watch sports and occasionally ask, "Daddy, can I use your treadmill while watching TV?" The television-exercise combination results in a good old enjoyable family fat burn. A family running or bicycling outing would be even better, but sometimes dad needs his football fix.

11. Send your child off to school with a good nutritional start. Studies show that breakfast skippers tend to overeat the rest of the day, so that the total number of daily calories goes up rather than down. Hunger triggers the neurotransmitters that stimulate eating, so a child who skips breakfast overcompensates in the afternoon and evening. (See the related discussions "The Chemistry of Cravings," page 44, and "Breakfasts for Growing Brains," page 310.) Get your child up early enough in the morning to eat a good breakfast. And pack a healthy lunch for him, too.

12. Water down the sodas. Children, especially teens, are more likely to head to the soda vending machine than the water fountain. Besides having no nutritional benefit (and in fact robbing the body of calcium), sodas (even diet sodas) can be a subtle cause of obesity. Soft drinks contain 5 to 10 teaspoons of sugar per serving, and they trigger the sugar-insulin-fat cycle. Offer your child healthy alternatives to soda: bottled water, diluted fruit juice, or fruit juice and soda water mixes.

13. Use positive motivators. You want to trim your child's fat, not her self-esteem. Rather than use phrases that focus on body image, such as, "so you don't get fat" or "to help you lose weight," use more positive messages that focus on fun and what her body can do. Offer healthful foods "to help you run faster," or "to help you play basketball better." Market carrots as "good for your eyes" and fruit as an energy food for playing after school.

14. Remove overeating cues. Foods that trigger overeating should be hidden, or maybe left in the supermarket. If a bag of fatty chips stimulates a child to plop down in front of the TV and eat until they're gone, don't have chips in the house. Most of us weaklings eat what we see. Out of sight keeps it out of the stomach. Buffets, except for salad bars, are off-limits for compulsive eaters.

15. Set realistic goals. If your child is overfat, an achievable goal is to stay the same weight for one year. For a growing child this amounts to a relative fat loss. Enlist your doctor's help in monitoring your child's progress with periodic "health checks," not "weight checks."

16. Serve nutrient-dense foods. Teach children which foods contain more for less. Nutrient-dense foods pack in more nutrition per calorie than junk foods, which are dense in calories but not in nutrition. (See page 352 for a discussion and examples of nutrient-dense foods.) A proven approach in teaching children about nutrient-dense foods is known as a "traffic light" approach (see page 335). It's more important to teach children what to eat differently than to get them to eat less. If you want your child to be lean, don't put her on a diet. Just change her diet.

35

Trimming Adult Fat: The L.E.A.N.® Program

WHEN I CHANGED MY LIFESTYLE after having surgery for colon cancer, I found myself feeling better and trimmer than I ever had before. So I began to ask myself, why am I feeling so good? The answer was summed up by the acronym L.E.A.N., which stands for *l*ifestyle, *e*xercise, *a*ttitude, and *n*utrition. These are the four keys to optimal health and well-being. Too bad I, like most others, waited to discover this until after I experienced a life-changing catastrophic event, such as a heart attack, a stroke, or, in my case, cancer. Ideally, people should get on the L.E.A.N. program before they get sick and use this rejuvenating program not only to prevent illness but simply to feel great!

This program uses the principle of "synergy." When you get all four facets of the program working together, the whole is greater than the sum of its parts. In this case, 1 + 1 + 1 + 1 = 5, or maybe even 10! Synergy is a principle employed both in biochemistry and in human relations. Think tanks put a group of people together in a room, each one with a different field of expertise, and they feed off one another, developing ideas together that none of them could have thought of alone. Put a group of nutrients together in a well-balanced meal, and the body absorbs the nutrients

better than it would if the same vitamins and minerals were isolated in a capsule. When you put all the four components together, each individual one works better.

Most diets fail because people tire of the program, get bored, or resent all the things they have to give up. The L.E.A.N. program works because the returns are so great that you don't feel you're giving up anything. Once you're into the L.E.A.N. program, it becomes self-motivating. You begin to feel so good that you want to do everything you can to perpetuate the feeling. Up to this point, this book has been concerned almost exclusively with nutrition, but practically speaking, you can't isolate what you eat from other parts of your life. That's why we've included this chapter about the L.E.A.N. program, so that you can maximize the benefits of eating wisely. Becoming a lean adult is about more than just the food you put into your body.

The great news is that once you become lean, you have a greater chance of staying lean if you are paying attention to lifestyle, exercise, and attitude, as well as good nutrition. You will have reprogrammed your mind and body, and your internal monitors will steer you to what's good for you and away from what's bad. You'll not only eat right but will also have a basic drive to continue eating right. You'll crave exercise, and you'll be satisfied with less food.

There are more should's than should not's in the L.E.A.N. program. And the results last, unlike other diet and fitness programs that promise quick results but don't deliver in the long run. You'll feel *fit*. You'll fit better not only into your clothing but also with your family, your job, and yourself. I am now two years into the L.E.A.N. program. It has enriched my life, and it will enrich yours. Let's get started.

LIFESTYLE

The L.E.A.N. program calls for a close look at your lifestyle, including your job, your relationships, the way you spend your leisure time, how much sleep you get, how you experience stress — even your spiritual life. Some of these things you may believe you can't change, but you can. We all know that smoking and excessive drinking are bad for health, and we won't belabor the obvious by listing the hazards of each. Cutting out these habits is an important part of a healthy lifestyle. A healthy lifestyle can also be defined in a positive sense: a life filled, as much as possible, with work, relationships, habits, and activities that contribute to your well-being.

Realize that no one is able to live a stress-free life all day every day. (That would be boring.) But you can make choices about how to cope with stress. Do the best you can. Pat yourself on the back for the positives and don't dwell on the negatives.

If you have a job that drives you to junk food, makes it impossible for you to exercise, and grinds you down with daily stress, you need to make some changes. You may not be able to run off and join a vegetarian monastery, but what can you do to improve your life? Walk to work? Keep an apple in your briefcase? Do deep-breathing exercises for five minutes at your desk? Put a little more energy into relationships that build you up? Shed

---

WHAT L.E.A.N. MEANS

Being lean does not mean being skinny. It means having the right amount of body fat for your body type. This means around 15 percent body fat for most men and around 18 percent for women. Individuals who are more muscular, athletes in training, or genetically slim people may lower this by two or three percentage points and still be healthy. Being lean involves more than just carrying around less fat. It means keeping an eye on all these factors that influence health:

L Lifestyle: This means healthy living without smoking, excessive alcohol, or other unhealthy substances.

E Exercise: One of the healthiest ways to stay lean is exercise. The more muscle you have, the more fat calories you can burn.

A Attitude: Trim the fat in your feelings by keeping your mind off counterproductive stuff.

N Nutrition: Emphasize a low-fat diet.

---

those that are tearing you down? Does your marriage need some enriching? There are always things you can change to make your life better. The L.E.A.N. program encourages you to go ahead and make these changes for the health of body, mind, soul, and spirit.

You may need to make some drastic lifestyle changes. Isn't your life worth changing jobs? The "L" in lifestyle could also stand for "love" and "laughter." If there are not enough of these two "L's" in your job, relationships, habits, or activities, some changes are needed. For some people, change is difficult, since the body and the mind often resist change, but remind yourself we're talking about change for the better, not for the worse.

EXERCISE

We have yet to see a diet work in which exercise is not at least of equal importance with healthy eating. In the L.E.A.N. program, exercise is nutrition's close partner. Why not just stay on the couch and eat less? Restrictions on calories, the basis of most diets, are the main reason most diets don't work. Years of taking in more calories slows your metabolism, sort of like a mechanic turning down an engine's idle speed. When you turn down your idle speed, you burn less fuel, and therefore less fat. Burning calories off by exercise boosts your metabolism. Combine this with a diet that emphasizes nutrient-dense foods without empty calories, and you are much more likely to stay lean than you would if you only cut back on calories. The good news is that the people who need exercise the most (the overweight, sedentary, poorly nourished, etc.) are the ones most helped by it. In a nutshell, exercise contributes to your health in these ways:

- burns fat
- increases muscle, which burns calories
- decreases the risk of nearly all major diseases
- releases "feel good" hormones that contribute to your overall sense of well-being

The Health Benefits of Exercise

Exercise will help you lose fat and become lean. But there are even more important reasons to exercise. Exercise not only for health but also for life. Here are the main health benefits of exercise:

RESETTING YOUR FAT POINT

Buried somewhere in the brain, physiologists believe, is a sort of *appestat,* which regulates how often and how much you eat. This appestat control is the *fat point* (also known as the "set point"), the fat level your body has gotten used to. Your body believes that it needs to maintain this fat level to protect you against the day when food may not be so plentiful. It believes this fat level is important to your well-being, and it will strive to maintain this level of body fat. So your body resists any attempt to lose fat or to lower the fat point, which is one of the reasons people who lose weight tend to regain it. If you suddenly start to eat less, your body thinks, "Oh, my goodness, it's a famine. Hoard the fat." Your metabolic rate slows (like a hibernating bear's), and your appetite increases. You may struggle to stay on your diet, but your fat point insists that you store fat rather than burn it. Losing weight becomes very difficult, but if you follow your appetite and eat more, you may push your fat point even higher.

What you have to do is trick the fat point by gradually easing down your daily calories. The fat point gradually lowers, and your body becomes more comfortable with the idea of burning fat stores, because there seem to be adequate amounts of food available. When your body gets accustomed to lower-calorie eating, it becomes more efficient, using more energy instead of storing it. *So, the key to getting and staying lean is to set your fat point to burn fat rather than to store fat.* How do you do this? By eating right and exercising more.

Exercise plays an important role in resetting your appestat. If you've been dieting and losing weight steadily but then reach a plateau, your body has probably decided this is a good fat balance for you. Stepping up the amount of exercise you do will push your body back into fat-burning mode and you'll continue to lose.

THE HAZARDS OF BEING A COUCH POTATO

Just sitting there on the couch will get you into trouble. Sitters are fat storers, and they're less healthy than people who move. When a couch potato sits there, eyes fixed on the TV, his breathing becomes more shallow. In time this reduces the vital capacity of the lungs, which means there is less oxygen available to the intestines, muscles, heart, and brain. The heart, like all the other muscles of the body, becomes weaker. This means it has to work harder to pump less blood, which further deprives the other parts of the body of oxygen. Inactivity raises the level of all the bad fats in the blood and lowers the level of good cholesterol. Even the muscles of the intestines slow down, increasing constipation, contributing to fatigue. The combination of a tired heart, tired brain, and tired gut motivates the couch potato to spend even more time on the couch. The sad result is that the couch potato is more likely to wind up in the permanent state of inactivity sooner than his lean friends.

Picture the difference: It's Monday night and Mr. Couch Potato is watching football. He lies on the sofa with a beer, potato chips, and onion dip. Mr. Lean Machine is outside on the lawn tossing a football with his kids after a brisk walk around the neighborhood. He comes in, grabs some fruit for a snack, and watches the second half of the game while doing some upper-body work with his weights. Obviously, Mr. Lean Machine is more likely to be rewarded with a longer life and more Monday night football games than Mr. Couch Potato.

GAIN MUSCLE — LOSE FAT

Here's the best nutritional deal in the body: The more muscle you put on, the more fat you're likely to take off. The reason is that muscle tissue, even just resting there, burns more calories than fat tissue, which essentially burns very little. Every pound of extra muscle you put on automatically burns 50 to 100 extra calories a day. So, just by adding an extra pound of muscle to your body, you could automatically burn as many as 10 pounds of fat a year. The cellular basis for the term "beef up" is that exercise causes an increase in fat-burning enzymes in the muscles, so that "beefing up" really means increasing the body's ability to burn fat. As you can see, one of the main goals of the L.E.A.N. program is to change body fat into muscle.

It reduces the risk and severity of adult-onset diabetes. Moderate exercise that burns just 200 calories a day, such as a brisk thirty-minute walk, can lower the risk of adult-onset (Type 2) diabetes. Exercise boosts the efficiency of insulin, helping it remove sugar from the blood before it can be stored as fat. (Insulin could be called the "unfair" hormone. It sees to it that excess sugar is stored as fat, yet it blocks the conversion of fat back to glucose.) Increased insulin efficiency has also been linked to lower blood pressure, higher levels of HDL (good) cholesterol, and a lower incidence of cardiovascular disease.

It boosts immunity. Regular, moderate exercise increases the white cell count, improving the body's ability to fight off infection. Exercise also increases the number of "killer cells," those special cells that are mobilized to fight serious diseases, and it increases the body's production of the antibody immunoglobulin A (IgA). Another way exercise boosts immunity is by reducing stress, which can itself depress the body's immune system.

It lowers cholesterol. When combined with a low-fat diet, exercise can reduce levels of LDL (bad) cholesterol twice as effectively as diet alone. Exercise also increases levels of HDL (good) cholesterol. Exercise is one of the few things that accomplish both these goals.

It improves sex life. One of the great perks of the L.E.A.N. program is that it should improve your sex life. A study showed that a group placed on a program of improved diet, stress management, and exercise had heightened sexual arousal and pleasure.

It builds stamina. People who begin an exercise program often discover they have so much more energy. At the muscular level, exercise improves the efficiency with which the muscles can use oxygen. Exercise also helps the body deliver more oxygen to vital organs, such as the lungs, brain, heart, and muscles. In a nutshell, exercise helps transport the oxygen through the body and into cells more efficiently.

It builds a healthy heart. Exercise builds muscle, and when you exercise, you build the heart muscle. A stronger heart is able to pump more blood per stroke, and thus it requires fewer beats to pump the same amount of blood. In a study of thirteen thousand men and women divided into categories of fitness ranging from sedentary to well conditioned, those who walked thirty minutes a day three to four times a week were half as likely to have a heart attack or develop cancer. In people with high blood pressure, regular exercise has shown to lower both systolic and diastolic blood pressure by an average of ten points. Exercise also reduces the tendency for the blood-clotting cells, called "platelets," to stick together, and thus prevents blood clots that reduce the blood supply to the tissues of the heart, brain, and other vital organs, causing strokes or heart attacks.

It slows aging. Nearly all the physiological changes that are associated with aging are delayed with exercise, including decreased muscle mass, increased body fat, reduced muscle strength and flexibility, decreased bone mass, decreased metabolic rate (which promotes fat storing), decreased cardiovascular fitness, sleep difficulties, reduced sexual performance, diminished oxygen utilization by muscle, and reduced mental acuity. Exercise acts like a tonic, delaying or diminishing many of the symptoms of aging.

It increases lifespan. A study of seventeen thousand male Harvard graduates aged thirty-five to seventy-four showed that men who exercise regularly live longer. The death rates declined as the number of calories burned in exercise increased, up to a weekly calorie expenditure of 2,000 calories (which would be an average of forty minutes of moderate exercise per day). The study suggested an increase in death rate among men expending more than 3,000 calories per week, leading the researchers to conclude that moderate exercise seems to be the healthiest for most people.

New studies have shown that reducing calories can also increase a person's lifespan, so the combination of a low-calorie diet with exercise to burn off calories brings double benefits. Between twenty and eighty years of age, the average male may lose a quarter of his total muscle mass, which leads us to conclude that the amount of exercise you do should *increase* with age rather than decrease. The L.E.A.N. program is likely to help you die young — but at an old age.

It builds muscle. Exercise builds muscle, and muscle is the biggest fat burner in the body. Muscle burns calories, not only during exercise but also while you are resting. It's automatic. The more muscle mass you have, the more calories (and therefore fat) you burn, even during your sleep. This is why one goal of the L.E.A.N. program is to replace fat with muscle. Consider these fat stats: With moderate exercise (you don't have to be an Olympic weight lifter), you can increase your muscle mass enough to automatically burn more than 100 extra calories a day, which translates into an automatic fat loss (or lack of fat gain) of a pound a month. So once you become lean, you increase your chances of staying lean. The best exercise for building muscles is resistance training, in which the muscles work against gravity, such as weight training with free weights or a resistance machine. Even senior citizens can build more muscle with resistance training. So we could say, "Lift weights to lose weight." Exercise enough to build the muscle and maintain the muscle, and it keeps right on burning the fat to keep you lean. *Exercise speeds metabolism.* Not only do you burn fat while you're exercising, but your metabolic rate remains elevated for six to twelve hours after you exercise. You're still getting the fat-burning benefit of your morning workout in the early afternoon.

It builds bone. Exercise also builds bone. Astronauts working in zero gravity in space lose bone mass. Weight-bearing exercise here on earth makes bones stronger. Weight-bearing exercise is a good way to prevent osteoporosis, or softening of the bone. One reason exercise helps build bone is that exercising bodies tend to excrete less calcium through the kidneys than sedentary bodies do.

It improves mood. Exercise releases endorphins, the body's own internal opiates, or mood-elevating, pain-relieving hormones. It's on the days when you least feel like exercising that you'll notice the endorphin effect the most. It relieves tension and soothes stress. Endorphins even curb food cravings. The neurochemicals that are released during exercise can not only calm you if you're anxious but also pull you out of a depression. In studies, depressive symptoms decreased in women who engaged in regular exercise, such as walking briskly, jogging, lifting weights, or dancing, three to four times a week for eight to ten weeks. Psychiatrists often prescribe exercise to combat depression. It's cheap, too, and the side effects are all good ones.

It sparks the brain. Because exercise increases blood flow to the brain, it's as good for the head as it is for the body. Exercise can help you concentrate and also helps your brain relax when it's time for sleep.

It gives a good "gut feeling." Exercise improves digestion and speeds the passage of food through the intestines. Chronically constipated persons often notice a return to regular bowel movements when they begin the L.E.A.N. program. So exercise regularly to stay regular.

It reduces the risk of cancer. A study of thirteen thousand men and women followed for fifteen years by aerobics expert Dr. Kenneth Cooper showed that the incidence of all forms of cancer was related to fitness. The fitter the subjects were, the less their risk of cancer.

Exercise and a low-fat diet are partners in health. Dieting without exercise leads to little or no permanent fat loss, and possibly a fat gain. Exercise without good nutrition equals little or no fat loss. Dieting plus exercise equals lots of fat loss. You don't burn off much fat while you're doing the exercise. While you exercise, you burn mostly carbohydrates. The fat burning occurs during the twelve hours after exercise, when your metabolic rate is elevated. This is why morning exercise is likely to yield a greater fat loss than exercise in the evening or before bed. Sleep depresses your metabolic rate. So, the best time for exercise is first thing in the morning. Late afternoon, before dinner, is also a good time to exercise; you'll eat less at dinner and burn calories all evening long. This metabolism speeding is especially important for the fortysomethings and older, since metabolism begins to slow down once you hit middle age, and exercise speeds up this natural slowdown.

ATTITUDE

Is there such a thing as mind over fat? Yes! You've heard the phrase "set your mind to it." The attitude part of the L.E.A.N. program is about using your mind to help you get a lean body. You can't just think fat away, but there are fascinating ways your mind can affect your body — for better and for worse.

How Stress Can Make You Fat

Stress gets in the way of good health. Your body can't reap all the benefits of nutrition and exercise if it's overstressed. And stress can get in the way of

---

MENTAL EXERCISE

Exercise is not only good for the body, it's great for the brain, too. The brain is an oxygen hog, which is why it takes 25 percent of the blood that the heart pumps (more in children). Exercise delivers more oxygen to the brain and helps all tissue, especially brain tissue, use oxygen more efficiently, which translates into better thinking. Pumping more blood to the brain stimulates the release of a group of neurochemicals, collectively called "brain growth factors," which increase the production of neurotransmitters and make more receptor sites for these brain messengers to land on.

Exercise is not only nature's smart drug, it's also nature's Prozac. By stimulating the release of endorphins, exercise beefs up the body's own "feel good" hormones. Endorphins are most stimulated by exercise and laughter. And the good-feeling effects of these hormones last about as long as a pill, four to six hours after exercise, and without the unpleasant medical side effects. Therapists have long prescribed exercise to pull people out of the pits of depression. So, exercise not only burns fat — it burns stress, too.

---

eating right and getting enough exercise. Stress hormones stimulate the neurotransmitters that increase your cravings for sugar-rich foods, stimulate your appetite, and foster overeating. (See "The Chemistry of Cravings," page 44.) Chronic, unresolved stress throws off the biochemical equilibrium of your body, making it difficult for your body to feel good and for you to recognize what makes you feel good.

Stressbusters

For the L.E.A.N. program to work best, it's important not only to cut out junk calories but also to cut down on your stress. Here are six tips that will show you how:

Stressbuster #1: You can't control situations, but you can control your reactions to them.
This is the basis of all successful stress-management programs. In real life you can't isolate yourself from stress-producing situations. Stress happens. Traffic lights turn red. Children get sick. And sometimes worse things happen. You lose your job, for example. You can, however, control your reaction. The stress may be involuntary, but your reaction, believe it or not, is voluntary. Here's an example:

Turn an accident into an opportunity. Most parents, when their children begin to drive, have mixed feelings. On the one hand, they're glad to be out of the car-pool scene and feeling like a family chauffeur. On the other hand, they're worried for their child's safety. When our son Peter first began to drive, he accidentally stepped on the gas instead of the brake while pulling into the garage, scraping one side of the car and damaging one wall of the garage. This was a stressor to me, and I overreacted. I yelled and complained. My worry and my griping about the inconvenience and the cost of repairs elevated my pulse and blood pressure and certainly didn't do my body any good. Three years later, our daughter Hayden, the latest addition to the list of family members with keys to the car, did the same thing, but to the other side of the car and a different wall in the garage. But by this time I had learned the importance of practicing stressbuster #1. So, instead of reacting in anger, I told Hayden, "I'm so glad that you didn't get hurt. Having your first accident in the garage is probably the best place. Now you'll be more careful. A car is easy to fix; your body isn't. Of course, you know you're more important than the car." I actually felt peaceful, as did Hayden after a while. I realized that the internal turmoil caused by an overreaction to stress would have been costly to my body — and to my daughter.

Stressbuster #2: Focus on solutions, not problems. This is a variation of #1. You can't change the problem by getting yourself all worked up with the usual "what ifs," but you can look for solutions. This is especially important in family dynamics. When children have problems, your first reaction may be to point out how their own faults created the situation. Soon everyone is feeling negative and hopeless. If you focus instead on solutions (and preventing the problem from happening again), you can pull up everybody's mood from negative to positive and teach your children a valuable lesson in life: Stress happens, but you quickly fix it before it takes its toll on your mind and body. The child says, "Dad, I messed up . . ." and the parent responds, "Okay, let's find a way to fix it." By offering a mature response, wise parents can lower the stress level of an entire family. It's a good approach to your own problems, too.

Practice what we call in our family the "Caribbean attitude" ("No problem, mon!"). Our family hobby is sailing, and we often charter a boat in the Caribbean for our family vacation. Part of the "fun" of boating is that something usually goes wrong and needs fixing. One day our engine died and we limped under sail into a marina on a remote island, hoping to find a mechanic to fix our engine. As the ship's captain, I was beginning to worry that this situation would ruin our whole family vacation, but we were greeted by a friendly mechanic who said, "No problem, mon!" Everyone relaxed, me most of all. We ended up enjoying the time we spent on that island and learned some lessons about Caribbean life while the locals fixed our boat.

Stressbuster #3: Focus on biggies and downplay smallies. Some stressors don't merit more than a minute of worry. Unfortunately, most of us learn that lesson too late. For our own survival as parents of eight, we've had to concentrate on the biggies and forget the smallies in disciplining our children. Otherwise, the constant annoyances (smallies) of childish behaviors would have driven us bananas long ago. For us, biggies are about respect for one another, values, responsibility, and serious threats to life and limb. Smallies are life's little annoyances that really don't hurt anyone. Yet the importance of concentrating on the biggies and letting go of the smallies didn't really come home to me until my recovery from cancer. The stress of cancer gave me a more mature outlook on life. After my recovery, one day I came into the office and our office manager greeted me with the news of "a serious problem." The computer had crashed. I thought to myself, "That's a smallie. Cancer is a biggie." So I responded, "Well, who do we get to fix it?"

Stressbuster #4: Learn to relax. Chronic, unresolved stress basically exhausts your brain's neurotransmitters so that you don't feel good and can't think clearly. Relaxation allows these neurotransmitters to recuperate from the exhaustion created by stress. An important part of the L.E.A.N. program is not only using our six stressbusters to learn to relax in response to stressful situations, but also setting aside some time each day for relaxation.

In the L.E.A.N. program, we focus on five important kinds of relaxation:

- *Daily meditation.* Morning meditation is a must, and evening meditation is a second must. Many spiritual disciplines teach that meditation is the key that opens the morning and closes the evening. The time spent in meditation allows you to become more aware of your thoughts and how your body and mind are supposed to feel. This is called being mindful. You learn to become more sensitive to your internal workings, which makes you more able to make necessary corrections in your course.

- *Relaxation exercises.* On the surface, it may seem that the terms "exercise" and "relaxation" don't go together, but this association is biochemi-

cally correct. Working at relaxation and acquiring disciplined relaxation techniques stimulate your brain to produce calming neurochemicals such as endorphins and encourage your body to shut off production of upsetting stress hormones. Meditation clears the mind, and the body, of internal stressors and allows the helpful neurochemicals to have their say.

- *Imagery.* Imagery fills your mind with pleasant thoughts, replays of pleasant scenes, and thoughts of happy relationships before negative thoughts, or unpleasant replays, overtake you. Imagery is an effective way to counteract external and internal stressors.

- *Music.* Listening to music relaxes the mind, and the body, by stimulating those "feel good" thoughts and hormones. This is known as "The Mozart Effect.®"

- *Relax before you respond.* Learn to quickly fill your mind with positive thoughts before negative ones get a foothold.

Stressbuster #5: Focus on what you have, not on what you don't have. An important lesson to learn in life — and in staying lean — is that you can control what goes on in your mind. This is very important to your well-being. What happens to you — to your body, your finances, and your relationships — is often beyond your control. But, like the food you put in your body, the thoughts and the scenes that fill your mind are, for the most part, completely within your control. Filling your mind with rich thoughts is often more satisfying than having external wealth. As Thoreau said, "A man is rich in proportion to the number of things which he can afford to let alone." A positive mental attitude has always been important in stress management. A truly lean person becomes an optimist rather than a pessimist. When you focus on what you have rather than on what you don't have, you'll enjoy what you have to a greater degree and waste less energy on unfulfilled wishes.

WHY DIETS DON'T WORK

The market is obese with calorie-restricted weight-loss diets, the great majority of which reduce more dollars than fat from the obese person. Crash diets try to fool the body, but the body doesn't buy it. Rapid-weight-loss diets invariably fail because they are metabolically unsound (and often unsafe) and just plain don't work for the following reason: They don't reset the fat point (see page 341). When a person suddenly goes on a crash diet and restricts his calorie intake, the body, fearing it's starving, rebels to protect its fat point by lowering the body's metabolism to click into the fat-storage mode rather than the fat-burning mode. The body, in its wisdom, interprets the sudden caloric restriction as threatening its nourishment and therefore protects itself by lowering its metabolism to resist the sudden change of diet. One way it does this is by increasing the production of the enzyme lipoprotein lipase (LPL), which promotes the storage and transfer of blood fats into body fats. In essence, your body is working against you. When you suddenly reduce the number of calories going into it, your body responds by taking those fewer calories and turning them into fat. Then when you start eating "normally" again, the body has already set itself to a lower level of calorie burning, so you gain back weight faster than you took it off. The key is to gradually trick the fat point, so that your body metabolically cooperates rather than fighting fat loss.

Crash diets (those that don't work, don't last, and are often downright unhealthy) often give you a rapid weight loss in what you see on the scale. For these diets, weight loss does not equate with fat loss, since you are often losing water weight (which you quickly gain back) or muscle weight. Both of these types of weight loss are potentially harmful to your well-being. The reason for this false weight loss is that during the first week or two on a crash diet, the body first loses protein and water, since the wisdom of the body tells it to hold on to the fat as its last reserve. This loss of protein and water is the reason most people feel lousy during the first week or two on a crash diet.

Another reason that crash diets are bad for your health is that they cut out not only the bad fats but the good fats, too, causing the dieter to have a deficiency in essential fatty acids, which can compromise a person's health. The key to fat control is not only eating less fat, but eating the right fats. In fact, essential fatty acids may also be essential to maintaining proper fat-burning metabolism. Not only are crash diets unhealthy, but many crash dieters eat more and regain more fat once they discard the diet. The body was used to the fat it had and wants it back.

Another reason that crash diets fail is they do not respect the interplay between insulin, carbohydrates, and fat storage. When you restrict your calories, your blood sugar may drop, causing you to get hungry and binge on carbohydrates, which in turn triggers your insulin, the hormone that also promotes fat storage. In essence, for some people, going hungry can promote fat storage rather than fat burning.

FAT LOSS: HOW FAST? HOW SAFE?

Be patient about fat loss. Achieving a lasting leaner you is well worth the wait. Because the goal is to change fat into muscle, in the L.E.A.N. program we prefer the term "weight change" to "weight loss." As a general guide, it is impossible to lose weight faster than 3 pounds a week without seriously endangering your health, and even this requires you to burn 1,500 calories more a day than you eat. There have been recent reports of teenage wrestlers who have gone on crash diets so that they can compete in a lower weight class, and in some cases, the rapid weight loss has resulted in death.

Begin with a fat loss of ½ pound a week for several weeks. This is a comfortable loss that won't force your fat point to compensate by slowing your metabolism. Then, progress to a fat loss of 1 pound a week, which can be accomplished with an average daily calorie deficit of 500 calories. This means you eat 300 to 500 calories less than usual and exercise 30 minutes a day. For most healthy individuals, the maximum fat loss we would recommend would be 2 pounds per week. Your personal comfort level for fat loss will probably fall somewhere between 1 and 2 pounds a week.

Stressbuster #6: Eat a stress-relieving diet. See "Mood Foods," page 298.

NUTRITION

The final feature of the L.E.A.N. program is nutrition, which carries equal weight with exercise in the process of becoming lean. No, we don't mean you should go on a diet, at least not in the way most people regard this four-letter word. Most of us enjoy eating. We look forward to our evening meal, and even more to dinner or a banquet. We don't eat to live, we live to eat. So, instead of a diet, let's call it a "change in eating style," meaning you focus more on eating well rather than on eating less. For some overfat and underlean individuals, this will probably also mean eating less, and I know this is not easy. I belong to the category of people who like to eat. Martha, on the other hand, is more likely to eat primarily for health than for enjoyment. To stay lean you have to do one of two things: either eat less or exercise more — or, preferably, do both. You can't have it both ways. I have chosen to eat more and exercise more; Martha has chosen to eat less and exercise less. She often teases me during one of my exercise binges, "Why don't you just eat less?" "Because that's no fun" is my answer. It's not just your body type that determines how many calories you need. It's also what type of attitude you have about food. So, the key is to eat right for your type. Here is how.

Figuring Out How Many Calories You Need

Determine how many calories you need for optimal health. Because of the concept of "biochemi-

NUTRITIP
The Yo-yo Diet

Periodic crash diets in which you lose a lot of weight, gain it back, and then try to lose it again may confuse your body to the extent that it becomes more and more difficult to take pounds off and easier and easier to put them back on. You end up weighing more instead of less. Add exercise to your diet plan and you greatly increase your chances of keeping the pounds off.

DOWNSIZING

Ever wonder why it's so hard to stick to a diet? The reason is your body naturally resists change, even when it's for the better. It's like a company that is overloaded with too many employees — inefficient, mismanaged, and downright unhealthy. The shareholders of the company, let's cal it Obese, Inc., vote for a buyout, so new management takes over. The overweight company had developed a complex network of extra staff to support one another, and because there were more people, more managers were needed, the payroll was high, and office space was at a premium. The new management wants to trim this redundant support system, but the workers fight to keep their jobs. The company resists downsizing.

The body acts in a similar way. In order to lug around 20 pounds of extra fat, the body develops a support network. The heart has to pump more blood, there are extra nerves, the hipbones widen to support the extra poundage around the middle, and extra calories are taken in to support this extra stuff. But the body is used to this extra stuff and looks for strategies that help it hang on to all of its "employees."

Back to Obese, Inc. In the early stages of trimming, company personnel are uncomfortable. There are pink slips, layoffs, early retirements, demotions. Yet the management realizes that this initial discomfort is important in order to turn the company around. After a few months the company is running more efficiently, employees are happier, the stockholders are satisfied, wages are higher, and bonuses abound. The company is now trim, efficient, and making a profit. Now the support system fights to keep the company trim — an easier task now that those who had caused the company to become obese in the first place have been weeded out.

The same kind of metabolic changes occur in the body. The body initially fights the effects of eating less by resetting its metabolic set point lower, so it burns fewer calories. The body is uncomfortable. It may occasionally feel hungry. But after a couple of months of resisting the change, the body realizes that it is now feeling better, leaner, trimmer, and is working more efficiently, with more energy. It has a new set point, a new way of working, and now it will fight to stay this way. Foods that it used to crave it now shuns. Habits it used to enjoy it perceives now as threatening. And it keeps working harder to retain its new self.

Wise management changes a company gradually, so there's less resistance. This is the best way to approach the L.E.A.N. program, too. It works better when you make wise changes slowly rather than trying to change your lifestyle, exercise habits, attitude, and nutrition completely and all at once.

cal individuality," the custom of calorie counting for weight control is becoming less correct nutritionally, but it's a place to start. Calories are simply a measure of how much potential energy a particular food can deliver to your body. It used to be thought that the calories eaten–to–calories used ratio was all you needed to know to take off body fat. However, new nutritional insights show that it's not only the caloric value of the food but also the type of food and the type of metabolism that are important in fat gain or loss. Since 3,500 calories equals 1 pound of fat, if you eat 3,500 calories more than you burn, you put on a pound of fat. If you eat 3,500 calories less than you burn, you burn off a pound. But the real situation is more complicated than this. The body is pro-

---

NUTRITIP
Veggie Up.

Eat lots of vegetables, since ounce for ounce they contain fewer calories and more fiber than most other foods. They tend to fill you up without putting on the fat.

---

grammed to burn carbs but store fat, and different metabolisms react differently to different kinds of food. Still, figuring out how many calories you need each day will give you a rough guide to what you should eat.

You need calories for three bodily processes:

1. **Basic metabolic needs.** You need calories to keep your body going. How many you need is determined by your basal metabolic rate (BMR) as well as your size and your body composition. To figure your basic caloric needs, follow these general formulas:

   - For women, add a zero to your weight in pounds or multiply your weight by eleven. Then add your weight to that amount. For example, a 120-pound woman's basic caloric needs would be 1,200 + 120 = 1,320 calories a day.

   - For men, multiply your weight by twelve. For example, a 160-pound man's basic

caloric needs would be 160 x 12 = 1,920 calories a day.

   - Because body type contributes to BMR, if you are genetically lean (i.e., an ectomorph; see page 326), add 5 percent to your daily caloric needs. If you are a round, plump endomorph (i.e., an apple), subtract 10 percent.

2. **Exercise.** If you're already a very active person *and* you exercise around half an hour a day, add another 300 to 500 calories to your basic caloric needs. So, the calorie needs of an average active woman would be around 1,700 to 1,900 a day; for the average active man, around 2,200 to 2,500 calories a day, depending on the person's age.

3. **Growth.** Your basal metabolic rate (BMR) naturally decreases around 2 percent for each decade above age twenty. As a rough guide, you could subtract 40 calories per decade from your BMR, so a man of sixty would need 160 fewer calories than a man of twenty. Women need extra calories during pregnancy and lactation. Caloric needs also increase when you are recovering from an illness, or during competitive sports.

   Growing children, especially during infancy and adolescence, need 25 percent more calories for growth. An adolescent girl may need as many as 2,400 calories a day, and an average adolescent male may need as many as 3,000 calories a day, depending on how active they are.

In the early weeks of the L.E.A.N. program, it helps to consult a calorie-counting book and meticulously add up the calories in everything you eat to get an accurate idea of how many calories you consume each day and how close this comes to your basic caloric needs. As you store your knowledge of food calories, you won't need to do this anymore. You'll know that a carton of

---

NUTRITIP
Hidden Calories

Be particularly careful of foods that taste yummy but pack a frightening amount of fat, such as coffee cakes, piecrusts, hot dogs, doughnuts, and croissants.

nonfat plain yogurt contains 80 calories. As you keep track of your calories, you'll learn how many average calories per day you need to keep yourself as lean as you want to be. When you begin your calorie reduction, do it gradually. Begin by cutting 20 percent off your usual intake and see what results you get.

Make Changes in Your Eating Patterns

Eat Nutrient-Dense Foods

Nutrient-dense foods are those that pack the most nutrition into the smallest number of calories. The opposite of nutrient-dense foods are calorie-dense foods, those that pack a lot of calories into a small amount of food and leave you craving more. Examples are fast foods, junk foods, and high-fat and high-sugar foods. Nutrient-dense foods are more likely to satisfy you, leaving you feeling full while contributing to your body's overall nutritional needs. An interesting study showed that when people were allowed to eat all they wanted but only of nutrient-dense foods, they consumed fewer calories than when they were allowed to eat highly refined and processed foods. Here are examples of nutrient-dense foods:

- cantaloupe
- papaya
- fresh fruits instead of juice
- whole-grain cereals
- wild rice
- brown rice instead of white rice
- yogurt
- nonfat or low-fat milk
- nonfat cottage cheese
- turkey and chicken, white meat
- egg whites
- salmon
- tuna
- shrimp
- sweet potatoes
- all vegetables and legumes
- avocados
- soy foods

Fill Up with Fiber

Fiber is calorie free and filling. When you eat foods high in fiber, you feel full without consuming a lot of calories. Fiber also slows the absorption of nutrients into the bloodstream, which in turn lessens insulin bursts and thus slows fat storage. Soluble fibers, such as psyllium, pectin, citrus fruits, legumes, and oat bran are the best weight-loss boosters. One study showed that an extra 5 grams of fiber a day (equivalent to one serving of fiber-rich cereal) resulted in a daily decrease in calorie consumption. And, when you eat fiber along with fat, you're liable to eat less of the fatty foods. Pies are my downfall. For an extra piece of pie I'll willingly spend an extra thirty minutes on the family treadmill. Yet I notice that I tend to eat less pie and feel just as satisfied when we make homemade piecrust with whole wheat flour or brown-rice flour. Breakfast is an important fiber-rich meal. One study showed that persons who ate a high-fiber breakfast cereal ate an average of 150 fewer calories per day than those who ate a low-fiber cereal. (For more on fiber, including a list of fiber-rich foods, see Chapter 9.)

Little Bites Add Up

Small changes in your eating patterns result in big changes in your waistline — for better or worse. Take a close look at the food you're eating and trim away those unneeded calorie-dense, nutrient-poor foods that stand between you and a trim body. You'll be surprised how little you have to change to get lean. For example, five to ten potato chips a day is an extra 50 to 100 calories, which amounts to 5 to 10 pounds of extra fat in a year. Lose the chips and you'll lose the pounds. Or, try substituting a lower-calorie food for a higher-calorie one. Try these tiny calorie cuts:

- canned fruits packed in water instead of syrup
- tuna packed in water instead of oil

- low-fat or nonfat yogurt instead of whole-fat yogurt
- low-fat or nonfat milk instead of whole milk

Trim the Fat in Foods

As we discussed on pages 13 and 328, fatty foods are more fattening than foods that are high in proteins and carbs. Cutting back on fat will help you get lean. Most of us have a preference for foods with fat in them, so it is wise to lower the fat in your diet gradually, because drastic changes are harder to maintain. Try these low-fat versions of everyday foods: low-fat or nonfat dairy products (milk, yogurt, and cottage cheese) and yogurt instead of sour cream on baked potatoes and in dips. Removing the skin of chicken before cooking the chicken (or at least before eating it) can cut the amount of fat by at least half.

You may wonder how much fat should be in your daily diet. An already lean person, especially a person who has been lucky enough to be born lean and remain lean, can safely consume around 25 or even 30 percent of his or her daily calories as fat and stay lean. For most of us rounder mortals, 20 percent of calories from fat is a goal to aim for to get and stay lean. This amounts to 45 to 60 grams of fat per day, depending on your calorie needs. And don't forget, it's not only important to have a low-fat diet; you have to take a close look at the type of fat you're eating as well (see below).

Remember to read labels and pay attention to the fat information given. To keep yourself lean, eat mostly foods that contain less than 20 percent of the calories in the food as fat. Here's a quick way to calculate if the fat calories are greater or less than 20 percent of the total. The label on the food lists both the total calories and the calories from fat. Divide all calories by the calories from fat, and if the answer is less than 5, leave the food on the shelf. For example, a food contains 120

> **NUTRITIP**
> **Beware of Movie Popcorn.**
>
> The popcorn in movie theaters may be called "buttered," but really it's soaked in the worst oils — saturated and hydrogenated — with only a bit of butter flavoring. Bowing to public and parental pressure, some theaters are now offering air-popped popcorn and popcorn popped in unsaturated oils, such as canola. If you're a popcorn lover, ask about the oil used at your local movie theater. Let the management know you're concerned and, who knows? — you may motivate the theater to change the fat in its popcorn.

calories per serving, with 40 calories from fat. Divide 120 by 40 and the answer is 3. You may not want to eat this food, since 33 percent of its calories come from fat. Stick to reading the Nutrition Facts for your information about fat and ignore the come-ons on the front of the package. Even though "reduced fat" under the new label laws means that the food contains 25 percent less fat than the original product, it may still contain too much fat. For example, if the original product was half fat, the new product is still 35 percent fat. Labels with the words "light" or "lite" have to be one-third less fat than the original, but again, if you start with a high-fat food, the lite version could still be high in fat.

Eat Fats That Can Keep You Slim

All fats are not created equal, and one of the dangers of crash diets is that you cut out not only the bad fats but the good ones, too. Your body needs fats. You can't live without them, especially those that are high in essential fatty acids, which, as we have discussed (see page 4), are just that — essen-

Right Fats: Fat Burners	Wrong Fats: Fat Storers
essential fatty acids fish flax oil unsaturated fats	hydrogenated fats saturated fats partially hydrogenated oils land animal–source fats

tial for life and health. Essential fatty acids, such as those found in fish and flax oil, are more likely to stimulate the body to burn fat rather than store fat. By consuming enough of the right fats, your body is less likely to crave other fats trying to make up deficiencies. (For more on fats that are good for you, see "Best Fats," page 4, and the "green-light" foods in "Rating Fats," page 18.)

Be especially sure that growing children have a diet high enough in the right fats.

NUTRITIP
Never Dine After Nine.

If you're accustomed to big dinners, eat them early in the evening to give your body a chance to burn off some of your indulgence before you retire.

Drink Up

The higher the water content of a food, the more filling it is, and water itself has no calories. Fiber-rich foods need to be eaten with a lot of water; otherwise, the fiber may contribute to constipation or soak up water and other nutrients needed elsewhere by the body. Drinking at least eight 8-ounce glasses of water a day, perhaps slightly flavored with a little lemon or fruit juice, is a lean person's best choice in the beverage department. (For a discussion of how much water you need, see page 74.)

V

FOODS FOR HEALTH

"Let food be your medicine," wrote Hippocrates. Little did the father of medicine know that centuries later the quality of our food would be so poor that we would have to take more medicine to treat the diseases caused by our nutritional deficiencies. At no time in history has the term "health foods" been so important. Food processing, busy lifestyles, and downright lack of nutritional awareness have resulted in an epidemic of common diseases, such as cardiovascular disease, that were rare a hundred years ago. "But we don't have time to shop for and prepare fresh, nutritious foods," you may think. Trading convenience for health, in the long run, doesn't save you time or money. If you don't have time to eat nutritiously, you'd better plan to spend time in the hospital. New studies are proving what our parents told us long ago: "Persons who consistently eat a more nutritious diet live better and longer." Eat more nutritious foods now and pay the doctor less later. We'll show you how.

36

Foods for Healthy Living

MOLECULAR SCIENCE IS FINALLY confirming what your mother always told you: "Eat your fruits and vegetables." As you will soon learn, the power-packed nutrients that give fruits and vegetables their many colors also provide a lot of Mother Nature's medicine.

FANTASTIC PHYTOS

Have you had your phytos today? That's nutri-talk for the millennium. Once upon a time it was thought that fats, proteins, carbohydrates, vitamins, and minerals were all the nutrients necessary for growth and health. Now we know there's another group of nutrients necessary for optimal health — phytonutrients. Despite its high-tech ring, "phytonutrient" (from the Greek *phyton* for "plant") simply means a "nutrient from a plant."

How Phytos Work

While many phytos have been identified, there are probably thousands more that remain to be discovered. The best known of the phytos are carotenoids, flavonoids, and isoflavones. Carotenoids include yellow, orange, and red pigment in fruits and vegetables. Dark green, leafy vegetables are rich in one of the carotenoids, beta carotene, but the usual yellow color is masked by the chlorophyll, the green pigment in the vegetables. Flavonoids are reddish pigments, found in red grape skins and citrus fuits, and isoflavones can be found in peanuts, lentils, soy, and other legumes. You're familiar with vitamins, but now we have "phytomins," which are less familiar, but equally important, health-promoting substances in food.

Phytos protect the body and fight disease. One day while I was watching my garden grow, I wondered how plants stay so healthy. They don't wear sunscreen or a raincoat; they don't go to the doctor. The answer: They make their own disease-fighting chemicals we call "phytonutrients" — "phytos" for short. The same phytos that help keep the plant healthy keep our bodies healthy. Phytos provide medicine for cell health. They help the cells repair themselves by stimulating the release of protective enzymes or those that rebuild damaged cells. Other phytos inhibit cancer-producing substances, reducing their ability to damage cells. When the repair squad can stay ahead of the damage, degenerative diseases, such as multiple sclerosis and arthritis, can't get started. Phytos also keep infections and cardiovascular disease in check.

FAMOUS PHYTOS

Currently these are the most popular phytos that are known for their powerful antioxidant, anti-cancer, and heart disease protective properties.

Phytomin	Food Source
Carotenoids (alpha carotene, beta carotene, and lutein)	yellow-orange fruits and vegetables: carrots, cantaloupe, papaya, pumpkin, squash, sweet potatoes, broccoli, dried apricots, asparagus, kale, green leafy vegetables, peppers
Lycopene	tomatoes, tomato paste, tomato juice, guava, pink grapefruit, watermelon
Beta cryptozanthin	tangerines, papaya, oranges, peaches, mangoes, nectarines
Flavonoids	soy, green tea, tomatoes, sweet potatoes, cruciferous vegetables, citrus fruits, red wine, red grapes, onions
Indoles	cruciferous vegetables*
Sulforaphane	cruciferous vegetables*
Isoflavones	legumes (beans, peas, lentils), soy products
Allicin	garlic, onions
Genistein	soy products (e.g., tofu)
Polyphenols	green tea
Anthocyanins	wild blueberries, bilberries, blackberries
Limonoids	citrus fruits
Sterols	cruciferous vegetables,* cucumbers, squash, sweet potatoes, soy foods, eggplants, whole grains, tomatoes
Capsaicin	chili peppers
Elegiac acid	strawberries
Lignans	nuts and seeds

* Cruciferous vegetables include broccoli, cabbage, brussels sprouts, mustard greens, kale, and cauliflower.

Phytos fight cancer. Cancer starts with a cell out of control. As cells wear out or get injured, they replace themselves with new and healthy cells. Within each cell a network of inner controls (the DNA) keeps this process working. But with this cellular cloning happening millions of times a minute, there are many opportunities for an occasional cell to defy the rules and get out of control. It may go on reproducing itself, eventually damaging the organ of which it is a part. Like a band of terrorists, the out-of-control cancer cells also try to infiltrate other organs by entering the body's blood vessels and traveling to places near and far, a process called "metastasis." Some cancer cells are probably formed in every person every day. Yet the body's own defense system recognizes these invaders and attacks. Almost always, the body wins the battle, so that these cancer cells either never have a chance to develop or are destroyed before they have a chance to spread or cause damage. Occasionally, the body's defenses aren't strong or effective enough to overcome these rebellious cells, and the person "gets cancer."

Phytos fight on the side of the body. Carcinogens (cancer-causing substances) can enter the body from all kinds of sources (e.g., tobacco smoke, pollution, pesticides). Carcinogens attempt to enter cells and change how they develop. But antioxidant phytos nab the carcinogens before they have a chance to cause cancer in the cell. If the carcinogen manages to infiltrate the internal controls of the cell, other kinds of phytos help to shut down the precancerous cell so it does not multiply into a gang and overrun the neighborhood. The phytos' protective mechanism explains why cultures whose diets are rich in plant foods have the lowest rates of cancer. The Mediterranean diet, for example, emphasizes garlic, tomatoes, onions, fruits, whole grains, and olive oil — all of which contain cancer-fighting phytos.

Phytos seem to be the most cancer protective against the cells that form the lining of organs such as the mouth, lungs, bladder, uterus, and digestive tract. These cells, called "epithelial cells," are the ones most exposed to carcinogens. They also have a rapid turnover rate, meaning they're replaced often. Even though there are anti-cancer phytos in all plant foods, those found in fruits and vegetables seem to be the most powerful. Of course, it's not only what fruits and vegetables contain that makes them effective cancer fighters, it's also what organic ones do not contain — the saturated fats and chemical pollutants frequently found in animal foods.

Phytos help hearts. Antioxidant phytos can interfere with LDL (bad) cholesterol's damaging effects on arteries. The LDL's become harmful after an encounter with a free radical, during which they are oxidized, in a process like rusting metal. And when artery walls are damaged by free radicals, it's easier for the oxidized LDL's to build up there. Antioxidant phytos, especially beta carotene, can block these free radicals and thus prevent cardiovascular disease.

Phytos boost immunity. Phytos such as carotenoids and flavonoids mobilize the body's immune cells, called "natural killer cells" and "T-helper cells." These act like a protective armor to keep invading pollutants and germs from entering the cell. (See "All About Antioxidants," page 362.)

Phyto Facts

Libraries of information exist about vitamins, but phytonutrients are newcomers to the health-food table. There is currently a sort of phyto information war going on. On the one side, pill makers are trying to package and promote phytonutrient supplements as the new magic cure-all. On the other side, researchers are trying to determine scientifically just what phytonutrients are in which foods and what good things they do for you. Here is information you need to know to separate the hype from the useful information:

Eat the real thing. Get your phytos from foods, not just from pills. Even reputable phyto-supplement makers offer this grandmotherly advice. Like other nutrients, phytos operate under the biochemical principle of synergy (1 + 1 = 3). For example, flavonoids and carotenoids have more health-promoting properties when they are eaten together in the same food rather than when they are taken separately in a supplement. Each one of the hundreds (perhaps thousands) of yet-undiscovered phytos helps others biochemically in the food — and presumably also in the body. Eating a whole tomato is better than popping a pill that contains a chemical isolated from a tomato. By eating a few florets of broccoli you're getting not only the beta carotene you could get in a pill but also the health benefits of probably hundreds or thousands of other phytos that don't even have names yet. And, of course, you're getting vitamin C, fiber, and calcium, too.

Eat variety. Because each class of phytos affects cellular well-being in different ways, the best way to take full advantage of the best medicine nature has to offer is to eat a variety of fruits and vegetables. One phyto may bind a carcinogen to keep it from latching onto a cell; another may whisk carcinogens out of the cells; still another may handcuff free radicals before they are allowed to roam in the body; still others stimulate the body's own enzymes to break up potential cancer-causing chemicals. Certainly, a multivegetable salad is more heart-healthy and cancer-protective than an apple. (Better still, eat the salad for lunch and have the apple for dessert.)

Specific phytos fight specific cancers. For example, the phytos in cruciferous vegetables (e.g., broccoli and cauliflower) are most protective against colon cancer; the phytos in garlic are most protective against stomach cancer; those in tomatoes fight against prostate cancer; and those in cruciferous and dark green, leafy vegetables reduce the risk of breast cancer. For optimal health, eat some of all of these foods regularly.

Food preparation affects the phytos. Usually raw vegetables have more phytonutrients than cooked ones, but sometimes this is not true with phytonutrients. Crushing or chopping garlic releases the enzyme allicinase to produce the active phytonutrient allicin.

FOODS FOR TEEN HEALTH

Healthy nutrition — or the lack of it — can affect the three A's of a teen: athletics, academics, and attitude. During teenage growth spurts, adolescents need extra calories, and they should be nutritious ones. Here are some tips on using wise nutrition to improve the growth and performance of your teen.

Teen Health Food Tips

The irony of teen eating habits is that at the very stage they need to eat very nutritious foods, they

HEALTH FOODS

While most foods are good for you, some are better for you than others. Besides being a good source of nutrition, the following foods are also good medicine.

Health Food	Nutrients It Contains	Health Benefits
Garlic	allicin, allylic sulfides, antioxidants	antibiotic, anti-fungal, anti-cancer; lowers cholesterol
Onions	similar to garlic	similar to garlic
Apples	quercetin, flavonoids, pectin	anti-cancer
Spinach	lutein	protects retina of eye
Tomatoes	lycopene, other carotenoids, vitamin C, coumaric acid, chlorophyll acid	anti-cancer, especially prostate cancer
Chili peppers	capsaicin, vitamin C, beta carotene	anti-cancer; binds carcinogens
Red grapes	resveratrol	anti-cancer; prevents sticky platelets, lowering risk of cardiovascular disease and stroke
Soy products (e.g., tofu)	isoflavones, genistein	anti-cancer; reduces cholesterol
Green tea	polyphenols	anti-cancer; lowers heart disease; prevents gingivitis
Cruciferous vegetables: broccoli, cauliflower, brussels sprouts, kale, cabbage	beta carotene, vitamin C, sulforaphane, indoles	anti-cancer
Fish (especially salmon and tuna)	omega-3 fatty acids, DHA	lowers triglycerides and cholesterol
Flax oil	omega-3 fatty acids	boosts immune system; lowers LDL (bad) cholesterol; promotes healthy skin; anti-cancer

HEALTH FOODS (CONTINUED)

Health Food	Nutrients It Contains	Health Benefits
Legumes: beans, peas, lentils	isoflavones	anti-cancer
Pink grapefruit	lycopene, pectin	anti-cancer
Strawberries	elegiac acid, quercetin	anti-cancer
Blueberries	anthocyanins	anti-cancer
Citrus fruits	limonene	anti-cancer
Nuts and seeds	omega-3 fatty acids, lignans, vitamin E	anti-cancer
Cantaloupe	carotenoids, vitamin C	anti-cancer
Watermelon	lycopene	anti-cancer
Papaya	carotenoids, vitamin C	anti-cancer
Sweet potatoes	beta carotene, vitamin C	anti-cancer
Olive oil	monounsaturated fatty acid	lowers cholesterol
Shiitake mushrooms	lentinin	boosts immune system
Cranberry juice	hippuric acid	Acidifies urine and prevents bacteria from adhering to lining of bladder, thus reducing urinary-tract infections

don't want to. Second to infancy, adolescence is the most critical time for nutritious eating.

Adolescent Eating Habits

Most teens are overfed but undernourished. Teens grow a lot, so they need to eat a lot, but they need not just more food but the right kinds of food. Several pressures unique to teens keep this from happening.

- Teens eat more of their meals away from home than previously, so that mother nutritionist is not always around to supervise their eating.

- Teens frequent fast-food outlets, where high-fat (and high in the most unhealthy fats, hydrogenated fats and oils) and nutrient-depleted food is the norm.

TOP TWELVE PHYTO FOODS

While nearly all plant foods contain health-promoting phytochemicals, the following are the most phyto-dense food sources:

1. Soy
2. Tomato
3. Broccoli
4. Garlic
5. Flax seeds
6. Citrus fruits
7. Melons: cantaloupe and watermelon
8. Pink grapefruit
9. Blueberries
10. Sweet potatoes
11. Chili peppers
12. Legumes: beans and lentils

Honorable mentions: green tea, red grapes, papaya, carrots, kale, nuts and seeds, eggplant, artichoke, cabbage, brussels sprouts, onions, apples, cauliflower, dried apricots, pumpkin, squash, spinach, mangoes, and shiitake mushrooms.

ALL ABOUT ANTIOXIDANTS

One of the most important roles of phytos is acting as antioxidants. Here's why your body needs antioxidants.

When the cells in your body burn fuel for energy, they burn oxygen as well, but when oxygen is burned, molecules called "free radicals" are released. Free radicals are like vandals loose in your body. They have at least one extra electron, giving them a negative charge, which drives them around the body looking for cells with which they can react. These reactions damage the DNA and other substances in cells. Much of the time the cells can repair themselves, but the cell neighborhood can't protect itself from these gangs of free radicals all by itself.

Enter the antioxidant "police." Antioxidant molecules have a positive charge, so when they meet up with the negatively charged free radicals, they neutralize them — handcuff them so they can't do any damage. Your body needs more antioxidant police officers as you get older, since the body's ability to repair itself diminishes with age. Antioxidants also help to prevent damage by carcinogens, such as ultraviolet radiation, tobacco smoke, and environmental pollutants.

- The adolescent boy is into bulk, erroneously believing that more food builds more muscle. The adolescent girl is into being thin, believing that eating less equates with being slim.

- Menstruation increases a girl's monthly iron loss, and it is often not replenished by an iron-rich diet.

- Tastes change at puberty. Teens, in general, increase their preference for fat. Boys also increase their cravings for protein-rich foods (the triple hamburger crowd), perhaps believing that meat builds muscle. Girls, most likely because of rising estrogen levels, crave sweets.

- Finally, as part of their declaration of independence, teens are resistant to any outside pressure telling them to do anything, especially what and how to eat.

Improving Your Teen's Nutrition

As we have stressed throughout this book, feeding children is a combination of good nutrition and creative marketing. Ditto this for feeding teens. Try these creative marketing and nutritional tips:

- As with all ages, model healthy eating habits rather than preaching them. Show your teens how to shop. Make each stroll down the supermarket aisle a nutrition lesson. Encourage your teens to help with shopping selections and meal planning so they learn the connection between good food and good health.

- Say no. When it comes to junk food, you are bound to hear, "But all my friends are eating it." Just because they have unhealthy and undernourished friends who are indulging in junk food doesn't mean your teens must be allowed to. Especially resist the pressure of packaged foods (which are nutrient poor and loaded with hydrogenated fats) and soft drinks, which are loaded with sugar, artificial colorings, and chemicals that rob the bones of the growing teen of calcium.

- Use teen thinking to your advantage. Teens want to grow, so you talk about foods that help them grow and foods that don't. For example, if your teen sees some of his peers growing at a faster rate (which is genetic, not nutritional), take this opportunity to talk with him about calcium-rich foods and how soft drinks contain phosphoric acid, which can rob him of calcium that interferes with bone growth. Adolescents are appearance conscious. Talk to them about the correlation between nutritious food and healthy-looking skin. Athletic teens are concerned about their sports performance. Teach them the connection between nutritious eating and optimal exercise performance. (See "Foods for Sport," page 367.)

This form of teaching uses the principle of "relevance." In order for a message to sink in, teens must believe the nutritional message has specific reference to them. Be specific. Tell them how it is going to affect their growth, their looks, their emotional feelings, their sports performance, or whatever seems to be the most important to the teen during that particular week.

Specific Extra Nutritional Needs of Adolescents

Encourage your teens to eat nutrient-dense foods. Adolescence is the most critical time for children to learn which foods are the most nutrient dense — those that pack the most nutrition in the fewest calories. (For a list of nutrient-dense foods, see page 352.) Here are the specific extra nutritional needs of your teen:

More iron. When entering adolescence, males need around 20 percent more iron during the phase of rapid muscle growth. Females need around 33 percent more iron once they begin menstruation. (For a list of iron-rich foods, see page 64.)

More protein. Teen males need around 25 percent more protein, at least 15 more grams than a pre-teen. Adolescent females, on the other hand, need less daily protein than males.

More zinc. Adolescent males need about a 33 percent increase in their daily requirements for zinc; adolescent females need about 20 percent more zinc than pre-adolescent females.

More calcium. Both adolescent males and females need around 33 percent more calcium than pre-adolescents (1,200 milligrams a day versus 800 milligrams).

More vitamins. Both males and females show at least a 20 to 30 percent increase in daily requirements of nearly all the vitamins as they grow from pre-teens to adolescents. Even though it is always best for an adolescent to get his or her increased needs for vitamins and minerals from food rather than from supplements, the erratic and nutrient-poor eating habits of most teens suggest that a daily multivitamin/multimineral supplement would be wise.

Finally, avoid the Barbie Doll syndrome. Teen magazines can be hazardous to your children's emotional and nutritional health, leading them to feel that they can never measure up to the perfect body and perfect skin on the perfect model shown in the magazine. Many teens equate their self-worth with what they look like — an unhealthy perception that is fostered by the unrealistic photos and messages in publications targeted to adolescents.

One of the ways that we have shaped the tastes of our adolescents is to have frequent one-on-one "dates" or "sports outings" with our teens. Either Martha or I take our teens to one of their favorite restaurants with the condition that it must have an exciting and nutritious salad bar. Watching how we carefully select a variety of fruits, grains, and vegetables will, we hope, have a lasting effect on the eating habits of our teens.

FOODS FOR SLEEP

What you eat affects how you sleep. One of the keys to a restful night's sleep is to get your brain calmed rather than revved up. Some foods contribute to restful sleep; other foods keep you awake. We call them "sleepers" and "wakers." Sleepers are tryptophan-containing foods, because tryptophan is the amino acid that the body uses to make serotonin, the neurotransmitter that slows down nerve traffic so your brain isn't so busy. Wakers are foods that stimulate neurochemicals that perk up the brain.

Foods That Help You Sleep

Tryptophan is a precursor of the sleep-inducing substances serotonin and melatonin. This means tryptophan is the raw material that the brain uses

---

NUTRITIP
A Goose Egg to Help You Sleep

One goose egg contains 400 milligrams of tryptophan, more than a serving of beef or poultry and five times the amount of tryptophan found in a chicken egg.

---

to build these relaxing neurotransmitters. Making more tryptophan available, either by eating foods that contain this substance or by seeing to it that more tryptophan gets to the brain, will help to make you sleepy. On the other hand, nutrients that make tryptophan less available can disturb sleep.

Eating carbohydrates with tryptophan-containing foods makes this calming amino acid more available to the brain. A high-carbohydrate meal stimulates the release of insulin, which helps clear from the bloodstream those amino acids that compete with tryptophan, allowing more of this natural sleep-inducing amino acid to enter the brain and manufacture sleep-inducing substances, such as serotonin and melatonin. Eating a high-protein meal without accompanying carbohydrates may keep you awake, since protein-rich foods also contain the amino acid tyrosine, which perks up the brain.

To understand how tryptophan and carbohydrates work together to relax you, picture the various amino acids from protein foods as passengers on a bus. A busload containing tryptophan and tyrosine arrives at the brain cells. If more tyrosine

---

NUTRITIP
Don't Worry, Be Sleepy.

Stress releases a hormone called "cortisol," which depletes the brain of tryptophan. This may be one reason stress keeps you awake.

SNOOZE FOODS

These are foods high in the sleep-inducing amino acid tryptophan:

- dairy products: cottage cheese, cheese, milk
- soy products: soy milk, tofu, soybean nuts
- seafood
- meats
- poultry
- whole grains
- beans
- rice
- hummus
- lentils
- hazelnuts, peanuts
- eggs
- sesame seeds, sunflower seeds

CAFFEINE AND KIDS

Many school-age children get squirrelly following a jolt of caffeine-containing cola. Kids who are already hyperactive may be bouncing off walls following a caffeine jolt. It is best to limit children's caffeine consumption to less than 50 milligrams a day, no more than one 12-ounce cola. Avoid beverages that have added caffeine, touted for their energy-boosting effects. Children should not be exposed to the addicting effects of a regular caffeine buzz.

"passengers" get off the bus and enter the brain cells, neuroactivity will rev up. If more tryptophan amino acids get off the bus, the brain will calm down. Along comes some insulin which has been stalking carbohydrates in the bloodstream. Insulin keeps the tyrosine amino acids on the bus, allowing the brain-calming tryptophan effect to be higher than the effect of the brain-revving tyrosine.

You can take advantage of this biochemical quirk by choosing protein- or carbohydrate-rich meals, depending on whether you want to perk up or slow down your brain. For students and working adults, high-protein, medium-carbohydrate meals are best eaten for breakfast and lunch. For dinner and bedtime snacks, eat a meal or snack that is high in complex carbohydrates, with a small amount of protein that contains just enough tryptophan to relax the brain. An all-carbohydrate snack, especially one high in

junk sugars, is less likely to help you sleep. You'll miss out on the sleep-inducing effects of tryptophan, and you may set off the roller-coaster effect of plummeting blood sugar followed by the release of stress hormones that will keep you awake. The best bedtime snack is one that has both complex carbohydrates and protein, and perhaps some calcium. Calcium helps the brain use the tryptophan to manufacture melatonin. This explains why dairy products, which contain both tryptophan and calcium, are one of the top sleep-inducing foods.

Best dinners for sleep. Meals that are high in carbohydrates and low to medium in protein will help you relax in the evening and set you up for a good night's sleep. Try the following "dinners for sleep":

- pasta with parmesan cheese
- scrambled eggs and cheese
- tofu stir-fry
- hummus with whole wheat pita bread
- seafood, pasta, and cottage cheese
- meats and poultry with veggies

THE EFFECTS OF ALCOHOL ON SLEEP

Contary to what many people believe, alcohol is more likely to disturb rather than induce a good night's sleep. While a drink before bed may help you fall asleep faster, alcohol interferes with sleep cycles, resulting in poorer-quality sleep. Indulging in alcohol within a couple of hours of bedtime may cause increased night waking, frequent urination during the night, indigestion, less time spent in delta (or deep) sleep, and less REM sleep. The end result is a restless night followed by a day of feeling sleep deprived. As with caffeine, the effects of alcohol on sleep vary greatly from person to person. Most people can handle a glass of wine, a bottle of beer, or one drink before bedtime and suffer no sleep disturbances.

- tuna salad sandwich
- chili with beans, not spicy
- sesame seeds (rich in tryptophan) sprinkled on salad with tuna chunks, and whole wheat crackers

Lighter meals are more likely to give you a restful night's sleep. High-fat meals and large servings prolong the work your digestive system needs to do, and all the gas production and rumblings may keep you awake. Some people find that highly seasoned foods (e.g., hot peppers and garlic) interfere with sleep, especially if they suffer from heartburn. (See the related discussion of gastroesophageal reflux, page 98.) Going to bed on a full stomach does not, for most people, promote a restful night's sleep. While you may fall asleep faster, all the intestinal work required to digest a big meal is likely to cause frequent waking and a poorer quality of sleep. Eat your evening meal early. Heed the sleep wisdom: "Don't dine after nine."

Best bedtime snacks. Foods that are high in carbohydrates, calcium, and tryptophan and medium to low in protein also make ideal sleep-inducing bedtime snacks. Some examples:

- apple pie and ice cream (my favorite)
- whole-grain cereal with milk
- hazelnuts and tofu
- oatmeal and raisin cookies, and a glass of milk
- peanut butter sandwich, ground sesame seeds

(It takes around one hour for the tryptophan in the foods to reach the brain, so don't wait until right before bedtime to have your snack.)

Foods That Keep You Awake

Caffeine-containing foods top the list of foods that wake you up. As a stimulant, caffeine speeds up the action of not only the nervous system but other major body systems, too. Within fifteen minutes of downing a cup of coffee, the level of adrenaline in your blood rises, which triggers an increase in heart rate, breathing rate, urinary output, and production of stomach acids. Basically, caffeine's effects are the reverse of what you want to happen as you go to sleep. Caffeine also prompts adrenal hormones to release sugar stored in the liver, which stimulates sugar cravings to replenish the stores. Caffeine heightens the rollercoaster effect of blood-sugar swings, producing a quick high after a morning cup of coffee, followed by a downturn in the afternoon. Caffeine's effects in the body are sort of like the law of gravity: What goes up must come down. The morning jolt is often followed by afternoon doldrums. Caffeine also makes it difficult to stay asleep.

Know your caffeine quota. Some persons are more caffeine sensitive than others. Many adults can take up to 250 milligrams of caffeine a day (the average amount in 2½ cups of coffee) and experience no sleep problems. Others get jitters after one cola.

Time your caffeine boost. For most people, the effects of caffeine wear off within six hours, so coffee in the morning will usually not interfere with sleep in the evening. Caffeine-containing beverages at lunch may not affect your sleep, but coffee, tea, or cola in the evening is likely to keep you awake.

Know what foods contain the most caffeine. As you can see from the chart, coffee, sodas, and tea rank highest in caffeine content.

Contrary to popular belief, chocolate is not high in caffeine. Two chocolate chip cookies may contain less than 5 milligrams of caffeine, a packet of cocoa mix contains 5 milligrams, and one chocolate candy bar contains only around 10 milligrams. In fact, many people find chocolate desserts that also contain dairy products are actually sleep inducers, because of the combination of tryptophan and carbohydrates.

To get the taste of tea with less of a caffeine jolt, recycle the tea bag. Discard the first cup of tea made from the tea bag, which contains the most caffeine, and make another cup. Also, don't squeeze the tea out of the tea bag, as these drops of tea contain more caffeine. Try grain-based hot beverages and caffeine-free herbal teas as alternatives to coffee and tea.

Some over-the-counter cold and headache remedies are high in caffeine. Check the labels or ask the pharmacist, especially if you are a caffeine-sensitive person.

FOODS FOR SPORTS

Young athletes burn a lot of calories, so obviously they need to eat more food than the average person. Yet, for optimal athletic performance, they need not only more food but the right kind of extra nutrition. Besides needing food to meet the body's basic nutritional requirements, the young athlete will need extra energy in proportion to the demands of the sport. For example, if an athlete in training uses 1,000 extra calories per day (the average amount used in two hours of vigorous exercise), she needs to add 1,000 extra calories of high-energy food to an already balanced diet. These foods should be primarily complex carbohydrates, foods such as fruits, juices, and grains. These additional energy requirements cannot be met by taking vitamins, protein powders, or mineral supplements, since these are not energy sources.

Get Your Stamina from Starch

Studies of athletes and the foods they eat have shown that complex carbohydrates are the best energy boosters. To appreciate the connection between what you eat and how your body uses the energy, it helps to understand a bit of muscle biochemistry.

Your body stores extra fuel in energy "banks." As you expend energy, you withdraw fuel from your bank. Your body's best bank — the one that provides the quickest service — is the carbo bank. The central carbo bank is in the liver, which stores a lot of carbohydrate energy in the form of

Food	Caffeine (mg.)
coffee, brewed, 6 ounces	105
coffee, instant, 6 ounces	55
Mountain Dew, 12 ounces	55
colas, 12 ounces	35–45
tea, 6 ounces	35

SPORTS DRINKS

Should you be lugging a bottle of commercial sports drink to your child's soccer game? What drinks provide the best nutrition for optimal performance? The answers to these questions depend upon how long and how strenuous the exercise is. If you or your child exercise moderately for *less than an hour,* plain water is the best source of fluids. Water is absorbed more rapidly than any other liquid, but once you begin adding stuff to water, the absorption slows. Drink ahead. Drink a few glasses of water before a game. During the game, drink enough to quench thirst, and after the game drink enough water to quench thirst and then drink at least two more glasses, since thirst is not a reliable indicator of adequate hydration. For high-endurance exercise lasting longer than sixty minutes, you will probably need a "carbo-lyte-hydration" drink (i.e., one containing sugar, salts, and water).

During strenuous exercise, lasting *more than one hour,* sports drinks help prevent dehydration, a major cause of muscle fatigue. The main nutritional elements in a commercial or homemade sports drink are water, carbohydrates, and electrolytes (sodium and potassium).

Try these carbo-hydration tips to enhance your performance and enjoyment of sports:

- Avoid junk juice "drinks," which contain a tiny bit of juice and a lot of added sweeteners. Instead, use "100 percent juice."
- Avoid carbonated drinks, which can leave the athlete feeling bloated.
- Before the game, instead of soft drinks, drink plain water. Besides slowing the absorption of much needed water, the sugar in the soft drink could trigger low blood sugar during the game — just what the athlete doesn't need.
- Instead of buying commercial sports drinks, make your own. Juices such as apple, orange, or grape are an excellent base for sports drinks, since they contain both glucose and fructose sugars, as well as potassium, which is lost with sweating. Fructose sugar is one of the best carbohydrates for replacing used-up muscle glycogen stores. Add 1 teaspoon of salt (to replace the sodium lost while sweating) to 1 quart of diluted juice, to taste, and you've made your own sports drink.
- The best time to drink commercial or homemade sports drinks is *during* exercise, since the carbs in the drink do not cause high blood-sugar fluctuations during exercise. (Drinking a high-sugar drink prior to exercise may trigger insulin release and lead to hypoglycemia in the middle of the game.)
- As a general rule, sip 1 quart of cool rehydration liquid per hour of strenuous exercise.
- It's better to drink liquid calories rather than eat solid food during exercise, since solids remain in the stomach longer and delay the absorption of the much-needed carbs and water.

A useful reference for eating and drinking wisely during exercise is *Nancy Clark's Sports Nutrition Guidebook* (Human Kinetics, 1996).

glycogen, long chains of glucose molecules linked together. Glycogen molecules are like stacks of money in the bank, ready to be withdrawn as needed. The carbo bank has branch offices located in the muscles throughout your body. The deposits in the branch offices are known as "muscle glycogen." When muscles need energy during exercise, they quickly withdraw muscle glycogen from the bank, like having a cash machine right there at the shopping mall.

Of course, you have to put money in the bank before you can take it out. So it is with depositing fuel into your carbo bank. Before a high-energy competition, you'll want to be sure you have enough extra energy stored so that you can withdraw it as needed. Depositing energy stores before the big game is called "carbo loading," which means you stock your carbo bank with extra fuel to burn on game day.

Best Foods for Carbo Loading

Starches, such as grains and legumes, are the best foods for building up muscle glycogen. A steady insulin level is necessary for stocking the muscles with glycogen, which is why complex carbohydrates, those with a low glycemic index, promote better glycogen storage than simple sugars, such as glucose or sucrose. Eating an increased amount of complex carbohydrates for several days before a major competition will build up stores of muscle glycogen. Best carbohydrates for carbo loading are fruits (e.g., apples and oranges), vegetables, legumes, and whole grains. Carbo loading does not mean overeating. It simply means increasing the percentage of carbohydrates in your diet to around 70 percent of your total daily calories for three days before the game. Immediately before or during a game it's best to eat foods with a high glycemic index, such as honey, bananas, raisins, carrots, and white rice. Corn flakes also have a high glycemic index.

Why not simply eat more complex carbs right before the game? Because of a biochemical quirk, stored muscle glycogen is a more readily available source of fuel than carbohydrates consumed right before the game. Muscle glycogen is like an automatic withdrawal system, releasing energy quickly as the muscles need it during exercise. The sugar consumed just before the game must go through some biochemical processing before it can be released for energy. That takes time, like depositing a check in the bank and then having to wait for the check to clear before withdrawing money. For maximal energy release, you load the muscles with glycogen for several days before the game.

Best Foods for Amateur Athletes

Carbo loading is not necessary or advisable for every sport. It is used mainly by participants in endurance sports, those that require continuous exertion for longer than ninety minutes. For most amateur athletes, extreme carbohydrate loading is not necessary. Instead, sticking to a balanced diet (approximately 60 to 65 percent complex carbohydrates, 15 to 20 percent protein, and 20 to 25 percent fat) in the days before the game is sufficient. If you are involved in an important competition and you think carbo loading might help you, consult a professional trainer or ask your coach about the right type of diet and training regimen for the week before your competition. For most amateur athletes, the following carbohydrate regimen is sufficient for optimal sports performance:

Make carbohydrates 70 percent of your calories three days before the game. A teen athlete consuming around 3,000 calories daily would need to consume around 500 grams of carbohydrates spaced in several meals throughout the day. Remember the sports axiom "Saturday's game is played on Thursday's food." Eating a high-energy, nutritious diet for several days before the game stores up energy.

Prehydrate your body for three days before the game. Drink extra water, approximately three-quarters of an ounce per pound (a 160-pound athlete would drink twelve 10-ounce glasses of water a day). Since muscle contains so much water, a slight degree of dehydration can greatly diminish muscle performance. Dried-up muscles become weak.

Enjoy a performance-boosting pregame meal. The pregame meal should be low in fat, since fatty foods take longer to digest and may leave an athlete still feeling full at game time. Ideally, the pregame meal is eaten three hours prior to the game. The best pregame meal is high in complex carbohydrates (about 70 percent of calories), with medium amounts of protein (about 20 percent of calories), and low in fat (around 10 percent of calories). Protein stimulates insulin to help the muscles use glucose more efficiently. Protein also helps to energize the brain. The small amount of fat slows the intestinal absorption of carbohydrates, so that the sugar enters the bloodstream at a steady rate.

For a teen athlete, the pregame meal should contain about 100 grams of complex carbohydrates. Here are some good foods to include:

- oatmeal (or cereal), fruit, and carrot juice
- peanut butter and jelly sandwich on whole-grain bread
- whole-grain pasta with a low-fat sauce
- low-fat yogurt and fruit

Eating and drinking just before and during the game. Studies show that taking sugars, such as candy, honey, or sucrose, before exercise results in reduced performance. Some research suggests that eating or drinking sweets within an hour of exercise may decrease performance, due to too much of an insulin rush and the roller-coaster effect of high and low blood sugar. While the amount of energy already in your body at the start of the game has the most influence on your performance, it's also important to replenish food and fluids during the game. Quick-energy carbohydrates are those with a high glycemic index (see page 35), carbs that raise blood sugar quickly, such as orange juice, bananas, raisins, and carrots.

Rehydrate your body after the game. After vigorous exercise, you need to replenish water, carbohydrates, and electrolytes that were used up during the game. As soon as the game is over, drink at least two full glasses of plain, cool water. Then eat and drink carbohydrate-rich foods. Remember to eat and drink *slowly* after a game to avoid nausea, heartburn, and cramps that may result from overloading your intestines with too much food and drink too soon. Rehydrating yourself with plain water first will often prevent after-game fatigue, cramps, and abdominal upset.

NUTRITIP
Foods for Skin

The best foods for healthy skin (especially for treating dry skin and eczema) are omega-3 fatty acids, such as flax seeds or flaxseed oil and salmon and tuna fish. The antioxidants vitamin C and vitamin E act like nature's own protection.

37

Feeding Your Immune System

AN ARMY OF MILLIONS of microscopic soldiers operates within you, each one ready to spring into battle against invading germs and to do sentry duty to prevent disease from occurring in the first place. How you feed these soldiers has a great influence on how well they protect you from germs and disease. Because of poor diets, many school-age children and adults have immune systems that don't operate at peak efficiency. They get sick more often. Here's how to have a well-nourished immune system.

HOW YOUR IMMUNE ARMY WORKS

Think of your immune system as an army in which each division has a specific job, depending on the enemy it is fighting. Let's meet the troops to see what each kind of defender does.

White Blood Cells

White blood cells are the body's infantry, the hardworking soldiers on the frontlines. These cells patrol the highway of the body's bloodstream, preventing germs from gaining a foothold. There are millions of these microscopic fighters in each drop of blood. There are also many specialized units. For example, when enemy cells try to hide from the main white-cell troops, specialized units of white cells called "macrophages" (the word means "big eaters") mount search-and-destroy missions, going into all the nooks and crannies of the body to gobble up harmful invaders.

Suppose a flu virus enters your body, mutliplies rapidly, and threatens to overwhelm the circulating white-cell army. The main troops can call out the reinforcements. These specialized cells include T-lymphocytes (white cells that originate in the thymus, a tiny gland in front of the heart) and even a special SWAT team called "killer lymphocytes."

Chemical Messengers and Fighters

The immune army has a magnificent communication system. If a germ enters the body, say, through a break in the skin or an infection in the throat, the white cells send out chemical messengers that quickly mobilize reinforcements and direct them to the area of infection. Once they reach the battle, these cells produce chemical fighters known as "cytokines" (meaning, "molecules that move to the cells"). These cytokines perform all kinds of functions around the infection site to surround the invaders and heal the havoc the enemy has created. They dilate the blood vessels, causing more blood flow, enabling more white-cell police to enter the

SNAKE OIL SCIENCE

How often have you heard herbal medicine or alternative therapy sneered at as "snake oil"? This term and the attitudes behind it are both unfair and unscientific. The original snake oil was not a hoax, but a real medicine. It came from a Chinese snake that in Oriental medicine was believed to have healing properties. Around the turn of the century there was a fight between the snake oil salesmen and the patent medicine salesmen, and as the big business of pharmaceutical patents began to dominate the practice of medicine, nearly all the medicines found in natural sources were dubbed "snake oil." Over the years, the public was swayed into trusting "scientific" prescription patent medicines and distrusting alternatives.

There were economic reasons for this shift. Stringent FDA regulations were designed to protect the public from drugs that make false healing claims. To comply with these regulations, pharmaceutical companies must spend millions of dollars to test both the efficacy and safety of their drugs. In order to protect their investment, companies patent their drugs, so that other companies can't steal their product and make a profit without having paid for the development of the drug. The potential profit is what motivates companies to spend huge sums of money for research and development of new medicines. Seems fair. It's the American way!

While this process may seem to be good economics, is it good medicine? Natural-source medicines can't be patented or tightly regulated, so there is little economic motivation for research on these alternative therapies. Under current laws in the United States, anyone can make just about any health claim about natural medicines or herbs without having the science to back it up. But the growing disillusionment with standard medicine and the soaring cost of prescription drugs have sent millions of health seekers to their local health food store for more easily available and less costly alternatives. So, it's back to the battle between the snake oil and the patent medicine salesmen. The modern difference is they're both making a huge profit.

---

infected area of battle. One well-known cytokine, interferon, even sends a signal back to command headquarters to tell the brain the body needs to rest. This allows the body to concentrate its energies on the battle against the disease. Another important cytokine is called the "tumor necrosis factor." It can gobble up cancer cells that are acting like traitors and weakening the body from within. Another task of these cytokine messengers is to tell the body to conserve supplies, such as important nutrients that are needed to win the infection battle. For example, the command center instructs the body to hold on to immune-boosting elements such as zinc rather than eliminating it through the kidneys.

Chemical Weapons

The army of white cells and chemical messengers has a number of chemical weapons available. They can shoot gamma-interferon into the enemy like a poisonous dart. This substance interferes with the germ's ability to reproduce itself. Another special group of white cells, called "B-cells," produces chemicals called "antibodies," which act like smart missiles, seeking out and attaching themselves to specific germs. Some of these antibodies, called "immunoglobulins," poke holes in the germs, so that in essence they "bleed" to death. Others act like a chemical glue, making the germs stick together so that they can be rounded up easily by the white blood cells. The immune army also guards strategic entry points to the body, such as the respiratory and gastrointestinal tracts. Within the mucus that lines these passages, specialized immunoglobulin antibodies called "secretory IgA" patrol the walls and prevent bacteria and allergens from invading the tissues.

The most fascinating aspect of this immune army is the remarkable memory it possesses. It remembers every past battle and learns from experience. If the same, or a similar, germ tries to attack again, the army is ready for it. It recognizes the invader and pounces on it, winning every time. This is the rationale behind immunizations. The small dose of killed virus given in an immunization sets up a training exercise for the immune army. It uses the lessons learned in training to overcome threats from the real germ.

Problems in the Ranks

While the immune system works well most of the time, some germs, such as the herpes virus, are particularly adept at evading attacks. Herpes can lie undetected in the tissues for long periods of time only to come out and spread when the army's defenses are down. Then it retreats back into its hideout, lying dormant for months or years before it wages another attack. Some viruses, such as HIV, can even hide within the immune system itself, infiltrating the ranks of the army and destroying it from within.

Cancer cells are another tough challenge to the immune system. These are cells whose internal control mechanism is damaged, allowing the cells to multiply out of control. Most of the time the immune army quickly recognizes these "criminal" elements and eliminates or jails them before they cause damage. Sometimes the cancer culprits go unnoticed for a while, and by the time they are detected, the immune system is powerless to stop them. The battle spreads to other parts of the body (a disease process called "metastasis").

Sometimes the immune army mutinies and attacks the very organs it is supposed to defend. Examples of such autoimmune diseases are arthritis (in which antibodies attack tissues of the joints), diabetes (in which antibodies attack insulin-producing cells in the pancreas), and perhaps multiple sclerosis (in which the immune system may be attacking the myelin sheath of the nerves).

Finally, there are times when the immune system overreacts, in effect, burning an entire village to kill a few terrorists. This happens in the case of allergy, a hypersensitive response. The army of white cells not only engulfs the invading allergen, such as a particle from a dust mite in the bedroom, but also releases enough chemicals in this battle to cause other problems, such as wheezing or rashes.

IMMUNE SYSTEM WEAKENERS

Certain foods and environmental influences can keep the immune system army from doing a good job. Watch out for these threats to your body's defenses.

An overdose of sugar. Eating or drinking 100 grams (8 tbsp.) of sugar, the equivalent of two and a half 12-ounce cans of soda, can reduce the ability of white blood cells to kill germs by 40 percent. The immune-suppressing effect of sugar starts less than thirty minutes after ingestion and may last for five hours. In contrast, the ingestion of complex carbohydrates, or starches, has no effect on the immune system.

Excess alcohol. Excessive alcohol intake can harm the body's immune system in two ways. First, it produces an overall nutritional deficiency, depriving the body of valuable immune-boosting nutrients. Second, alcohol, like sugar, consumed in excess can reduce the ability of white cells to kill germs. High doses of alcohol suppress the ability of the white blood cells to multiply, inhibit the action of killer white cells on cancer cells, and lessen the ability of macrophages to produce tumor necrosis factors. One drink (the equivalent of 12 ounces of beer, 5 ounces of wine, or 1 ounce of hard liquor) does not appear to bother the immune system, but three or more drinks do. Damage to the immune system increases in proportion to the quantity of alcohol consumed. Amounts of alcohol that are enough to cause intoxication are also enough to suppress immunity.

Food allergens. Due to a genetic quirk, some divisions of the immune army recognize a common everyday food (e.g., milk) as a foreign invader and attack it, causing an allergic reaction. Before the battle, the intestinal lining was like a wall impenetrable to foreign invaders. After many encounters with food allergens, the wall is damaged, enabling invaders and other potentially toxic substances in the food to get into the bloodstream and make the body feel miserable. This condition is known as the "leaky gut syndrome."

Too much fat. Obesity can lead to a depressed immune system. It can affect the ability of white blood cells to multiply, produce antibodies, and rush to the site of an infection.

Stress. While periodic stress can help the body mobilize its resources to fight off threats to its well-being, chronic stress or unresolved anxiety can wear out the immune system. This is called "stress-induced immune suppression," a condition that explains why people often get sick after a divorce, death of a loved one, loss of a job, or some other stressful life event. Stress hormones, such as cortisol, decrease the immune response. Also, because the brain and the immune system communicate with one another by neurohormones, your state of mind can affect your state of immunity.

Stress control is especially important as we age. Repeated exposure to stress gradually wears out the immune system, which may explain why older people get sick more often. The older you are, the more careful you need to be about feeding your immune system well.

IMMUNE SYSTEM BOOSTERS

Feeding your immune system well boosts its fighting power. Immune system boosters work in many ways. They increase the number of white cells in the immune system army, train them to fight better, and help them form an overall better battle plan. Boosters also help to eliminate the dead wood in the army, substances that drag the body down. Below are the top nine nutrients to add to your family's diet to cut down on days missed from work and school because of illness. Over the years, numerous nutrients have been touted to boost immunity, but there is some scientific basis for believing that the following substances can improve your health.

Vitamin C. Vitamin C tops the list of immune boosters for many reasons. There has been more research about the immune-boosting effects of vitamin C than perhaps any other nutrient. Vitamin C supplements are inexpensive to produce,

---

NUTRITIP
Partners in Health

The three top immune-boosting antioxidants, vitamins C and E and beta carotene, work better together. This is the principle of synergy: 1 + 1 + 1 = 4. Either take a multivitamin supplement that is rich in all three of these antioxidants or eat a variety of foods that contain significant amounts of these three antioxidants.

THE IMMUNE SYSTEM—BOOSTER SMOOTHIE

Children and adults don't feel like eating following a cold or illness. Their nutrition and their immune system suffer. This accounts for the common occurrence of getting one infection after another. It's best to keep so well nourished that the nutritional reserves can withstand several days of poor eating. Drink this smoothie for two weeks after an illness to bounce back from poor nutrition during an infection. As a preventive measure, drink this smoothie daily upon school entry in September, upon beginning day care, upon exposure to a contagious illness, or when you or your child feel a cold coming on.

½ cup each high vitamin C–containing fruits: strawberry, papaya, cantaloupe, guava

8 ounces plain yogurt (Be sure it contains live and active cultures, which replenish the bacteria of the bowels, especially after taking antibiotics.)

¼ cup flaxseed meal

500 mg. echinacea (drops or powder)

a multivitamin formula (see "School-Ade," page 309)

10 mg. zinc

100 mcg. selenium

50–100 IU vitamin E

Mix the above ingredients with the rest of the School-Ade recipe according to the instructions listed on page 309.

and it's available naturally in many fruits and vegetables. Also, you can buy a vitamin C–fortified version of just about anything. Here's what the research shows about how this mighty vitamin protects your body.

Vitamin C increases the production of infection-fighting white blood cells and antibodies and increases levels of interferon, the antibody that coats cell surfaces, preventing the entry of viruses. Vitamin C reduces the risk of cardiovascular disease by raising levels of HDL (good) cholesterol while lowering blood pressure and interfering with the process by which fat is converted to plaque in the arteries. As an added perk, persons whose diets are higher in vitamin C have lower rates of colon, prostate, and breast cancer.

You don't have to take in massive amounts of vitamin C to boost your immune system. Around 200 milligrams a day seems to be a generally agreed-upon amount and one that can be automatically obtained by eating at least six servings of fruits and vegetables a day (see "Top Seven Vitamin C–Containing Fruits," page 52, and "Top Vitamin C Veggies," page 164). If you take vitamin C supplements, it's best to space them throughout the day rather than taking one large dose, most of which may end up being excreted in the urine.

Vitamin E. This important antioxidant and immune system booster doesn't get as much press as vitamin C, yet it's important to a healthy immune system.

Vitamin E stimulates the production of natural killer cells, those that seek out and destroy germs and cancer cells. Vitamin E enhances the production of B-cells, the immune cells that produce antibodies that destroy bacteria. Vitamin E supplementation may also reverse some of the decline in immune response commonly seen in aging. Vitamin E has been cited as lowering the risk of cardiovascular disease. In the Harvard School of Public Health study of eighty-seven thousand nurses, vitamin E supplementation was shown to cut the risk of heart attack by 50 percent.

The richest sources of vitamin E are listed on page 71. It's not difficult to get 30 to 60 milligrams every day of vitamin E from a diet rich in seeds, vegetable oils, and grains, but it's difficult for most people to consume more than 60 milligrams a day consistently through diet alone. Supplements may be necessary to get enough vitamin E to boost your immune system.

You need 100 to 400 milligrams per day, depending on your general lifestyle. People who don't exercise, who smoke, and who consume high amounts of alcoholic beverages will need the higher dosage. Those with a more moderate lifestyle can get by with lower levels of supplementation.

Carotenoids. Beta carotene increases the number of infection-fighting cells, natural killer cells, and T-helper cells, as well as being a powerful antioxidant that mops up excess free radicals that accelerate aging. Like the other two of the Big Three antioxidants, vitamins C and E, it reduces the risk of cardiovascular disease by interfering with how the fats and cholesterol in the bloodstream oxidize to form arterial plaque. Studies have shown that beta carotene can lower the risk of cardiovascular disease, especially strokes and heart attacks, lending scientific credence to the belief that a carrot a day can keep the heart surgeon away. Beta carotene also protects against cancer by stimulating the immune cells called "macrophages" to produce tumor necrosis factor, which kills cancer cells. It has also been shown that beta carotene supplements can increase the production of T-cell lymphocytes and natural killer cells and can enhance the ability of the natural killer cells to attack cancer cells.

Beta carotene is the most familiar carotenoid, but it is only one member of a large family. Researchers believe that it is not just beta carotene that produces all these good effects, but all the carotenoids working together. This is why getting carotenoids in food may be more cancer-protective than taking beta carotene supplements.

The body converts beta carotene to vitamin A,

> ### NUTRITIP
> #### Color Means Carotenoids.
>
> Dr. Bill would like to add an addendum to grandmother's wise principle that the more colorful the diet, the more nutritious it is: The deeper the color, the more nutrients there are. Don't settle for pale iceberg lettuce; eat deep green spinach instead. Try bright orange sweet potatoes.

which itself has anti-cancer properties and immune system–boosting functions. But too much vitamin A can be toxic to the body, so it's better to get extra beta carotene from foods and let the body naturally regulate how much of this precursor is converted to the immune-fighting vitamin A. It's highly unlikely that a person could take in enough beta carotene to produce a toxic amount of vitamin A, because when the body has enough vitamin A, it stops making it. (For a list of carotenoid-containing foods, see page 69.)

Bioflavonoids. A group of phytonutrients called "bioflavonoids" aids the immune system by protecting the cells of the body against environmental pollutants. Bioflavonoids protect the cell membranes against the pollutants trying to attach to them. Along the membrane of each cell there are microscopic parking spaces, called "receptor sites." Pollutants, toxins, or germs can park here and gradually eat their way into the membrane of the cell, but when bioflavonoids fill up these parking spots, there is no room for toxins to park. Bioflavonoids also reduce cholesterol's ability to form plaque in the arteries and lessen the formation of microscopic clots inside arteries, which can lead to heart attack and stroke. Studies have shown that people who eat the most bioflavonoids have less cardiovascular disease. A diet that contains a wide variety of fruits and vegetables, at least six servings per day, will help you get the bioflavonoids needed to help your immune system work in top form.

Zinc. This valuable mineral increases the production of white blood cells that fight infection and helps them fight more aggressively. It also increases killer cells that fight against cancer and helps white cells release more antibodies. Zinc supplements have been shown to slow the growth of cancer.

Zinc increases the number of infection-fighting T-cells, especially in elderly people, who are often deficient in zinc and whose immune system often weakens with age. The anti-infection hype around zinc is controversial. While some studies claim that zinc supplements in the form of lozenges can lower the incidence and severity of infections, other studies have failed to show this correlation. A word of caution: Too much zinc in the form of supplements (more than 75 milligrams a day) can inhibit immune-system function. It's safest to stick to getting zinc from your diet and aim for 15 to 25 milligrams a day.

For infants and children, there is some evidence that dietary zinc supplements may reduce the incidence of acute respiratory infections, but

---

NUTRITIP
More Is Less.

If some is good, more is better, right? Not necessarily. Sometimes more is less. The body works best with an optimal amount of nutrients. Too little can make you sick, but so can too much. Take care when adding vitamin and mineral supplements to your diet, particularly vitamin A, and the metal-minerals, namely, zinc, iron, and copper.

---

this is controversial. The best source of zinc for infants and young children is zinc-fortified cereals.

Garlic. This flavorful member of the onion family is a powerful immune-system booster that stimulates the multiplication of infection-fighting white cells, boosts natural killer cell activity, and increases the efficiency of antibody production. The immune system–boosting properties of garlic seem to be due to its sulfur-containing compounds, such as allicin and sulfides. Garlic also acts as an antioxidant, reducing the buildup of free radicals in the bloodstream. Garlic may protect against cancer, though the evidence is controversial. Cultures with a garlic-rich diet have a lower incidence of intestinal cancer. Garlic may also play a part in getting rid of potential carcinogens and other toxic substances. It is also a heart-friendly food since it keeps platelets from sticking together and clogging tiny blood vessels.

Selenium. This mineral increases natural killer cells and mobilizes cancer-fighting cells. Best food sources of selenium are tuna, red snapper, lobster, shrimp, whole grains, vegetables (depending on the selenium content of the soil they're grown in), brown rice, egg yolks, cottage cheese, chicken (white meat), sunflower seeds, garlic, Brazil nuts, and lamb chops.

Omega-3 fatty acids. A study found that children taking ½ teaspoon of flax oil a day experienced fewer and less severe respiratory infections and fewer days of being absent from school than children who did not. The omega-3 fatty acids in flax oil and fatty fish, such as salmon, tuna, and mackerel, act as immune boosters by increasing the activity of phagocytes, the white blood cells that eat up bacteria. (Perhaps this is why grandmothers used to insist on a daily dose of unpalatable cod liver oil.) Essential fatty acids also protect the body against damage from overreactions to infection. When taking essential-fatty-acid supple-

RICH SOURCES OF ZINC

Food Source of Zinc	Serving Size	Zinc (in milligrams)
Oysters	6 medium	76
Zinc-fortified cereals	1 ounce	0–15
Crab	3 ounces	7
Beef	3 ounces	6
Turkey, dark meat	3 ounces	3.8
Beans	½ cup	1.2–1.8

ments, such as flax or fish oils, take additional vitamin E, which acts together with essential fatty acids to boost the immune system. One way to get more omega-3 fatty acids in your diet is to add 1 to 3 teaspoons of flax oil to a fruit and yogurt smoothie (see School-Ade recipe, page 309).

Echinacea. Echinacea is one of the top-selling herbal remedies throughout the world. It also is one of the oldest. Not only has this healing herb enjoyed long popularity, it also has been the subject of much scientific research. These are the questions you may have about about this valuable addition to your home pharmacy.

What is it, and how does it work?

Echinacea is a native American plant that was recognized over a century ago as a natural infection fighter. It is an *immunostimulant,* a substance that boosts the body's immune system. Unlike traditional antibiotics that kill bacteria directly, echinacea works indirectly, killing the germ by strengthening your immune system. While the entire echinacea story is still being researched, there is some evidence that it stimulates the body to produce more infection-fighting white blood cells, such as T-lymphocytes and killer white blood cells. It may also stimulate the release of interferons, one of the body's most potent infection-

fighting weapons. Interferon kills germs and also infiltrates their genetic control center, preventing them from reproducing. Besides helping the body produce more infection-fighting cells, echinacea helps these cells to produce more macrophages (germ-eating cells), and it helps these cells eat the germs more voraciously, a process called "phagocytosis." Echinacea also prevents bacteria from secreting an enzyme called "hyaluronidase," which enables them to break through protective membranes, such as the lining of the intestines and respiratory tract, and invade tissues. Echinacea also seems to search out and destroy some viruses, such as the common cold and flu viruses.

Is there proof that echinacea works?

Absolutely, but the research is not well known in America. The best research on echinacea comes from Germany, a country that is far ahead of the United States in the scientific study of over-the-counter herbal medicines. Echinacea has been studied in Germany using double-blind, placebo-controlled studies, the gold standard for scientific research on drugs. In this type of study, one group gets the real pill and the other group, the control group, gets a look-alike dummy pill. Neither the researcher nor the research subjects know who has gotten which pill until data collection is completed and the data are analyzed. This kind of research is especially necessary in studying herbal medicines to correct for the well-known placebo effect in which even a dummy pill can produce healing effects because of the power of suggestion. A double-blind, placebo-controlled study has shown that echinacea users experienced less frequent and less severe virus infections (colds and flus) by one-third to one-half compared to the group that took dummy pills (which, it's interesting to note, also reported a decrease in severity of flu symptoms).

Is echinacea safe?

Studies have not shown any toxic effects of echinacea. The occasional person may experience some GI disturbances, such as diarrhea.

How should echinacea be taken, and what is the proper dosage?

When and how much echinacea to take depends on your individual immune system and the medical reason you want to take it. It's best to seek dosage and timing advice from a naturopath or medical doctor knowledgeable about herbal medicines. For example, there are conditions in which you wouldn't want to hype up your immune system, such as illnesses presumably caused by an overactive immune system, called "autoimmune diseases."

Studies on the safety and efficacy of echinacea in adults suggest the following dosage: 300 milligrams three times a day for a total of 900 milligrams a day. The dosage in children has not been studied as much, but a sensible amount would be one-half the adult dose for children aged six to thirteen, and one-quarter the adult dose for children under six.

Some people take echinacea all the time to prevent colds and flu, and others take it just for a couple of weeks when they feel the first signs of a cold coming on or if they have been exposed to a contagious viral infection. While there is no scientific evidence that taking echinacea daily for months helps or harms, theoretically, taking any immune booster for too long could cause it to lose its punch or could stress the immune system. Another theoretical concern is that any drug that tampers with the genetic material of a virus cell (as echinacea does) could also affect the genetic material of cells in the body or could cause a few viruses to change genetically and become more resistant and more virulent.

Because of these concerns, taking echinacea as a preventive medicine during the cold and flu season (two weeks, then two weeks off) may be unwise, as there is no scientific basis for this popular regimen. Instead consider the following:

1. when you feel a cold coming on or have been exposed to a contagious virus, take echinacea for two weeks, then stop;
2. when you are under stress because of life changes (positive as well as negative), pressures at work or at home, travel, or any other situation that affects your emotional or physical health, take echinacea for a couple of weeks;
3. when entering a situation that challenges the immune system, such as the beginning of school in September, entering a new day-care situation, or any other new group of people that increases your contact with germs, take echinacea for two weeks.

Feeding your immune system each day is one way to help your medical bills go away.

38

The Anti-Cancer Diet

CANCER IS A PREVENTABLE disease in many cases. The Harvard Report on Cancer Prevention lists the relative risk factors as the following:

Cancer Risk Factors	Percent of Cancer Deaths
• Smoking	30
• Diet (animal-food based)	30
• Lack of exercise	5
• Carcinogens in the workplace	5
• Family history of cancer	5

Since one-third of cancers are diet related, change your diet and you drastically decrease your chances of getting cancer.* Each year the United States spends billions of dollars on cancer research, and our country excels in the treatment of cancer. We have some of the best cancer specialists and cancer treatment centers in the world. Yet, the United States is pitifully inadequate when it

comes to cancer prevention. After battling and surviving colon cancer, my main concern was how to keep from getting cancer again. As part of my treatment program, I consulted top cancer specialists and visited one of the top cancer centers in the world. When I asked what I could do nutritionally to lower my chances of having, shall we say, a "return visit," the oncologist glibly said, "Don't eat too many hamburgers." Such was the extent of nutritional counseling for cancer prevention. That's when I realized that a cancer survivor is more motivated than even the top cancer specialists to do his homework on preventive medicine. After all, cancer centers and cancer specialists make their living on treatment, not prevention, and while there is no lack of money for cancer research in America, research money is targeted primarily at developing new understandings and treatment of cancer, with a pitifully small proportion of government research funds directed toward prevention. Cancer research is a glaring example of funding the wrong end: too much money spent on treatment, too little spent on prevention.

No one in the world is more motivated to seek out an anti-cancer regimen than a cancer survivor who wants to be sure he remains a survivor, but I was also motivated by concern for my children. There is a strong hereditary tendency in our fam-

---

* A link between diet and cancer is difficult to study because of the many factors that contribute to the development of disease. For example, persons with healthier diets tend to have healthier overall lifestyles. Researchers use various statistical methods to factor in these variables when drawing diet-cancer correlations.

NUTRITIP
Nasty Nitrates

Nitrates and nitrites, preservatives added to foods, especially processed meats, form carcinogenic nitrosamines in the intestines. Fortunately, many of the phytonutrients in fruits and vegetables can fight against these nitrosamines. It's even better to keep them out of your bowel in the first place.

NUTRITIP
**An Apple a Day May Keep
the Cancer Doctor Away.**

Pectin, the fiber in apple skin, is fermented in the intestines, producing short-chain fatty acids that prevent the growth of harmful bacteria. They also nourish the cells of the intestinal lining, making them a more

---

ily for cancer. Both Martha's mother and my father died of colon cancer. Some people have genes that give cells an increased chance of mutating, or becoming malignant. These are called "oncogenes," meaning, "cancer-risk genes." The influence of these genes does not become apparent unless they are activated by certain carcinogens. If you inherit oncogenes for a particular cancer, there are three ways to lower your risk of getting that cancer:

1. Decrease your exposure to carcinogens — cancer-causing irritants, pollutants, or substances in your diet.
2. Boost your immune system so it can fight against and eliminate cells that have become precancerous by mutation.
3. Consume a diet that decreases the formation, or growth, of potentially malignant cells.

THE LINK BETWEEN DIET AND CANCER

While there is ongoing debate in many fields of preventive medicine, the diet-cancer link is no longer controversial, thanks to a monumental six-year study called the "China Project," conducted by universities in America, China, and Great

Britain. This study concluded that the standard American diet contributes greatly to the high incidence of cancer and cardiovascular disease. The most influential studies linking cancer and diet showed the following significant correlations:

- A plant-based diet instead of an animal-based diet lowers the rate of breast, prostate, and colon cancers.

- Lung, breast, prostate, and colon cancers (the "big bad four") account for more than half of all cancer deaths. The good news is these are also the cancers for which dietary changes can lower the risk.

- Diet can be implicated in at least one-third of all cancers.

- Increasing your daily consumption of fruits and vegetables can greatly lower your cancer risk.

- Diet probably plays more of a role in cancer development than genes. It is well known that the incidence of most cancers is less in Asian cultures. Studies have shown that when Asians moved to the United States and switched from primarily a plant-based diet to an animal-based diet, their cancer rates increased to approach those of Americans.

During my recovery from surgery, chemotherapy, and radiation therapy for colon cancer, I

THE ANTI-CANCER TEN-STEP PROGRAM

1. Reduce stress.
2. Stay lean.
3. Increase exercise.
4. Limit dietary fat to 20 percent of total calories, with less than 7 percent of total calories from saturated fats. Eliminate hydrogenated fats.
5. Increase fiber to between 25 and 35 grams a day.
6. Eat lots of fresh fruits and vegetables.
7. Eat foods high in the antioxidants beta carotene, vitamin C, and vitamin E.
8. Switch from red meat to seafood and soy products.
9. Eat foods high in calcium.
10. Consider daily supplements of the following:

- vitamin C, 500 mg.
- calcium, 500 mg. (elemental)
- flaxseed meal (ground flaxseed), 30 grams
- acidophilus powder, 1 tsp.
- vitamin E, 200 IU
- selenium, 100 mcg.

With trillions of cell duplications occurring inside you every day, it stands to reason that a few of those cells will become out-of-control renegades. If your body's immune system is strong enough to search out and destroy these cells, you don't "get cancer." If the cells win the battle with your body, you do get cancer. Good nutrition is one of many ways you can help your body fight this daily battle. If you think of phytonutrients in plant foods as *chemo-prevention,* you may someday spare yourself chemotherapy. Enjoy your food and your health!

thoroughly researched many claims about diet and lifestyle in relation to cancer risk. The anti-cancer regimen in this chapter is based on scientifically valid studies about cancer risk.

You don't all of a sudden "get cancer." Chances are great that you, and even your children, have a few cancer cells lurking in your body, but an efficient immune system is eliminating these threatening cells before they have a chance to multiply. This is why we emphasize beginning the anti-cancer regimen, especially the anti-cancer diet, in early childhood, since cancer cells develop very slowly over decades and may not be detected until decades later.

I shared this information and everything that follows with my children, wanting to inform them, not scare them, and, if possible, spare them the incredible pain of surgery, chemotherapy, radiation therapy, and the possibility of a shorter life.

Judging from all the research I have read, if I follow the anti-cancer regimen in this chapter, I have a 95 percent chance of beating this cancer. I wish somebody had given me this information when I was thirty.

TWELVE DIETARY CHANGES THAT WILL LOWER YOUR CANCER RISK

Some foods actually contribute to the development of cancer; other foods lessen the risk. The following anti-cancer diet greatly lowers your risk of colorectal cancer and nearly all other types of cancers. It can also help prevent cardiovascular disease. It is basically the diet all people should follow anyway. For people with a genetic tendency to colorectal cancer, it is not just an option, it's a lifesaving necessity.

1. Keep Your Diet Low in Total Fat and Very Low in Saturated Fats

There are at least two ways in which dietary fat contributes to cancer. First, tumor cells need low-density lipoproteins (LDL's) to grow. Therefore, a diet that helps to lower LDL (bad) cholesterol levels could keep potentially cancerous cells from growing. Eating fat also stimulates the production of bile, which is needed to digest fat. If a lot of bile is allowed to stagnate in the large intestine for a long period of time, bacteria convert the bile into a proven carcinogen, apcholic acid. Here are some tips for eating not only less fat but the right fats:

Eat less total fat. Limit your daily fat intake to no more than 20 percent of your total food calories. (I shoot for 15 percent.) This means that if you average 2,500 calories a day, fat should provide no more than 500 of these calories. This means you should eat around 55 grams of fat per day — maximum. (On a 2,000-calories-per-day diet, you would eat about 45 grams of fat.)

Eat the right fat. Eating the wrong kinds of fat may be even more cancer causing than eating too much fat. Cancer researchers became aware of this fat fact when they noticed that the incidence of most cancers is less in some cultures that actually

have a high-fat diet, such as Eskimos (who eat a lot of seafood rich in omega-3 fatty acids) and the Mediterranean diet (which is plant based, but high in monounsaturated oils). These fats do not contribute to cancer and may in fact have some anti-cancer properties:

- unsaturated fats, found in plant foods, such as legumes
- vegetable oils that are high in monounsaturated fats, such as olive oil (Greek women who tend to eat a diet rich in olive oil have a very low incidence of breast cancer) and canola oil. A 1998 study showed that men who ate less animal fat and more vegetable fat in their diets had less prostate cancer.
- seafood, such as salmon and tuna, that is high in omega-3 fatty acids
- oils that contain more omega-3 than omega-6 fatty acids, such as flaxseed, pumpkin seed, canola, soybean (not hydrogenated), walnut, safflower, sunflower, sesame, and virgin olive oils. (Heating vegetable oils at high temperatures can change fatty acids and make them carcinogenic. Peanut oil and extra virgin olive oil stand up best to cooking, but try not to overheat them. It helps to keep stirring stir-fries so the oil does not get burnt.)

Studies in experimental animals showed that fish oil–supplemented (i.e., high in omega-3 fatty acids) animals had significantly fewer colorectal tumors. In addition to being the heart-healthiest fats, omega-3 fatty acids may have anti-cancer properties. Eskimo women who have a high concentration of omega-3 fatty acids in their diet have a negligible incidence of breast cancer. It is thought that omega-3 fatty acids may block the effect of estrogen on breast cells, thus lowering the risk of their becoming cancerous.

Don't eat bad fats. Avoid oils high in saturated fats, such as palm, palm kernel, coconut, and cottonseed oils. Hydrogenated fats, those that have been chemically changed from unsaturated to saturated fats, are potentially carcinogenic. Adding hydrogen to a fat molecule may enable the molecule to interfere with the normal metabolism of cells in the body, setting the cell up for cancerous

changes. So get used to reading labels. If any food contains "hydrogenated" or "partially hydrogenated" fats, leave it on the shelf. Most fast-food outlets use hydrogenated fats. (Ask! If they do, don't eat the food.) Nearly all packaged foods, such as potato chips, contain hydrogenated fats, since these allow a longer shelf life.

2. Increase Your Fiber Intake

In all the research on the connection between food and cancer, the evidence for a relationship between a high-fiber diet and lower chances of colorectal cancer is the most conclusive. It follows common sense as well. Fiber moves potential carcinogens through the intestines faster, decreasing the contact time between carcinogens and the intestinal wall. The less exposure to carcinogens, the less chance of colon cancer. Besides pushing them through faster, fiber binds carcinogens, keeping them away from the intestinal wall. Fiber also absorbs bile acids, keeping them from acting on bacteria to produce cancerous substances that are formed by decaying foods within the colon called "fecapentanes." There are about twenty of these compounds that can mutate colon cells into cancerous cells. Fiber also promotes the growth of healthy bacteria in the intestines, which crowd out the undesirable bacteria that produce fecapentanes. A high-fiber diet seems particularly protective against cancer in persons who have a hereditary risk of developing precancerous colorectal polyps. In a study of persons who were at high risk for developing colorectal cancer, those who ate at least 13 grams of wheat bran fiber a day (All-Bran is a good source) for eight weeks showed less growth of potential cancer cells in the colon. Besides lowering the risk of colorectal cancer, a high-fiber diet can lower the risk of breast cancer by binding estrogen in the bowels, thereby lessening the estrogen effect in the cells of breast tissue.

Based on both these scientific and common-sense findings, we suggest you eat at least *25 grams of fiber a day.* Best anti-cancer fiber sources are: wheat bran, kidney beans, chickpeas, navy beans, whole wheat, whole grains, legumes, whole-grain bread, and prunes. Get used to looking at package labels to find the fiber content of foods. Simple modifications in your diet can increase the amount of fiber you eat. Use whole-grain breads instead of white bread (white bread is junk bread). Eat beans regularly (try a salad composed of kidney beans, chickpeas, broccoli, and other raw vegetables). Have a big bowl of high-fiber bran cereal for breakfast.

3. Eat Lots of Raw Fruits and Vegetables

The consensus of the hundreds of studies exploring the link between diet and cancer is that eating more fruits and vegetables reduces the risk of all types of cancers. Eating more fruits and vegetables decreases your appetite for fatty foods, which themselves increase the risk of cancer. Also, plants contain phytochemicals, which are substances that have evolved as part of the plant's natural defense mechanism against its own diseases. These substances may help your body fight cancer. Five major classes of compounds that occur in fruits and vegetables are natural blocking agents against carcinogens: phenols, indoles, flavones, and isothiocyanates. These neutralizing agents prevent carcinogens from reaching critical target sites within the cell. The vegetables most important to reducing the risk of cancer are the cruciferous vegetables: broccoli, cabbage, brussels sprouts, mustard greens, kale, and cauliflower. These vegetables contain three cancer-protective biochemicals: sulforaphane, which not only boosts immunity but blocks enzymes that draw carcinogens into healthy cells; compounds that prevent the formation of carcinogenic nitrosamines in the intestines; and indoles, which lessen the risk of

breast cancer. Researchers estimate that by eating lots of cruciferous vegetables you could lower your risk of breast and colon cancer by 40 percent (Think: Crucifers against cancer). Making your main meal, such as lunch, a huge salad from a salad bar (no more than a tablespoon of vegetable oil as a dressing if you must) would be one of the healthiest habits you could get into. Best salad sources of anti-cancer nutrients are dark green leafy spinach (instead of iceberg lettuce, which is nutritionally useless), broccoli, tomatoes, red peppers, kidney beans, and chickpeas. Sprinkle on a little chopped garlic, which has also been shown to have health-promoting and possibly anti-cancer properties. Also, phytoestrogens from plant foods, especially soy and cruciferous vegetables, can lower the risk of estrogen-dependent cancers, such as breast cancer. The phytoestrogens fill estrogen receptor sites on cells, keeping the cancer-causing estrogen from promoting the growth of malignant cells.

4. Switch from Red Meat to Seafood

Populations who eat the most red meat and fat in their diet have the highest incidence of colon cancer. My fifty years of eating steaks, cheeseburgers, and french fries were not worth the price of getting cancer. Instead of eating red meat as the main course, let it be an accent in a dish based on vegetables or grains, such as a stir-fry or pasta.

NUTRITIP
Sleep to Prevent Cancer.

Melatonin, the hormone that is naturally produced when you sleep, has been shown to inhibit tumor growth. It causes immune cells to produce anti-cancer proteins called "phytokines," which activate other immune cells in the fight against cancer.

Anti-Cancer Vegetables	Anti-Cancer Fruits
broccoli	apricots
brussels sprouts	blueberries
cabbage	grapefruit
carrots	grapes
cauliflower	lemons
eggplant	mangoes
green beans	oranges
kale	papayas
onions (red)	peaches
peppers	persimmons
radishes	strawberries, organic
soy	tangerines
squash	
sweet potatoes	
tomatoes	
yams	

NUTRITIP
Foods Protect Against Cancer Better Than Pills.

It's better to get your anti-cancer nutrients from foods rather than supplements. One study showed that a combination pill of vitamin C, vitamin E, and beta carotene offered no greater protection against colon cancer than a placebo. It seems that something other than these specific nutrients in foods may be responsible for the cancer-protective effects of fruits and vegetables.

Beginning in 1976 a group of researchers at the Harvard School of Public Health set out to study the role of dietary factors in colon cancer and test some of the theories suggested by earlier studies. They followed eighty-eight thousand healthy women, ages thirty-four to fifty-nine, and discovered these correlations:

- The risk of colon cancer was 2.5 times higher in women who ate beef, pork, or lamb as a main dish every day, compared with those eating it less than once a month.

- The risk of developing colon cancer correlated with the amount of animal fat in the diet.

- Eating meat, especially processed meats, was highly associated with increased risk of colon cancer. Eating fish and chicken without skin was related to a decreased risk.

- A low intake of fiber from fruits was also a risk factor for the development of colon cancer.

No association was found between the risk of colon cancer and vegetable fat or linoleic acid (the most abundant polyunsaturated fat) in the diet.

The reason for the red meat–colon cancer connection is still being studied. Current research suggests a combination of factors. High-fat diets increase the excretion of intestinal bile acids, which act as tumor promoters. Some processed meats contain nitrates and nitrites, which can be carcinogenic to colons. Also, compared with vegetarians, meat-eating persons have different colonic flora (see "Bugs in the Bowels," page 100). The effects of the meat diet may cause the intestinal bacteria to transform bile acids into potential carcinogens. Research shows that reducing the intake of beef fat decreased the ability of colonic flora to make these changes.

In a fourteen-year study of sixteen thousand Swedish men and women, the foods that were associated with the highest risk of colon cancer were beef and lamb. As a lamb chop lover, I took this study personally. Whenever our local meat market got in a shipment of lamb chops, I used to stock up. A month after my colon cancer was diagnosed, Martha took the 30 pounds of lamb chops that were in our freezer back to the market and traded them for salmon. Proud of her healthy swap, she announced, "You've eaten your last lamb chop."

Not only can red meat itself be carcinogenic but how you prepare it can elevate the cancer risk. Grilling over high heat (such as searing or flame-cooking meat so it is well done) can release carcinogens into the meat called "heterocyclic amines," which can damage cellular DNA. Poaching, stewing, microwaving, or slow low-heat cooking releases fewer carcinogens.

5. Switch from an Animal-based to a Plant-based Diet

The most compelling research linking diet to cancer are studies of groups of people who have primarily plant-based diets, such as vegetarians and Seventh-Day Adventists, and who have a much lower risk of cancer. One of the theories about the high incidence of cancer in modern times is that the switch from plant- to animal food–based diets correlates with the increase in cancer. The correlation between more plant food and less cancer is primarily due to three health-promoting factors of plant foods: less fat, more fiber, and more phytonutrients. Besides providing the anti-cancer properties of fiber, legumes (e.g., soybeans, beans, and chickpeas) contain anti-cancer chemicals called "protease inhibitors," which have been shown to reduce the growth of breast, colon, and skin cancers in experimental animals. (See the list of anti-cancer plant foods on page 361.)

6. Eat More Soy Products

Soy is a more healthful source of protein than meat. (This whole soy story is explained in Chapter 21.) The primary anti-cancer value of soy probably comes from phytonutrients, such as

isoflavones, which inhibit the growth of new blood vessels necessary for tumor survival, a process called "angiogenesis." Soy also protects against colon cancer by blocking the carcinogenic effects of bile acids. Isoflavones also help regulate the production of sex hormones, which could affect the risk of prostate and breast cancers. Studies have shown that women who eat more soy foods have a lower risk of breast cancer. American women, especially those whose diet is low in soy products, are four times more likely to die of

---

GENISTEIN CONTENT IN SOY

The isoflavone in soy that has the most potent anti-cancer properties is genistein. The highest content of genistein is found in these soy foods, ranked from highest to lowest:

Soy Food	Genistein Content (milligrams/100 grams)
soy flakes	156
soy nuts	94
soy flour	94
soybeans, roasted	87
soy protein isolate	56
tempeh	40
miso	26–38
tofu, firm	5–30
soy burgers	20 (varies)
soy milk	4–10

Be sure to consume soy products from a manufacturer that uses a water-extraction process, not an alcohol-extraction process, which can remove much of the genistein from the soy. Check the label or call the manufacturer.

LESS STRESS — LESS CANCER

Stress affects your immune system's ability to respond to foreign cells. Many oncologists believe that everyone has some precancerous cells. It stands to reason that of the trillions of cells within the body undergoing daily change, some of these will go astray and begin multiplying out of control. Normally the body's immune system detects these cells as foreign cells and sends out mainly macrophages to eliminate them from the body. Anything that depresses your immune-system response increases the risk of cancer, and stress does affect your immune responses. The good news is you don't have to be a victim of the stress in your life. Throughout your life you will encounter many circumstances that are beyond your control, yet the attitude you take toward these circumstances is always within your control. In fact, the circumstances themselves are not going to be as detrimental to your body as your attitude toward these circumstances. If you can maintain a positive attitude during stressful times, your body will react physiologically in a positive way. Do whatever you can to reduce chronic stress in your life. Don't sweat the small stuff.

breast cancer than Japanese women whose diet is plentiful in soy. This fact is attributed mainly to soy and not to genes. Even in their own country those Japanese who eat the most soy foods get the least cancer. Soy seems to protect against the most common types of cancer, including lung, rectal, colon, stomach, prostate, and breast. Experimental animals who are fed high-soy diets and then given a chemical that causes cancer develop fewer tumors than the animals who are not fed soy. And you don't need to eat much. One serving of soy (equal to a ½ cup of cooked soybeans), tofu, tempeh, or 1 cup of soy milk a day can lessen the risk of cancer. But don't rely on highly processed soy foods, such as soy burgers, soy sauce, and possibly some soy beverages to contain a lot of cancer-fighting isoflavones.

7. Change Your Oils

Oils that are rich in omega-3 fatty acids (i.e., fish and flax oils) have anti-cancer properties. Studies in experimental animals have shown that fish oil–supplemented animals develop significantly fewer colorectal tumors. Omega-3 fatty acids, such as those found in oily fish and flax seeds, help produce cancer-fighting phytochemicals, and flax oil also contains the anti-cancer

phytonutrient lignan. The best protection against cancer is a diet that contains more omega-3 than omega-6 fatty acids, just the reverse of the typical American diet. Cold-water fish, such as salmon and tuna, are high in omega-3 fatty acids. Most vegetable oils, except flax oil, contain little omega-3 and a lot of omega-6 fatty acids. I take 1 tablespoon of flaxseed oil or 2 tablespoons of ground flaxseed meal a day, which mixes beautifully in a yogurt shake or in a salad dressing (see "Fabulous Flax," page 211).

Monounsaturated oils, such as olive oil, also play a role in cancer prevention. Populations with an olive oil–rich diet, such as those in Mediterranean countries, have a lower incidence of cancer. Greek women, who tend to have an olive oil–rich diet, have a much lower risk of breast cancer. One study found that the incidence of breast cancer correlated with the amount of hydrogenated oils in the women's diets. As much as possible, avoid saturated and hydrogenated oils. (For more information, see Chapter 22, "All About Oils.")

8. Eat Foods Containing Calcium

Studies have shown that populations with a high intake of calcium (e.g., Swedes) have a lower incidence of colorectal cancer. Calcium controls the multiplication of epithelial cells lining the colon. When these cells proliferate at a fast rate, the risk of cancer increases. Calcium also binds cancer-producing bile acids and keeps them from irritating the colon wall. One study showed that an average intake of 1,200 milligrams of calcium a day was associated with a 75 percent reduction in colorectal cancer. In another study of persons with an increased risk of colorectal cancer, a daily supplement of 2,000 milligrams of calcium carbonate significantly decreased the risk by suppressing the uncontrolled growth of the cells that line the colon. To lower your risk of colorectal cancer, consider taking between 500 and 1,000 milligrams of calcium carbonate or calcium citrate daily, depending on how much calcium you get from food each day. Best sources of calcium are dairy products, such as yogurt, and bony fish.

9. Eat a Diet High in Antioxidants

While there are many unsubstantiated claims about the benefits of antioxidants, there is reliable

MORE LEAN — LESS CANCER

Too much body fat is one of the leading risk factors for cancer, especially colorectal cancer. Obesity is also a risk factor for breast cancer; increased fat tissue raises circulating estrogen levels, which increase the risk of breast cancer. Vegetarian women who typically consume a low-fat, high-fiber diet tend to have lower blood levels of estrogen, excrete more estrogen in their stools, and therefore are less prone to breast cancer. Obese men have a higher rate of prostate cancer. The two ways to stay lean are to exercise and to maintain healthy eating habits. (For more information, see Chapter 35, in which you will notice the similarity between the L.E.A.N. program and this anti-cancer regimen.)

scientific evidence that beta carotene, vitamin C, and vitamin E lower the risk of colorectal cancer. Fruits and vegetables are the main sources of these naturally occurring antioxidants. Antioxidants protect against cancer in several ways:

- They protect the membrane of intestinal cells.
- They prevent free-radical reactions that can cause bowel contents to be carcinogenic.
- They prevent faulty metabolism in the cell, which can predispose a cell to becoming carcinogenic.

Beta Carotene

Beta carotene fights against cancer by both boosting the immune system and releasing a specific chemical called "tumor necrosis factor." Beta carotene can block the growth of potentially cancerous cells. The recommended cancer prevention dose of beta carotene is 15 to 25 milligrams per day (around 30,000 IU). This is about ten times the amount in the average American diet, but it's actually easy to get enough beta carotene in your diet without taking supplements. Best sources of beta carotene are sweet potatoes, carrots, cantaloupe, pumpkins, butternut and other types of winter squash, spinach, broccoli, mango, and papaya. Eating pink grapefruit (which contains beta carotene) instead of white grapefruit gives you a beta carotene boost. You could get enough protective beta carotene each day by eating a few servings of beta carotene–rich foods. Best sources of beta carotene are these:

- carrots — 1 carrot contains 4.4 milligrams
- sweet potatoes — 1 medium contains 12 milligrams
- butternut and other types of winter hard-shell squash — ½ cup contains 2.4 milligrams

Tomatoes contain lycopene, which enhances the absorption and utilization of beta carotene, so eating tomatoes with beta carotene–rich foods provides an added boost. Carrots and tomatoes are a good combination.

Vitamin C

A big dose of vitamin C fights "the big C." Studies have shown that persons with the highest intake of vitamin C have the lowest incidence of intestinal cancers. Vitamin C blocks the formation of nitrosamines in the gut. These are potent carcinogens made from nitrates and nitrites found in food, especially processed meats. Vitamin C also boosts the immune system by increasing the production of lymphocytes. Best sources of vitamin C are fresh fruits and vegetables. Taking 1,000 to 2,000 milligrams of vitamin C daily may have anti-cancer benefits.

Vitamin E

The anti-cancer properties in vitamin E are similar to those in vitamin C. In a ten-year study that followed twenty-one thousand men, those with high levels of vitamin E in their diet showed a 30 percent lower risk of all types of cancer. Women with low blood levels of vitamin E and selenium had ten times the risk of breast cancer in one study. In another study at the University of Toronto, researchers gave colon cancer patients vitamin C and vitamin E supplements after surgery and found two years later that the supplements reduced the recurrence of precancerous colon polyps by 20 percent. Some studies suggest vitamin E supplements (around 75 IU per day) may reduce the risk of prostate cancer. Other studies suggest a dose of 200 to 400 IU a day, which is nearly impossible to get from foods. You may get less than 10 percent of this amount from even the best diet.

10. Don't Forget Your Flax

Flax seeds contain two cancer risk–reducing compounds: omega-3 fatty acids and lignans, which may reduce the risk of breast cancer and colon cancer. Ground flax seeds, because they contain

---

NUTRITIP
Natural vs. Synthetic E

Whether or not natural vitamin E from foods or the factory-made vitamin E is biologically better is still a subject of debate, but the natural vitamin E may be more biologically active. Natural vitamin E is identified on the package label by the "d" prefix, or "d-alpha tocopherol"; the synthetic compound will have a "dl" prefix.

NUTRITIP
An Anti-Cancer Smoothie

If you are undergoing chemotherapy and/or radiation therapy for cancer, you will find the smoothie called School-Ade (see page 309) to be a particularly nutritious food during these debilitating treatments. The combination of flaxseed oil, dairy products, and whey protein has been found experimentally not only to increase energy levels but to shrink tumors.

---

both the fiber and the oil, have more potent anti-cancer properties than flax oil alone. Cancer researchers suggest 25 grams (approximately ¼ cup) of ground flax seeds a day. You can grind your own in a coffee grinder or purchase pre-ground flaxseed meal, which mixes well in smoothies or can be eaten sprinkled like bran flakes over yogurt and cereal.

11. Drink Less Alcohol

Alcohol consumption slightly increases the risk of colorectal cancer, and the alcoholic beverage with the strongest link to colon cancer is beer. Beer is thought to produce nitrosamines, a carcinogen or pre-carcinogen that is activated in the intestines. While red wine is touted to have health-promoting properties, due to the natural phytonutrients that are found in the grape skin, you're better off simply eating the grapes.

12. Eat Other Anti-Cancer Nutrients

Increasing several other daily nutrients can also lower your risk of cancer.

Vitamin D. Vitamin D, which you get from exposure to sunshine (around 10 to 15 minutes a day) and from vitamin D–fortified milk and other foods, has anti-cancer properties. It suppresses angiogenesis, the formation of new blood vessels that nourish the growth of tumors. The rates of breast, prostate, and colon cancer are lower in climates that have the most sunshine. Low levels of vitamin D have been found in some people with colon cancer. Women whose diets are high in vitamin D have a lower risk of breast cancer.

Selenium. This overlooked mineral is a potent antioxidant or scavenger of carcinogenic free radicals. Studies have shown a lower incidence of colon cancer in people taking selenium supplements in the range of 100 to 200 micrograms a day. In other studies persons who had lower levels of selenium in their blood were more likely to have colon polyps, and those with higher levels of selenium had a much reduced chance of getting cancer. Men with the highest level of selenium in their diet were found to have the least chance of prostate cancer. Selenium is most effective when taken along with foods or supplements that are high in vitamin E. Consider taking 100 micrograms of selenium a day as a supplement. Best sources of selenium in food are Brazil nuts, fish (especially tuna, red snapper, lobster, and shrimp), whole grains, and vegetables, depending on the selenium content of the soil they're grown in. Other sources include brown rice, cottage cheese, egg yolks, lamb chops, chicken (white meat), sunflower seeds, and garlic.

Acidophilus. These intestines-friendly bacteria have been shown to have anti-cancer properties. They promote the growth of healthy bacteria in the colon and reduce the conversion of bile acids into carcinogens. Studies have shown that consuming dietary supplements of *Lactobacillus acidophilus* greatly diminishes the level of colon

EXERCISE CANCER CELLS AWAY

Moving your body moves your bowels, which reduces the risk of colon cancer. Many scientific studies have shown that people who exercise regularly have a much lower incidence of cancer than people who don't exercise much. In a study that tracked seventeen thousand Harvard alumni for twenty-five years, the group of men who were highly active (burning at least 2,500 calories in exercise each week, the equivalent of 45 minutes a day) had half the incidence of colon cancer compared with their sedentary peers. In another study, men who had sedentary jobs had a 1.6 higher risk of developing colon cancer than their more active colleagues. Cancer researchers believe that a high-fat diet (especially a diet high in saturated fats) coupled with inactivity accounts for as much as 60 percent of all colorectal cancers in men and 40 percent in women.

Exercise moves waste products through the intestines more quickly, thereby reducing the time that the intestinal walls are exposed to carcinogens. Exercise promotes insulin efficiency, which decreases the risk of all diseases, thus accounting for a common warning of cancer researchers: "If you have no time for exercise, you'd better reserve a lot of time for disease."

Exercise boosts your immune system by increasing the number of lymphocytes, interleukin 2, neutrophils, and other immune substances circulating in your body. One study showed that exercise more than tripled the circulating level of T-killer cells. Exercise also raises the level of high-density lipoproteins (HDL), the good cholesterol that sweeps excess cholesterol off the walls of your arteries. When you build muscle mass through exercise, the muscle itself burns more fat and therefore helps the body maintain its leanness. Once you're lean it's easier to stay lean. Increasing your muscle mass actually enables you to consume more calories without increasing your body fat. A study of thirteen thousand men and women followed for fifteen years by aerobics expert Dr. Kenneth Cooper showed that the incidence of all forms of cancer closely correlated with a lack of physical fitness and that the combination of a high-fat diet and inactivity accounted for as much as 60 percent of all colorectal cancers in men and 40 percent in women. Unfit men and women were 300 percent more likely to develop cancer. The study concluded that a half-hour of exercise several days a week can dramatically lower your risk of cancer. In another study of eight thousand men over twenty-one years old, those with the lowest resting heart rate had the lowest risk of colorectal cancer.

---

enzymes that produce carcinogenic decomposition products from food. In studies on experimental animals, 75 percent of the animals tested showed slower tumor growth when fed yogurt containing live bacterial cultures.

Populations such as the Finns, who have a diet relatively high in fat but who also eat a lot of fiber and a lot of yogurt, have a relatively low incidence of colon cancer. In an experiment in which car-

cinogens were given to rats, those animals that were fed large amounts of *Lactobacillus acidophilus* developed less colon cancer compared with those who were not given doses of these health-promoting bacteria. Take 1 to 2 teaspoons daily of live *Lactobacillus* — the one that is in the refrigerated section of the nutrition store. This can be added to a smoothie or a shake. Or eat yogurt with the LAC (live and active cultures) seal.

Garlic. Whether or not garlic has health-promoting and anti-cancer properties is controversial, but it's possible that garlic may have some anti-cancer benefits. The Kyolic brand of garlic supplements seems to be the most thoroughly tested and one that is often used in research studies.

Green tea. Green tea has been shown to inhibit the growth of cancer cells, possibly because of a phytochemical it contains called "catechins."

VI

FAVORITE RECIPES

Even the healthiest intentions of parent nutritionists go for naught if their children won't eat their painstakingly prepared meals. For children to enjoy the foods you fix, it must taste good and look inviting. Children are more likely to eat what they have helped create. Make meal preparation a family affair.

There are countless excellent cookbooks available at your bookstore, with hundreds of appealing and nutritious recipes the whole family will enjoy. Try, for example, La Leche League's classic *Whole Foods for the Whole Family,* by Roberta Johnson, ed. (1993), and *Whole Foods from the Whole World,* by Virginia S. Halonen, ed. (1997), both filled with hundreds of healthy recipes from mothers all over the world. The recipes in Penny Warner's *Healthy Snacks for Kids* (Bristol, 1996) are nutritious and easy to prepare, and each one includes a nutritional analysis. In addition to providing over one hundred recipes, *Sugar-Free Toddlers,* by Susan Watson (Williamson, 1991), gives you sugar ratings for popular store-bought foods. *Whole Foods for Kids to Cook,* by Judy Torgus (Cookbook Marketplace, 1997), is designed specifically for children to use; most of the recipes are meant for children who already have some basic cooking skills, but some are easy enough for preschoolers to prepare.

The following pages contain some of the most popular and nutritious recipes from the Sears family kitchen, plus a few selections from our friends. Enjoy!

Penne Rigate Casserole

Serves 6

Serve this nutritious casserole with a tossed green salad and Italian bread.

1 lb. penne pasta
12 ounces soft tofu
1 bunch parsley, finely chopped
1 egg
1½ cups grated parmesan cheese
2 cups marinara sauce
½ cup shredded mozzarella cheese

Boil pasta in salted water. Cook it until it is firm to the bite. Drain. Mix the tofu with the parsley, egg, and 1 cup of the parmesan cheese. In a 13" x 9" casserole dish, layer the sauce, pasta, tofu mixture, and mozzarella cheese. Sprinkle on ¼ cup parmesan cheese. Repeat the layering. Bake at 350° until the casserole bubbles.

PAMELA WOOLEY
FALLBROOK, CALIFORNIA

Gourmet Chili

Serves 12

Lengthy simmering brings out the full flavor of the spices in this delicious chili.

2 onions, chopped
4 cloves garlic, minced
2½ lb. lean ground turkey
4 ounces Italian turkey sausage
4 tbsp. chili powder
2 tsp. ground cumin
2 tsp. paprika
½ tsp. cayenne pepper
¼ tsp. turmeric
¼ tsp. ground coriander
¼ tsp. ground cardamon
2 tbsp. unsweetened cocoa powder
2 8-ounce cans tomato sauce
1–2 cans pinto beans
1–2 cans kidney beans
1 tbsp. dark molasses
2 cans beef broth
2 tbsp. balsamic vinegar
12 ounces beer (the alcohol evaporates during cooking)

Sauté the onions and garlic. Add the meat and sauté until it is no longer pink. Add the remaining ingredients and bring to a boil. Simmer for 2 hours. Serve with corn bread (see page 399).

Tofu Pot Pie

Serves 6

2 cans reduced-fat cream of celery soup
1 can reduced-fat cream of mushroom soup
1 can reduced-sodium chicken or vegetable broth
2 lb. firm tofu, cut into ½-inch cubes
1 large package (16–20 ounces) frozen mixed vegetables (or peas and carrots)

Mix all the ingredients together in a large bowl. Pour into a buttered 13" x 9" casserole dish. Pour the biscuit topping (below) on top. Bake at 350° for 1 hour or until bubbling.

BISCUIT TOPPING

2 cups whole wheat flour
1¼ tbsp. baking powder
½ tsp. sea salt
⅓ cup dry milk powder or soy powder (optional)
⅜ cup softened butter
1 cup milk or water

Combine the dry ingredients. Cut in the oil using your fingers or a food processor to get the texture of fine crumbs. (This mix can be made in larger quantities and stored in an airtight container in the refrigerator.) Add the milk or water and stir just until moistened.

PAMELA WOOLEY
FALLBROOK, CALIFORNIA

Tofu Enchiladas

Serves 6

1 pound firm tofu
juice from ½ lime
½ cup cilantro, chopped
3 cloves garlic, minced
8 ounces soy cheese, shredded
sea salt and pepper
16 ounces enchilada sauce
12 corn tortillas
1 small onion, chopped (optional)
olive oil (optional)
garlic seasoning

Blend the tofu in a blender or food processor until smooth. Pour it into a bowl. Add the lime juice, cilantro, garlic, and one handful of soy cheese. Season the mixture with salt and pepper.

Spread half the enchilada sauce on the bottom of a baking dish. Heat the tortillas slightly in a pan. Fill each tortilla with about 2 tablespoons of filling. Roll them burrito-style, and place them side-by-side in the baking dish. Cover them with the rest of the sauce and the remainder of the cheese. Sauté onions in oil and add them to the top (optional). Sprinkle with garlic seasoning. Bake at 350° for 25 minutes.

STEPHANIE MAYO
SAN JUAN CAPISTRANO, CALIFORNIA

Turning Island Baked Fish

Serves 4–6

We first used this recipe twenty-five years ago to prepare fish caught from the dock at our cottage on Turning Island in Georgian Bay, Ontario.

1½–2 lb. fish fillets (preferably salmon or tuna)
1 tbsp. onion, minced
½–¾ cup canola oil–based mayonnaise
½ tsp. marjoram
½ tsp. mustard powder
1 tbsp. lemon juice
fresh ground pepper to taste
paprika

Place the fillets in a buttered baking dish. Mix the remaining ingredients except paprika and spread over the fillets. Bake at 475° for 17 to 20 minutes or until browned. Sprinkle with paprika.

Dr. Bill's Tuna Salad

Serves 2–3

This tuna salad truly meets our definition of a nutrient-dense food. It packs a lot of nutrition in a small volume with a taste every family member will enjoy.

8 ounces tuna fillet, fresh or fresh-frozen
2 chopped hard-boiled eggs
¼ cup diced dill pickle
⅓–½ cup canola oil–based mayonnaise
1 tbsp. Dijon mustard
¼ cup sunflower seeds
1 tbsp. lemon juice
1 tsp. minced garlic or onion, or to taste
½ tsp. ground pepper
½ tsp. dried dill weed

1 tbsp. olive oil
1–2 tbsp. fresh red chili peppers, or to taste (use bell
peppers if serving to small children)
¼ cup chopped tomato
whole wheat pita or tortilla
½ cup bean sprouts, broccoli, or alfalfa sprouts

Grill, bake, or poach the tuna fillet. Chop it into small pieces or flake it with a fork. Mix it in a bowl with other ingredients except the pita and sprouts. Chill the salad and serve it in a pita pocket or burrito-style on warmed whole wheat tortillas. Garnish with sprouts. For added nutriton and taste, spread a layer of hummus on the bread first.

Bok Choy Chicken Soup

Serves 6

This is a nutritious way to get lots of calcium and phytonutrients into children who are not fond of greens.

CHICKEN MIXTURE

1 large, boned, skinless chicken breast cut into very thin
slices (cut while half frozen)
1 egg white
¼ tsp. sea salt
2 tsp. cornstarch
1 tsp. sesame oil
⅛–¼ tsp. white pepper

4 cups reduced-sodium chicken broth
⅔ cup straw mushrooms
½ lb. bok choy, cut into bite-sized pieces
¼ tsp. sugar
1 tsp. sesame oil

Combine all the chicken mixture ingredients in a bowl and refrigerate before use.

Pour the chicken broth into a 3-quart pot and bring to a rapid boil. Add the straw mushrooms and bok choy. Cook uncovered over medium heat for 2 minutes. While broth is cooking, stir in the chicken mixture. Stir to separate chicken pieces and cook until chicken is done (10–20 seconds). Stir in the sugar and sesame oil. Serve hot.

Lentil Supper Soup

Serves 4–5

1½ cups washed lentils
3 tbsp. butter
3 cloves garlic, minced
2 small onions, finely chopped
1 large celery stalk, chopped
¼ cup celery leaves, chopped
2–3 carrots, thickly sliced
⅓ cup raw brown rice
2 tbsp. fresh parsley or cilantro, chopped
1 tsp. sea salt
all-purpose, natural seasoning, to taste
fresh-ground black pepper, to taste
2 cups shredded spinach (optional)

Place lentils in a bowl and cover with cold water. Let them soak while you prepare the other vegetables.

Heat the butter in a large pot. Add the garlic, onion, celery, and celery leaves, and cook while stirring for 5 minutes over medium heat or until onions have wilted. Add the carrots, rice, parsley, and lentils. Add 1½ quarts of water and seasonings. Bring the soup to a boil. Cover it and simmer until the lentils, rice, and vegetables are tender (around 1½ hours). Add the spinach 20 minutes before serving.

Zucchini Pancakes

Serves 2

A long-standing Sears family favorite that even our toddlers enjoyed. The recipe makes one thick 8-inch pancake, or several smaller ones.

1 cup (or more) shredded zucchini
1 egg
1–2 tbsp. whole wheat flour
½ tsp. baking powder
dash of sea salt
1 tbsp. sunflower or sesame seeds (for children over four)
fruit spread or mild salsa

Stir ingredients together just until mixed. Pour the batter onto a preheated buttered griddle. Before flipping the pancake, sprinkle on sunflower or sesame seeds, if desired. Serve with fruit spread or salsa topping.

Wheat-Free and Dairy-Free Corn Bread

Serves 6

1⅓ cups cornmeal
⅔ cup brown rice flour
2 tbsp. soy powder (optional)
4 tsp. baking powder
½ tsp. sea salt
1 egg, slightly beaten
1 tbsp. dark molasses
¼ cup softened butter
1½ cups soy beverage or rice beverage

Preheat oven to 425°. Place all the dry ingredients in a bowl. Add the remaining ingredients and stir just until moistened. Pour into a buttered 9" x 9" baking pan. Bake 20 to 25 minutes or until done. Serve warm.

Almond-Strawberry Yogurt

Serves 1

Any fresh fruit (or combination of fruits) can be used in this recipe. Try blueberries, chopped apple, pear, peaches, or pineapple.

1 cup vanilla or plain yogurt
⅓ cup sliced fresh strawberries
slivered almonds (for children over four) or flaxseed meal

Layer the yogurt and strawberries in a parfait glass, or serve the yogurt in a small bowl with the berries arranged on top. Drizzle honey over the top if plain yogurt is used. Sprinkle with almonds or flaxseed meal just before serving.

Tofu Pudding

Serves 6

1 lb. soft tofu
1 can mandarin oranges, drained
½ cup honey
1 cup orange juice
2 tsp. grated orange peel
several drops almond extract
¼ cup toasted almond slivers

Cut tofu into half-inch cubes and place them in a bowl. Add the oranges. Combine the honey and juice and cook it until it is reduced to 1 cup. Add the orange peel and almond extract and pour the mixture over the tofu and oranges and stir. Cover and chill for 2 hours. Spoon the pudding into dessert dishes and sprinkle with almonds.

Tofu-Pumpkin Pie

Serves 8

A combination of soy and pumpkin makes this a nutritious alternative to traditional fat-laden cheesecake.

2 cups firm tofu
2 cups canned or cooked fresh pumpkin
½ cup honey or maple syrup
1 tsp. vanilla extract
½ tsp. nutmeg
1 tsp. cinnamon
½ tsp. ginger
¼ tsp. ground clove
one unbaked 9-inch deep-dish pie shell (recipe follows)

Blend the tofu in a blender or food processor until smooth. Add the remaining ingredients except pie shell and continue blending until mixed thoroughly. Pour the ingredients into pie shell. Bake at 350° for 1 hour, or until the crust is done. Chill it in the refrigerator for at least 1 hour. Serve chilled.

Martha's Easy Wheat-Free or Whole Wheat 9" Deep-Dish Piecrust

This piecrust makes a perfect shell for our "Tofu-Pumpkin Pie." The recipe makes two 9-inch single-crust pie shells or one 9-inch double-crust pie shell.

1½ cups brown rice flour or whole wheat pastry flour
½ tsp. sea salt
1 stick butter, chilled
1 egg yolk
2–3 tbsp. ice water

Blend the flour and salt in a food processor. Add butter cut into eighths and process until the mixture is evenly coarse, like cornmeal. Add the egg yolk and water while processor is running. The dough will gradually clump together to form a ball. You may need to add another ½–1 tablespoon of cold water if a ball doesn't form. Remove the dough, divide it into two balls, one slightly larger than the other. Wrap them and chill them in the refrigerator for at least 30 minutes.

Roll the dough out to the desired size between two sheets of waxed paper. The dough will be thinner than usual. Use the slightly larger ball for the bottom crust. (Hint: Wet the rolling surface first to keep the waxed paper from slipping around as you roll the dough.) For two single-crust pies (e.g., Tofu-Pumpkin), make the balls of dough the same size.

Granola Cookies

Makes around 2 dozen

These cookies will be different each time you make them, depending on the flavor and style of the granola you use. Be sure to choose granola that is not made with hydrogenated or partially hydrogenated oils or too much sugar.

1 egg, beaten
⅓ cup softened butter or peanut oil
⅓ cup honey (or barley malt)
½ tsp. vanilla
1 cup whole wheat pastry flour or brown-rice flour
½ tsp. sea salt
½ tsp. baking soda
1¼ cups granola

Preheat the oven to 325°. Mix the egg, butter or oil, honey or malt, and vanilla. Mix the flour, salt, and baking soda. Combine the wet and dry mixtures. Add the granola and mix thoroughly. Place dough by spoonfuls on a buttered cookie sheet. Bake 10 minutes or until browned around the edges.

APPENDIX: DAILY VALUES (DV'S)

Nutrient	DRV
Total Fat	65 g
Saturated Fat	20 g
Cholesterol	300 mg
Total Carbohydrates	300 g
Dietary Fiber	25 g
Sodium	2400 mg
Potassium	3500 mg
Protein	50 g

Nutrient	RDI (Adults and Children 4 or more years of age)	Infants	Children under 4	Pregnant and/or Lactating Women
Vitamin A	5000 IU	1500 IU	2500 IU	8000 IU
Vitamin C	60 mg	35 mg	40 mg	60 mg
Vitamin D	400 IU	400 IU	400 IU	400 IU
Vitamin E	30 IU	5 IU	10 IU	30 IU
Vitamin K	80 mcg	*	*	*
Thiamin (Vitamin B-1)	1.5 mg	0.5 mg	0.7 mg	1.7 mg
Riboflavin (Vitamin B-2)	1.7 mg	0.6 mg	0.8 mg	2.0 mg
Niacin	20 mg	8 mg	9 mg	20 mg
Vitamin B-6	2.0 mg	0.4 mg	0.7 mg	2.5 mg
Folate (Folacin, Folic Acid)	400 mcg	100 mcg	200 mcg	800 mcg
Vitamin B-12	6 mcg	2 mcg	3 mcg	8 mcg
Biotin	300 mcg	50 mcg	150 mcg	300 mcg
Pantothenic Acid	10 mg	3 mg	5 mg	10 mg
Calcium	1000 mg	600 mg	800 mg	1300 mg
Iron	18 mg	15 mg	10 mg	18 mg
Phosphorus	1000 mg	500 mg	800 mg	1300 mg
Iodine	150 mcg	45 mcg	70 mcg	150 mcg
Magnesium	400 mg	70 mg	200 mg	450 mg
Zinc	15 mg	5 mg	8 mg	15 mg
Selenium	70 mcg	*	*	*
Copper	2.0 mg	0.6 mg	1.0 mg	2.0 mg
Manganese	2.0 mg	*	*	*
Chromium	120 mcg	*	*	*
Molybdenum	75 mcg	*	*	*
Chloride	3400 mg	*	*	*
Sodium	2400 mg	*	*	*
Potassium	3500 mg	*	*	*

Bold Type = DV's based on 2,000-calorie diet for Adults and Children 4 or more years of age.

* = DV not established

DV's (Daily Values): New dietary reference term made up of two sets of references, DRV's and RDI's.

DRV's (Daily Reference Value): Set of dietary references that applies to fat, saturated fat, cholesterol, carbohydrate, fiber, protein, sodium, and potassium.

RDI's (Reference Daily Intakes): Set of dietary references based on RDA's for essential vitamins and minerals (and protein in select groups). "RDI" replaces "U.S. RDA."

RDA's (Recommended Dietary Allowances): Set of estimated allowances established by the National Academy of Sciences. Updated periodically to reflect current scientific knowledge.

Index

Page numbers in boldface type refer to main discussions.